*I wrote this book to be a source of hope to all those
mired in the misery of chronic Lyme disease.*

UNLOCKING LYME

UNLOCKING LYME

Myths, Truths, and Practical Solutions for Chronic Lyme Disease

William Rawls, M.D.

FirstDoNoHarm
PUBLISHING

Printed in the United States of America

First Printing, 2017

ISBN-13: 978-0-9823225-2-9 (FirstDoNoHarm Publishing)

ISBN-10: 0-9823225-2-6

Library of Congress Control Number: 2016919806
Vital Plan, Inc., Morehead City, NORTH CAROLINA

FirstDoNoHarm Publishing
13000 Weston Pkwy, Suite 100-B
Cary, NC 27513

RawlsMD.com

The information provided by this book is for informational purposes only. It should not be used to diagnose or treat any illness. Therapies discussed in this book potentially carry risks that are undisclosed. All health decisions should be made in conjunction with advice from a qualified healthcare practitioner.

Contents

Introduction 1

PART ONE Understanding Chronic Lyme Disease. 7

1 Lyme Disease and *Borrelia burgdorferi* · · · · · · · · · · · · · · · · · · 9
  An Enigma to Medical Science · · · · · · · · · · · · · · · · · · · 10
  Is Lyme Disease Actually New? · · · · · · · · · · · · · · · · · · · 11
  Borrelia, a Newly Emerging Microbe? · · · · · · · · · · · · · · · 14
  Essential Lyme Disease Facts · 17

2 After the Bite · 18
  Nature in Balance · 20
  Essential Lyme Disease Facts · 22
  Borrelia, the Ultimate Stealth Microbe · · · · · · · · · · · · · · 24
  How Borrelia Causes Symptoms · · · · · · · · · · · · · · · · · · 26
  A Healthy Immune System Is Not Naive · · · · · · · · · · · · · · 27
  Stages of Lyme Disease · 30
  Typical Presentation of Chronic Lyme Disease · · · · · · · · · · 31
  Essential Lyme Disease Facts · 33

3 *Borrelia burgdorferi* et al · 34
  Essential Lyme Disease Facts · 36
  Other Borrelia-Associated Illnesses · · · · · · · · · · · · · · · · 37
  Beyond Borrelia · 38
  Tick-Borne Microbe Sampler · 40
  Essential Lyme Disease Facts · 45

4 Why Virulence Matters · 46

The Virulence Pyramid · 52

The Virulence Factor · 55

The Microbiome and Stealth Microbes · · · · · · · · · · · · · · · · · 55

Stealth Microbe Characteristics · 57

5 Chronic Immune Dysfunction · 58

"Pot Boiling Over" Symptoms · 60

The Age of Chronic Immune Dysfunction · · · · · · · · · · · · · · 63

The Many Faces of Chronic Lyme · 67

Beyond Lyme · 69

A Closing Word on Parasites · 72

PART TWO Gathering Information **75**

6 A Holistic Approach to Evaluation · 77

Quest for a Diagnosis · 77

The Lyme Test · 79

Lyme Specialists · 80

Diagnosis from a Holistic Perspective · · · · · · · · · · · · · · · · · 81

7 Self-Assessment · 84

Measuring Wellness · 87

Monitoring Body Functions · 88

Measuring Your Vital Signs · 91

8 Making Best Use of the Medical System · · · · · · · · · · · · · · · 95

What You Need from Your General Provider · · · · · · · · · · · · · 96

Establishing a Good Relationship with Your General

Provider · 97

When to Consider a Medical Specialist · · · · · · · · · · · · · · · · 98

When to Consider a Lyme or Alternative Specialist · · · · · · · 99

Types of Providers · 99

9 Laboratory Evaluation · 103

Basic Testing That Everyone Needs · · · · · · · · · · · · · · · · · · 104

Advanced Testing · 109

Testing Beyond the Laboratory · 117

10 Testing for Microbes · 119

    Specialty Labs · 121

    Reasons to Test · 122

    Limitations of Testing · 122

    Types of Testing for Microbes · · · · · · · · · · · · · · · · · · · 124

    Accuracy of Testing · 125

    Diagnosing Borrelia · 126

    Diagnosing Coinfections and Related Microbes · · · · · · · · · 131

    Transmission Vectors · 136

    Hallmark Symptoms · 137

PART THREE Therapies for Getting Well. **141**

11 A Holistic Approach to Recovery · · · · · · · · · · · · · · · · · · 143

    Restorative Therapy · 144

    Symptomatic Therapy · 145

    Heroic Therapy · 145

    Looking Ahead · 147

12 Antibiotics and Lyme Disease · 149

    Current Recommendations for Antibiotics in Lyme Disease · · 154

    Antibiotics for Other Tick-Borne Infections · · · · · · · · · · · · 157

    General Guidelines for Antibiotic Use in Lyme Disease · · · · · 159

13 Herbal Medicine 101 · 161

    Modern Herbology · 162

    Antimicrobial Properties of Herbs · · · · · · · · · · · · · · · · · 164

    Herbal Preparations · 165

    Evidence for Herbal Therapy · 170

    Antimicrobial Herbs and Lyme Disease · · · · · · · · · · · · · · 171

    Beyond Herbs — Natural Bioidenticals · · · · · · · · · · · · · · 173

14 Core Herbal Protocol · 175

    Primary Supplements · 177

    Herbal Antimicrobials · 180

    Adaptogens for Immune Modulation · · · · · · · · · · · · · · · 185

    Supportive Supplements · 188

General Health and Blood Flow · 192

Intestinal Parasites · 195

Chronic Yeast · 195

15 Establishing a Supplement Routine · · · · · · · · · · · · · · · · 197

Core Protocol, Abbreviated · 197

Antimicrobial · 197

Adaptogens for Immune Modulation · · · · · · · · · · · · · · · · 198

Protecting Mitochondria and Cellular Functions · · · · · · · · · · 198

General Health and Blood Flow · 199

Tips For Taking Supplements · 199

Start with Good Products · 199

Getting into a Routine · 201

Dealing with Adverse Reactions · · · · · · · · · · · · · · · · · · · 204

16 Advanced Support · 207

Curbing Inflammation · 207

Rebuilding Collagen · 211

Restoring Brain and Nerve Health · · · · · · · · · · · · · · · · · · 213

Eye Health · 215

Mast Cell Hypersensitivity · 215

Enhanced Immune Support · 216

When to Consider Anti-Inflammatory Drugs · · · · · · · · · · · · 217

17 Sleep, Anxiety, and Depression · · · · · · · · · · · · · · · · · · · 220

Quick Tips for Better Sleep · 221

Medications for Sleep and Anxiety · · · · · · · · · · · · · · · · · 223

Guidelines for Safe Medication Use · · · · · · · · · · · · · · · · 225

Drug Habituation · 226

Medications for Depression · 227

Natural Options for Anxiety and Depression · · · · · · · · · · · 228

An Electrical Alternative · 229

18 Dealing with Pain · 232

Medications for Pain · 232

Natural Therapies for Pain · 233

Cannabis · 234

Low-Dose Naltrexone (LDN) · 238

Non-Pharmaceutical Devices· 239

Acupuncture · 240

19 Heroic Therapies and Other Alternatives · · · · · · · · · · · · · · 241

Chemical Warfare · 242

Oxidative Therapy · 243

Electrical/Energy Therapies· 248

Natural Heroic Therapies· 251

20 Setbacks and Relapses · 254

Herxheimer Reactions · 256

Bacterial and Viral Flare-ups · 257

Tolerance to Therapy· 257

Acute Viral Infections· 258

Food Reactions · 258

Flu Vaccine · 258

Drug Reactions · 259

Allergic Reactions to Herbs or Drugs · · · · · · · · · · · · · · · 259

Inadequate Sleep· 259

Travel and/or Stressful Events · · · · · · · · · · · · · · · · · · · 259

Complacency· 260

General Guidelines for Setbacks and Relapses· · · · · · · · · · · 260

21 Turn up the Heat on Your Recovery! · · · · · · · · · · · · · · · · 264

22 Understanding Biofilm · 267

What Exactly is a Biofilm? · 267

Common Biofilm Diseases· 268

Biofilm and Lyme Disease · 269

How to Overcome Biofilms · 270

PART FOUR Essential Support **273**

23 Mindset for Getting Well · 275

Making It Happen · 277

24 Digestive Dysfunction· 280

Is Lectin-Loaded Food Making You Sick? · · · · · · · · · · · · · 280

More Food Hazards To Avoid · 283
Details Of Digestive Dysfunction · · · · · · · · · · · · · · · · 289

25 Gut Restoration Protocol · · · · · · · · · · · · · · · · · · · 295
Additional Support for Gut Healing · · · · · · · · · · · · · 304

26 Curbing Toxic Threats · 311
Cleaning Up the Inflow · 312
Heavy Metal Concerns · 314
Detox Your Home and Workplace · · · · · · · · · · · · · 316
Protection from Artificial Radiation · · · · · · · · · · · · 317

27 Mold and Mycotoxins · 320
Finding Mold Where You Live and Work · · · · · · · · · · 321
Mold in Food · 322
Eliminating Mold from Your Environment · · · · · · · · 323
Eliminating Mold from Your Body · · · · · · · · · · · · · · 324

28 Adrenals, Thyroid, and Menopause · · · · · · · · · · · · · 327
Solutions for Adrenal Dysfunction · · · · · · · · · · · · · 329
The HPA Axis · 332
Thyroid Dysfunction · 332
Menopause · 335
Andropause · 336

29 Active the Right Way · 337
Boosting Endorphins · 340

30 Conclusion · 341
Expectations · 342
Personal Journey · 343

Appendix A: More Herbs, Bioidenticals, and Essential Oils. 345
Alternative Herbs · 345
Antimicrobial and Immunomodulating Herbs · · · · · · · · · · · 346
Other Beneficial Herbs · 353
Other Bioidenticals · 357
Essential Oils · 361

Appendix B: Protect the Integrity of Your Microbiome! · · · · · · · · · · 363
Acknowledgements · 369
Resources · 371
References· 375

Introduction

The status quo is the accepted norm that most everyone follows. While it isn't always correct, it's assumed to be correct, and most people never veer from it for their entire lives. When it happens not to be correct, changing it is like swimming against a stiff current.

People typically don't volunteerily choose to swim against the current because it's difficult and sometimes even hazardous — the choice is often made for them by life's situations.

And so, it was for me. If I hadn't encountered Lyme disease, I would have probably continued practicing conventional medicine, much like my colleagues, not bucking the system, and living out a relatively ordinary existence.

Like many others affected, however, Lyme disease changed everything about my life. In the beginning, I didn't understand Lyme disease. It took years of struggle for me to comprehend the true nature of the illness and years more to figure out how to overcome it.

With time, I came to see the illness very differently than the mainstream view. Lyme disease is widely accepted as a wolf at the door. In actuality, it's more like a cupboard full of rats. Both can do significant damage, but one is acute, and the other is insidious.

As such, if you bring high-powered guns to deal with a cupboard full of rats, you're more likely to destroy your cupboard than anything else.

In the beginning, because of my conventional medical background, I pursued conventional solutions, but I quickly found out that the "big guns" approach was not a good fit — antibiotics made me sicker, and I didn't tolerate drug therapies. Though there is a place for such potent therapies, I came to appreciate that their value in the treatment of chronic illnesses, such as the chronic form of Lyme disease, is somewhat limited.

As I came to know Lyme disease better, intuition led me to a better fit — I chose to restore my body with herbs.

At first, I used herbal therapy very tentatively; my medical training had biased me against herbs. But after reading Stephen Buhner's book, *Healing Lyme*, shortly after it was published in 2005, I fully embraced herbal therapy.

For dealing with the cupboard full of rats, herbs made sense. **With herbal therapy, I could suppress a wide range of potential offending microbes all at once, reduce the inflammation that was making me sick, enhance the healing systems of my body to repair damaged tissues, and, most importantly, restore normal immune function.**

I came to appreciate that the most commonly used herbs have very low potential for toxicity, so they can be taken at high doses for long durations. In effect, the strategy is wearing the microbes down and eliminating them slowly, rather than killing them all at once. Against a cupboard full of rats, this is how you ultimately win.

It was about that time that I first realized that I was swimming against the current. Herbal therapy is not accepted by the mainstream medical community. The deeper I immersed myself into herbal therapy, the harder I swam upstream.

By then, I had already given up my job practicing obstetrics and gynecology. I couldn't tolerate the 24-hour shift on call several times a week along with a regular work schedule. Not being able to take call like a "normal" doctor *and* embracing herbal therapy caused me to be an outcast in my local medical community. They simply didn't understand my situation.

I ended up opening a new medical practice with the intention of promoting wellness. Instead of just writing prescriptions, I routinely recommended herbs and other natural therapy options. The approach was truly holistic. Programs I developed to help people overcome chronic illness were a key part of the new practice. It was very different than the managed medical care found in a standard medical practice.

With this new approach, however, I found myself swimming upstream harder than ever. The system simply isn't designed to offer this kind of care; the current medical system is designed to manage illness, not restore wellness.

The way the system is set up, doctors are rewarded financially for ordering procedures and penalized financially for spending time with patients. Because I was routinely spending lots of time with patients and not doing procedures, it was sometimes hard to keep the doors of my practice open.

Having the knowledge and skills to help people, but not being able to use that know-how because of a dysfunctional healthcare system is frustrating. I found an outlet for my frustrations in writing. Through writing, I could share my story with others who were experiencing similar frustrations. My first book, *Health First* (later renamed *The Vital Plan*) was written in the early stages of my recovery. It was an exploration of why chronic illness happens and what can be done to prevent it. At that point, I was still trying to figure out why I was ill. I had just started to embrace herbal therapy.

By the time my second book, *Suffered Long Enough*, was written, my personal recovery was well advanced. It chronicled my recovery up until that point. By then, I felt very proficient with herbal medicine and concepts of holistic health. Through my medical practice, I had helped many people with a variety of chronic illnesses get their lives back, and, in the process, had restored my own health. At that point, I was still going by the label of fibromyalgia (Lyme testing had been ambiguous), but I felt strongly that I had Lyme disease.

In this book, I take a deeper dive into understanding this complex illness we call Lyme disease. I address the wide variety of concerns and questions that patients and others have expressed to me over the years. The primary goal of this book is to provide comprehensive information any sufferer would need to get well, respecting that Lyme disease is different for every individual. Your personal path to wellness will be different than mine. This book will help you create your unique pathway.

By reading this book, you will:

- Examine myths and misconceptions surrounding Lyme disease
- Find out how Lyme disease is linked to many other chronic illnesses
- Appreciate why fibromyalgia and chronic Lyme are often one and the same
- Understand the nature of the many microbes that surround Lyme disease

- Become familiar with current testing for Lyme disease and understand why testing for specific microbes isn't always necessary to become well

- Appreciate the limitations of antibiotic therapy, but know when antibiotics or other heroic therapies might be indicated

- Understand why modern herbal therapy is such a good fit for chronic Lyme disease

- Become acquainted with a comprehensive holistic protocol for getting well

I invite you to dive in and swim against the current with me. We're all in this together anyway, and together, we might even be able to change the direction of the stream!

I've put a lot of great information in this book, so take your time reading it. By the end of the first five chapters, you will likely have a very different impression of Lyme disease than you do now. That information is the key to getting well. The remainder of the book provides all the information that you will need to make a successful recovery. You can get your life back and live like a normal person again!

PART ONE
Understanding Chronic Lyme Disease

1

Lyme Disease and *Borrelia burgdorferi*

Most everyone who is familiar with Lyme disease has heard the story. In November of 1975, 51 people (39 children and 12 adults) mysteriously became ill in Lyme, Connecticut, and a new illness was born (Lloyd 1976).

The event became newsworthy because a cluster of people, all bitten by ticks, suddenly became ill simultaneously. Interestingly, it was a time when people were moving out of cities and into the suburbs built in the tick-filled, wooded countryside.

The illness, typified by arthritis and an unusual rash around the tick bite, was first thought to be viral. By 1981, however, a researcher named Dr. Willy Burgdorfer and his colleagues had isolated the now well-known, corkscrew-like bacteria (called a spirochete) from the blood of victims. The microbe[1] was named in his honor, **Borrelia burgdorferi**, and the illness was named for the place of origin (Burgdorfer 1984, 1993).

Once people became aware of the new microbe and the illness it caused, cases started popping up all over New England and beyond. Lyme disease seemed to be the newest plague.

---

1 Microbe is a general term that includes bacteria, viruses, protozoa, and certain species of fungi.

AN ENIGMA TO MEDICAL SCIENCE

From the very beginning, *Borrelia burgdorferi* frustrated both doctors and scientists. Medical science during that era was focused on snuffing out all the horrible poxes and plagues that threatened the lives of every person on the planet. Great progress was being made with new vaccines and synthetic antibiotics, and optimism was high that someday all threatening infectious diseases would be eradicated from the planet.

Borrelia hindered that optimism.

Borrelia simply didn't behave like other microbes and other illnesses that medical science was used to dealing with. It made people sick, but not deathly sick. And some people exposed to it didn't get sick at all.

The microbes were hard to grow in the lab and extremely difficult to isolate from the blood of people who displayed symptoms (making a definitive diagnosis a real challenge, even today). Though the bacteria were sensitive to most antibiotics in the lab, people often ended up chronically and miserably ill despite antibiotic therapy.

Today, *Borrelia burgdorferi* and Lyme disease are as much of a mystery as ever before. Public awareness about Lyme disease is at an all-time high, but concern from the medical community is at an all-time low. If something is difficult to diagnose, difficult to treat, difficult to understand, and rarely causes life-threatening illness, doctors simply don't have time in their busy practices to deal with it.

At the heart of this dilemma is a fundamental lack of understanding of the true nature of *Borrelia burgdorferi* (and possibly microbes in general).

IS LYME DISEASE ACTUALLY NEW?

When Lyme disease first debuted, medical science was just beginning to connect the dots between specific microbes and specific illnesses. Doing so was relatively easy with terrible illnesses that had well-defined symptoms, but Lyme disease was anything but well-defined. It took a cluster of similar cases for science (and the media) to take notice at all.

At the time, Lyme disease was labeled as a brand-new illness. It was assumed that new infections with Borrelia spread outward from the point of origin in Lyme, Connecticut. Information that has accumulated in the following years, however, strongly suggests that Borrelia is anything but new.

Even Dr. Burgdorfer and his colleagues suspected they were not dealing with a brand-new illness.[2] Physicians in Europe and North America had been describing a tick-borne illness associated with a bull's-eye rash (then called **erythema migrans**, for the rash emanating from the tick bite) for hundreds of years. Because the illness typically resolved without treatment, it had received little notoriety.

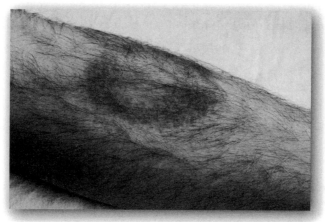

Figure 1 - Bull's-eye rash (erythema migrans)

---

2 Even before Lyme disease, Dr. Burgdorfer, a prominent researcher of tick-borne diseases, was familiar with other species of Borrelia and Rickettsia. *Rickettsia rickettsii*, the cause of Rocky Mountain spotted fever was already known, as were several other species of Borrelia that had been associated with human disease in other parts of the world (Burgdorfer 1993).

As it turns out, Borrelia is even much older than hundreds of years... Borrelia is truly ancient.

Borrelia species have been found inside ticks trapped inside amber dating back 15-20 million years[3] (and it may be even older). Over that period, Borrelia has developed host-microbe relationships with a huge variety of creatures. In fact, this extremely adaptable microbe can infect most anything with blood. Today, the microbe commonly infects mammals, birds, and even some reptiles[4].

Because ticks have been biting humans since there have been humans, it would be logical to assume that humans have been on Borrelia's list of hosts for a very long time as well. Recently, this fact was conclusively confirmed by a bit of evidence found frozen in a glacier for over 5,000 years.

In 1993, the remains of an ancient human were recovered from a glacier in the Italian Alps. Remarkably well-preserved, the 5,300-year-old mummy yielded a wealth of information to forensic scientists and anthropologists. Findings at a formal autopsy in 2011 revealed a surprise: the genetic signature of *Borrelia burgdorferi*.

At the time of his death, the mummy was in his mid-forties and showed signs of arthritis and degenerative disease, but was murdered with an arrow in the back. He did not die from Lyme disease (Hall 2011).

---

3 Ticks trapped in amber from the Dominican Republic dating back 15-20 million years contained Borrelia species very similar to modern *Borrelia burgdorferi* microbes (Poinar 2015).

4 It was once thought that the white-tailed mouse was the single primary reservoir for Borrelia and that most all other hosts, including humans, were dead-end hosts. A dead-end host is one in which the microbe cannot complete its reproductive cycle and cannot be transmitted to other hosts. It is now apparent that Borrelia can adapt and spread through a wide range of hosts and is not solely dependent on the white-footed mouse (Levy 2013, Radolf 2012).

This is the most intriguing part about the discovery — the 5,300-year-old man wasn't severely debilitated. He harbored the microbe[5], but was still mobile and functional. At the time of his murder, the man was actually traversing treacherously high mountain terrain in the European Alps (he apparently carried sacks of goods from one community to another).

This is a fundamental point for understanding Borrelia and tick-borne microbes in general. **Making the host deathly sick is not Borrelia's mission**. In fact, a bedridden host works against the microbe's primary purpose.

To complete its life cycle, Borrelia microbes must infect a new host via a tick bite, reproduce within that host (which only requires maintaining a simple presence of the microbe in the host's tissues, not an overwhelming infection), and then get on board a new tick when the host is bitten again. That last step, re-boarding a new tick, is crucial. If the host is never bitten by another tick, the microbe reaches a dead end. It can't spread to new hosts.

In other words, the microbes need a mobile host to fulfill their purpose. **The more mobile the host is and the more tick bites the host receives, the better it is for the microbes**.

A severely debilitated host is the sign of an imbalanced host-microbe relationship. It suggests that the host's **immune system has been unnaturally compromised**.

---

5 The iceman was carrying more than just Borrelia. Intestinal worms were identified, and his total burden of microbial parasites was likely much greater than a person living today in the developed world. Even with a greater microbial burden, however, he could accomplish physical tasks that someone suffering from chronic Lyme disease today would find nearly impossible. His body was, to a certain extent, tolerating the burden of microbes.

BORRELIA, A NEWLY EMERGING MICROBE?

Borrelia is often compared to HIV as a "newly emerging microbe." Newly emerging implies that such microbial infection is new to the scene and rapidly expanding.

Human immunodeficiency virus (HIV), the cause of acquired immune deficiency syndrome (AIDS), fits the definition of "newly emerging" perfectly. HIV first crossed over into human populations from monkeys in the early mid-twentieth century. It was first recognized in the United States in 1981. Over a very short period, HIV rapidly spread across the entire globe.

Most people infected with HIV become severely ill and often die (before drug therapies, most died). Symptoms of HIV are very recognizable; it's easy to tell who's sick and who isn't. Because the virus causes overwhelming infection in the host, testing for HIV is very reliable. The incidence of infection within any population of people has always been easy to define.

Infection with Borrelia is the exact opposite. We now know that Borrelia isn't at all new to humans, and that it's been infecting humans for many thousands of years. Symptoms related to infection are highly variable, and many people infected with Borrelia never get sick. People carrying the microbe without having symptoms are unlikely to be tested.

Testing for *Borrelia burgdorferi* wasn't done before 1981, so we have no idea how common it was for people to be infected prior to that date. Testing that has been done over the past 40 years has generally been poor and sporadically performed, certainly not enough to establish a reliable estimate of the true rate of infection.

Though more Borrelia diagnoses are made every year (especially over the past five to ten years), it may be a factor of improved testing (though testing is still far from being ideal) and the fact that more people with symptoms are being tested. Increased awareness artificially skews the data, making it appear that the rate of infection has increased, though it may or may not have.

No doubt, tick populations and the microbes they transmit are being affected by **environmental changes, global warming, loss of large animal species, reforestation of farmland, and mobility of human populations**, but how this affects the actual rate of Borrelia infection in humans is truly unknown.

Maybe there are a lot more ticks, but are people getting bitten more often? A hundred years ago, before industrialization, many people spent a good portion of their lives working outside in fields and woodlands. Tick bites were an everyday fact of life. Today, most people spend most of their time indoors. Tick bites are much less common for the average person.

Now that researchers are finally getting around to looking for Borrelia in tick populations, they are finding that the microbe is quite prevalent. Borrelia has been found in tick populations from the Arctic to the tropics and everywhere in between; it's present wherever there are ticks (Hvidsten 2015 and Masuzawa 2004). Because the relationship between Borrelia and ticks is so ancient, it can be assumed that Borrelia has had a widespread presence in tick populations worldwide for a very long time.

All of this leaves a very cloudy picture for Borrelia. At this moment, **no institution or individual in the world has any idea of how many people are infected with Borrelia, past or present** (no matter what they might say) — the rate of people harboring Borrelia without having symptoms may be much higher than presently estimated. Without knowing how many people are presently infected with Borrelia or have been in the past, it is impossible to classify Borrelia as a newly emerging microbe.

An overriding question, one that's more important than knowing the actual rate of Borrelia infection, is: **Are people getting sicker from Borrelia today than they did in the past?**

If the iceman of the Italian Alps provides any sort of example, Borrelia wasn't causing severely debilitating illness 5,000 years ago.

And before 1975, Borrelia wasn't making people sick enough to even get noticed.

Today, however, almost everyone knows someone who has been touched by the chronic, debilitating side of Lyme disease. It's in the headlines almost every day.

It does appear that **debilitating chronic illness associated with Borrelia infection is becoming much more prevalent** (or at least much more noticed), even though the *rate* of infection with Borrelia within human populations may or may not have changed much throughout history.

This is potential cause for concern. For an ancient bacterium that has been causing low grade infection in humans for thousands of years to suddenly start causing widespread, debilitating illness suggests an imbalance in nature. **It suggests that factors unique to the modern world are making people more vulnerable to becoming chronically ill.**

This concern, and how it affects our relationship with *Borrelia burgdorferi* and microbes with similar characteristics, will be thoroughly explored in upcoming chapters. It's the key to understanding Lyme disease and similar chronic illnesses that have become the plagues of modern times.

ESSENTIAL LYME DISEASE FACTS

- Borrelia is spread primarily by ticks, but also by other biting insects.

- Borrelia can adapt to a huge variety of natural hosts, including mammals, reptiles, and birds.

- Borrelia has been infecting humans for a very long time.

- *Borrelia burgdorferi* is widely distributed in ticks worldwide.

- Because of environmental disruption and mobility of people, tick-borne diseases may be changing, but whether this translates into an increase in human infection rate is unknown.

- Because infection with Borrelia is hard to diagnose and difficult to define, no organization has any idea how many people worldwide are infected.

2

I t's waiting for you.

Motionless, it remains perched on a twig extending across your foot-path. All it needs is a warm-blooded creature like you to come along. Time is of the essence, however, as it has great risk of drying out and falling dead to the ground — that is the fate of most ticks.

To gain protection from temperature changes and drying out, a tick spends most of its life under leaf litter. In desperate need of a blood meal, it makes the arduous climb up and out onto the twig, even though the chance of completing its mission is extraordinarily small.

When you happen along and brush against the twig, the tick makes a great leap of faith, hoping to connect with skin, hair, or clothing. After a successful landing, it makes a spectacular dash to a soft, hidden place and immediately buries itself into your flesh.

On penetration, chemicals present in the tick's saliva numb your skin and inactivate the first-response portions of your immune function, protect-ing both the tick and the microbes it carries. *All* ticks carry microbes. The possibility it's carrying some form of Borrelia is relatively high. After all, Borrelia has honed a working relationship with ticks over millions of years.

Simultaneously, blood floods into the tick. Borrelia microbes present in the tick assess the blood to determine which type of host the tick has bitten. Borrelia can adapt to a wide variety of hosts, but each host is different. By sensing the blood, Borrelia can alter its genetic profile to adapt to the environment inside your body.

When Borrelia microbes enter your bloodstream, they're ready and able. But because your human ancestors were well acquainted with Borrelia, your immune system is well prepared to fight them off. Though immune inhibitors present in tick saliva briefly give the microbes a slight advantage, they immediately find the first-responder cells of your immune system hot on their trail.

For this reason, Borrelia microbes clear the bloodstream quickly and penetrate deeply into tissues. With its corkscrew shape, Borrelia drills into joint cartilage and brain tissue. It can also enter and thrive inside many types of cells, thus gaining protection from immune functions and antibiotics.

It's during this transition that symptoms of initial infection can occur. Typically, most people have a benign flu-like syndrome that lasts a week or more, but often, noticeable symptoms don't occur at all. Rarely is acute infection with Borrelia ever enough to make someone bedridden. The fact that symptoms are typically mild is a strong indication that the human immune system is very familiar with Borrelia and immediately takes measures toward controlling it.

Common Symptoms of Acute Infection

- Low-grade fever

- Occasional chills

- Fatigue

- Stiff neck

- Rash around tick bite

- Transient muscle aches

Antibiotics taken during this period are known to reduce symptoms, but whether antibiotics eliminate Borrelia microbes is unknown. Borrelia is a master of penetrating spaces in the body where it's shielded from the immune system and antibiotics. All too numerous reports of people developing chronic symptoms months after taking antibiotic therapy attest to the persistence of this insidious microbe.

NATURE IN BALANCE
What happens next depends on the health of your immune system. If your immune function is robust, you and the microbe enter a balanced host-microbe relationship. Overtly symptomatic illness does not occur — this is nature in balance.

The potential for Borrelia to cause illness is dependent on how well adapted the host's immune system is to the microbe. In a well-adapted host, such as the white-footed mouse, illness almost never occurs; the mouse-tick-microbe relationship is many millions of years old. Though humans are not as well adapted as the mouse (therefore the potential for illness is higher than in the mouse), the relationship is still very well established.

If you think about it, **a balanced relationship works best for the microbes.** Consider the microbes' motives for survival. To complete their lifecycle, an infected host must be bitten by another tick. This allows Borrelia microbes to enter a new tick. When that tick drops off and later bites another host, microbes are transferred to the new host and Borrelia's mission becomes complete. The ongoing survival of the microbe species is secure.

In other words, Borrelia's primary objective is **turning its host into a mobile Borrelia-dispensing machine** — not making the host sick.

Each time a tick bites an animal, the tick's saliva circulates throughout the animal's body. Chemicals present in saliva send the "all aboard" signal for any Borrelia microbes present in tissues. Upon sensing these chemicals, the microbes mobilize from deeper tissues, flood into the bloodstream, and get on board the new tick.[1] Allowing the host to live for a full and mobile lifetime allows for unlimited opportunities.

To survive, Borrelia needs only to exist quietly inside a host's body until another tick comes along. **Low concentrations of the microbes are adequate** to complete the mission; overwhelming the host with infection is not required. In fact, an overwhelming infection is counterproductive. If the host is deathly ill, then it is less likely to go wandering through the woods. This decreases the chances of new tick bites. If the host doesn't get bitten by another tick, then Borrelia has failed; the life cycle has reached a dead end.

---

1 It was once thought that humans were dead-end hosts for Borrelia, that ticks that have bitten humans are not infective, but current information may suggest otherwise. Borrelia is very well adapted to a variety of hosts, including humans. When ticks engage in partial feeding (they feed on one creature, drop off, and later bite and feed on another creature), ticks that have bitten humans carrying Borrelia are likely infectious to other humans. In addition, after a nymph tick completes feeding on a human carrying Borrelia, it molts into an adult and is infectious to other creatures, including humans (Levy 2013, Cook 2015).

ESSENTIAL LYME DISEASE FACTS

- Ticks require a blood meal during each of their three stages (larva, nymph, adult). Borrelia can be transferred at any stage, but transfer during the nymphal stage is most common in humans because nymph ticks are so small (the head of a pin) that they go unnoticed.

- Female ticks lay about 2,000-3,000 eggs in spring, which take a month to hatch into larval ticks no bigger than a pinpoint (fortunately most eggs and larvae are eaten by other insects).

- Ticks require a blood meal during each of their three stages (larva, nymph, adult). While Borrelia can be transferred at any stage, the nymphal stage is most common in humans because nymph ticks are so small (the head of a pin) they go unnoticed.

- Female ticks lay about 2,000-3,000 eggs in spring, which take a month to hatch into larval ticks no bigger than a pinpoint (fortunately most eggs and larvae are eaten by other insects).

- Borrelia microbes can be transferred into eggs about 1% of the time (Though some sources suggest up to a quarter of larval ticks are infected at birth, Buhner 2015).

- Peak feeding for larval ticks occurs in August, primarily on small animals closer to the ground, such as mice (but humans can still be bitten).

- After engorgement, larval ticks molt into nymphs, hibernate over winter, and awaken hungry in the spring. Peak nymph activity is in spring through summer, when most Borrelia infections occur.

- After engorgement, nymph ticks molt into adults, with peak feeding activity in October through November. Adult ticks overwinter and then lay eggs in spring, making the cycle complete.

- Ticks routinely engage is partial feeding; they partially engorge, drop off, bite another creature, and feed again. Partially fed ticks transmit Borrelia microbes much more rapidly (Cook 2015).

- Ticks infected with Borrelia microbes are much less prone to dehydration, can take larger blood meals, have larger fat stores, are more cold tolerant, can climb higher, and are faster (Buhner 2015).

- Tick lifespans and life cycles are typically longer in very southern or tropical locations.

- Borrelia has also been found in other biting insects, including mosquitos (Melaun 2016).

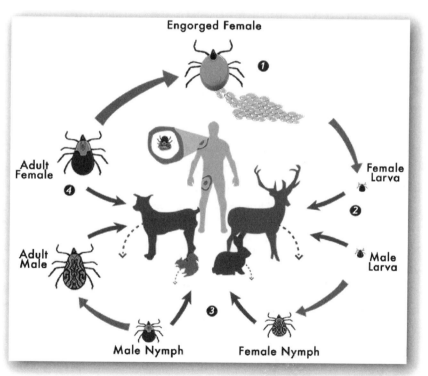

Figure 2 - Tick Life Cycle

BORRELIA, THE ULTIMATE STEALTH MICROBE

Borrelia has very sophisticated mechanisms for manipulating the immune system to allow it to exist indefinitely. It's always trying to stay one step ahead of immune functions.

A master of disguise, it can modify its surface proteins almost continually to keep the immune system guessing. Borrelia can shift its genes to adapt to any environment within a host. It can adapt to different tissues (heart, joints, brain, skin, etc.) such that different strains of the microbe often occur within the same host. Because every person's internal ecology is slightly different, a **Borrelia infection is different for every person**.

Borrelia microbes are very adept at using their corkscrew shape to penetrate cells, where they form vacuoles that fill with new microbes, one of the ways the microbe reproduces. Unlike most bacteria, however, they **grow very slowly**, creating new generations only every 8-12 hours (unlike other pathogenic bacteria that typically produce a new generation every 20 minutes).

Cell types that Borrelia microbes can infect include white blood cells. This enables the microbes to catch a ride to established sites of inflammation, such as arthritic joints. There, they will find abundant collagen, a favorite food source, already broken down and ready to be scavenged.

They can also penetrate between cells and slip into the space between layers of cells that make up tissues (called the extracellular matrix). There, they not only find substances that can be used for food (collagen, chondroitin, hyaluronic acid, and other substances), but also find protection from the immune system.[2]

---

2 The ability of Borrelia (and other microbes) to live inside cells may contribute to autoimmunity. To live inside cells, the microbes must turn off the ability of the immune system

If things really get hostile, individual microbes can curl up inside protective outer membrane sheathes and form **antibiotic resistant dormant cysts** (also referred to as round forms or persister cells).[3] When under extreme assault from the immune system or confronted with antibiotics, Borrelia microbes progressively shift from spirochetes to round forms (cysts).

In other words, the harder Borrelia microbes are hit with antibiotics or immune function, the more they encyst. As the microbes shift from active to encysted, symptoms decrease...but the relief is only temporary. After the hostile environment resolves, cysts quickly form new active spirochetes.

And then...there are biofilms. Borrelia, like most other bacteria can join with other microbes to form colonies shielded by a protective coating. Biofilms are extremely common in nature. The ring around your toilet bowl and the plaque on your teeth are prime examples.

Though you hear a lot about biofilms in Lyme disease forums, Lyme disease is not a primarily a biofilm disease. Biofilms require a surface on which to form (teeth, heart valves, joint linings, lumen of blood vessels, lining of the intestinal tract,[4] ventricles in the brain). Symptoms related to biofilm occur because of obstruction or damage to the surface. Though Borrelia may persist in biofilms (making it resistant to antibiotics and immune function), the symptoms of Lyme disease are primarily related to manipulation of the immune system by the microbe to generate inflammation.

---

to recognize the cell as abnormal. Eventually, however, the cell is recognized, and the immune system makes antibodies to that cell type.

3 Cyst forms occur in a wide range of atypical forms in a variety of shapes. Also, granules composed of budded-off cell wall containing cellular components, surface proteins, and linear/circular DNA that can form into active spirochetes (Buhner, Brorson 2009, Meriläinen 2016).

4 Biofilms in the large colon protect the lining of the gut and are important for normal health.

HOW BORRELIA CAUSES SYMPTOMS

To survive, Borrelia microbes must scavenge essential nutrients from the host. To get at these resources, they manipulate chemical messengers of the immune system called cytokines. **Using cytokines, they can shift immune functions away from attacking microbes and toward causing inflammation in tissues**. Inflammation breaks down tissues and releases vital nutrients to the microbe's ultimate benefit.

Because collagen is the primary nutrient Borrelia requires for survival, the microbes prefer collagen-rich tissues, such as joints, brain, muscle (heart muscle especially), eyes, and skin. Most symptoms associated with chronic Borrelia infection originate in these areas.

The microbes are also fond of myelin, a fatty substance that forms a sheath around nerves. Myelin is like the plastic coating on a copper wire; it insulates the nerve from other nerves and allows impulses to be conducted properly. Without it, nerve function is impaired, causing a wide range of neurological symptoms (symptoms like those seen in multiple sclerosis are common).

Symptoms associated with Borrelia infection are more related to cytokine-generated inflammation than direct damage by the microbe. Inflammation at specific tissue sites causes local symptoms such as arthritis. Cytokines circulating throughout the body are responsible for nonspecific symptoms such as fatigue.

For the most part, the intensity of **the immune reaction (cytokine production) dictates the intensity of a person's symptoms, not the concentration of microbes**. In other words, it doesn't take a high concentration of microbes for someone to be very sick. The fact that Borrelia microbes typically exist in very low concentrations in the body is one reason why Lyme disease is so difficult to properly diagnose.

A HEALTHY IMMUNE SYSTEM IS NOT NAIVE

If the immune system had never encountered Borrelia before, all the microbe's fancy maneuvers would be absolutely devastating. But Borrelia's complex adaptations did not occur overnight. It is the result of Borrelia and host immune systems "one-upping" each other; the microbes finding new ways to outsmart the host immune system, and the host immune system responding with innovative solutions to counteract the new threat — on and on for thousands upon thousands of years, one adaptation matched by another. Each adaptation is recorded in host genes and passed from generation to generation.

In this regard, the human immune system is very savvy to Borrelia's tricks and eminently qualified to deal with them. This is an old game, and the human immune system is an equal or better match for Borrelia. A healthy immune system can seek out and destroy it, wherever it may hide.

Then is even true of cysts (round forms) and biofilm. Borrelia is not the only microbe that forms cysts, and the human immune system is well equipped to deal with them. **Neutrophils, one of the champions of all immune cells, are very adept at killing cysts**. These white blood cells create a net that captures all types of microbes (big and small) and cysts. Once captured, the neutrophil secretes enzymes and substances to kill and digest the foreign invader (Menten-Dedoyart 2012). A healthy immune system is the best answer to Borrelia cysts.

The same is true of biofilm; **advanced life forms wouldn't be able to exist without effective mechanisms of breaking down biofilm**. Microbes of many varieties are constantly trying to form biofilms in the body, and a healthy immune system is constantly breaking them down. A healthy immune system is also the best answer to biofilms.

The immune system will make every effort to eradicate the microbes completely, but **often the tug-of-war between the microbes and the immune system ends in a stalemate** (the host becomes a carrier). Despite not being able to eradicate the microbes completely, however, a healthy immune system can keep the microbes marginalized such that harm is minimized, and symptoms do not occur.[5]

This is nature as intended; a balanced relationship works well for microbes such as Borrelia (but not necessarily the host). All creatures have balanced relationships with a huge variety of microbes, even some that have potential to cause harm.

Illness only arises when the immune system is in a weakened state and is unable to suppress the natural aggressiveness of the microbe. How sick someone becomes is dependent on how weak the immune system is and the natural aggressiveness of the microbe. Borrelia is more aggressive than microbes that are considered normal flora, but much less aggressive than many microbes that can cause severe acute illness.

Once infection with Borrelia becomes established, however, a vicious cycle of immune compromise is perpetuated by the microbes, and chronic misery can set in for a lifetime.

The degree and types of symptoms associated with chronic infection are highly variable; **Borrelia infection is different for every person**. The range of symptoms is **dependent on the species or strains of Borrelia present** in the host, the **host's total of microbes**[6] (other potential pathogens present), the **weakness of the host's immune sys-**

---

5 The microbial mix of the body, called the microbiome, is a complex mix of several thousand-possible species. Though most are friendly flora, there are always opportunists in the mix that can cause disease if unrestrained (potential pathogens). When totaled, a healthy host can support 100 trillion microbes, about three pounds of body weight, without having noticeable symptoms.

6 Borrelia adds to the total burden of potential pathogens in the microbiome. There are many species of microbes with similar characteristics to Borrelia. Having an infection with

tem, and the **genetic makeup of the host** (some people may be more susceptible to Borrelia than others).

Symptoms of Chronic Borrelia Infection

- Chronic fatigue
- Migrating arthritis/joint pain
- Muscle pain
- Chronic back pain and disc degeneration
- Chronic flu-like symptoms
- Headache/neck stiffness and creaking
- Bell's palsy
- Brain fog/decreased cognitive function
- Noise and sound intolerance
- Ringing in ears
- Disturbed sleep
- Blurry vision/floaters/eye discomfort
- Eye pain
- Tooth pain
- Dizziness and instability
- Muscle twitching
- Paresthesia (burning, tingling in feet and hands)
- Tremor (head and hands)
- Chest pain/irregular heartbeat
- Shortness of breath/difficulty catching breath

---

multiple microbes at once can tip the balance toward symptomatic illness (more on this in upcoming chapters).

- Unstable bladder
- Gastrointestinal dysfunction

STAGES OF LYME DISEASE

Classically, Lyme disease is divided into three phases: **Early Localized Disease**, **Early Disseminated Disease**, and **Late Disseminated Disease**.

The Centers for Diseases Control (CDC) and the Infectious Diseases Society of America (ISDA) also recognize **Post Lyme Treatment Syndrome** (PLTS), in which individuals who have been "adequately treated" with antibiotics remain symptomatic. **Neither of these groups recognize the term "chronic Lyme disease".**

Some experts are starting to use the term, **Lyme Borreliosis** instead of Lyme disease, but that determination depends on a positive lab test for Borrelia — false negative tests are common, and many people who carry Borrelia do not have a positive test. They may also harbor a variety of other microbes.

As with so many things in the world, **Lyme disease is hard to put into black and white**. It is mostly a big gray zone when it comes to definitions, and nothing about Lyme disease can be considered classic.

People with early localized disease often do not experience a rash or any symptoms, and symptoms associated with early disseminated disease are highly variable. Symptoms of Lyme disease in general vary widely between individuals because the microbe acts differently in every person it meets.

Many people experience late-stage symptoms despite being treated with antibiotics. Because testing is far from being one hundred percent accurate, it's virtually impossible to define whether antibiotics eradicate the microbe from the body.

Amidst all the confusion, most people who think they have Lyme disease refer to themselves as having **chronic Lyme disease**. They don't care about definitions...they're just sick and want to be well.

Because most people reading this consider themselves as having *chronic Lyme disease*, that term will be used for the remainder of this book.

TYPICAL PRESENTATION OF CHRONIC LYME DISEASE

There are a lot of people out there who consider themselves as having chronic Lyme disease, and the numbers are growing every day. Some of them have had a positive test indicating Borrelia infection, but many of them base the diagnosis on having all the symptoms of chronic Lyme disease, but have a negative test. **Testing for Borrelia is notoriously unreliable.**

The typical person claiming chronic Lyme disease (negative or positive testing) does not remember a tick bite and did not experience (or at least remember) acute symptoms. This is because the vast majority of people who are bitten by ticks carrying Borrelia are healthy.

Most Borrelia infections are transmitted by nymph ticks, which are very small and often unnoticed. If the person bitten does have a healthy immune system, initial symptoms are mild (if present at all), and the microbe and the host end up in a stalemate situation — the microbe persists in the person's tissues, but doesn't do enough harm to cause easily recognized symptoms (they become asymptomatic carriers).

Knowing how many people worldwide are harboring Borrelia without having symptoms is impossible; the number may be quite high. (Remember, a non-debilitated mobile host works best for the microbe.)

The **asymptomatic carrier state can last indefinitely.** If immune function remains robust, symptoms do not occur. If immune function starts breaking down for any reason, however, the infected individual gradually develops symptoms associated with chronic Lyme disease.

This is how it happened for me. I spent most of my youth in the woods; I loved the outdoors. Considering the number of tick bites I encountered, the chance that I didn't pick up something is remote.

But I didn't get sick...at least initially. I was healthy until my mid-forties when stress caught up with me. By then, I had been doing night call delivering babies (the worst type of call a doctor can take) for 24- to 36-hour shifts every second to third night for many years. I was also balancing a growing family and community involvement. Sleep became so much of an afterthought that I finally lost the ability to sleep altogether. Everything crashed. Over several years, I progressively developed every symptom of chronic Lyme disease.

In the beginning, I talked myself out of it being Lyme disease because all the experts said that Borrelia didn't exist in ticks in eastern North Carolina where I grew up. They were wrong.

The most convincing evidence suggesting Borrelia has been in North Carolina for a long time came from a gentleman I met years later. He was about 10 years my senior when I saw him as a Lyme disease patient. He related a story of knowing the exact day he was infected with Borrelia.

He had been hunting in eastern North Carolina 23 years prior to the day. He came out through heavy brush, and the next day picked off over 150 "seed" ticks embedded in his skin. From that point on, his health gradually deteriorated. Years later, he had a definitive positive test for Borrelia along with a variety of other tick-borne microbes. He had never been out of North Carolina. This period in his life would have corresponded to the time that I was very active outdoors and being bitten by ticks regularly.

ESSENTIAL LYME DISEASE FACTS

- Symptoms are associated primarily with inflammatory cytokines and not the bacteria itself. Borrelia has no genes coding for toxins that can harm the host (Tilly 2008).

- Borrelia does not rely on overwhelming the host with infection to be successful; significant illness can be caused by low concentrations of microbes.

- Lyme disease is often **divided into three stages: early localized, early disseminated, and late disseminated**, but the difference between the latter two stages is often arbitrary. Clinically, separating Lyme disease into initial infection associated with acute tick bite and chronic Lyme disease is more useful. The longer a person has had symptoms of Lyme disease, generally the more difficult the recovery process.

- If Lyme disease becomes chronic, it can make you miserable for a lifetime and will cause you to age faster, but it is unlikely to kill you directly. "Lyme disease was listed as an underlying or multiple cause of death on (only) 114 death records during 1999–2003. Upon review, only 1 record was consistent with clinical manifestations of Lyme disease. This analysis indicates that Lyme disease is rare as a cause of death in the United States" (Kugeler 2011).

3

Borrelia burgdorferi et al

As you get to know Lyme disease, you come to appreciate that the illness is much more complicated than an infection with bacteria known as *Borrelia burgdorferi*. Since 1981, many other species of Borrelia bacteria have been discovered worldwide, many of which have the potential to cause Lyme-disease-like syndromes.

This has led to the terms **Borrelia burgdorferi sensu stricto** and **Borrelia burgdorferi sensu lato**. The former refers to microbes that are similar enough genetically and structurally to the microbes discovered by Dr. Burgdorfer in 1981 to be called the same species. The latter are species of Borrelia that cause Lyme-like syndromes, but are not similar enough to be defined as the same species.[1]

As of 2015, there are over 20 known species of Borrelia worldwide and an uncountable number of different strains of each species. At least a dozen of them can cause Lyme-disease-like syndromes. (Current medical textbooks still only provide an outdated discussion of three species, and most doctors have received little education about Lyme disease.)

---

1 It was once thought that *B. burgdorferi* s.s. was the primary species causing Lyme disease in the United States, and *B. afzelii* and *B. garinii* were the primary species in Europe, with only *B. burgdorferi* s.s. causing Lyme disease both in the United States and in Europe, but that assumption is no longer valid. Many species of Borrelia have been associated with Lyme-disease-like syndromes.

And this may just be scratching the surface; the more researchers look, the more they find. New species are popping up all over the world.

If you consider the nature of the microbe, this shouldn't be surprising. Borrelia is an extremely adaptable microbe. It has been adapting to a wide range of different hosts and different environments over millions of years. With each adaptation, it changes ever so slightly. The potential for new variations is almost infinite.

If one group of Borrelia is only slightly different than another group, then the two are considered different strains of the same species. If differences are more significant, they are considered different species.[2]

Note that "newly discovered" does not necessarily imply that any of them are just emerging (coming onto the scene and rapidly expanding). The species present today have likely been present for a long time; it's simply that researchers are looking harder and getting better at looking.

Before 1981, researchers were hardly aware of any of them. Gradually, as other species were identified worldwide, and it became apparent that Borrelia is much more widespread in tick populations than originally thought.

Now, 35 years later, it is well accepted that Borrelia is widely distributed worldwide (WHO). And that's just the Borrelia species that we know about. With every year that goes by, new species of Borrelia are identified.

Despite all the species and all the variations, however, the method of operation for all Borrelia microbes causing Lyme disease is the same:

---

2 Separating life-forms into groups, species, and strains is the job of taxonomists (people who name life- forms). These people have a very challenging job, especially when it comes to separating and naming different species of bacteria.

transmit to a susceptible host via a tick bite, adapt to that host, fool the host's immune system enough to persist in low concentrations, wait for another tick to come along, spread to new host…and then do it all over again.

In other words, Lyme disease is Lyme disease, but because Lyme disease can be caused by different species and strains of Borrelia, it can vary in presentation. Some people with chronic Lyme disease have more pronounced neurological symptoms, and some people have more arthritis…or possibly a different presentation altogether.

Lyme disease also can vary geographically. Contracting Borrelia in Europe can be slightly different than contracting it in Australia or the United States. And Lyme disease in California may be slightly different than Lyme disease in Wisconsin or the Southeast.

ESSENTIAL LYME DISEASE FACTS

- Borrelia is found wherever there are ticks.

- There are many species of Borrelia that cause Lyme-disease-like syndromes.

- In the US, there are four geographic "islands" of different strains of *B. burgdorferi*: Northeast, upper Midwest, California, and Southeast, but further research may find more species of Borrelia in each of these areas and more overlap between areas.

- Different species of Borrelia have always been well distributed because ticks can be carried by birds (Scott 2010 and 2016, Klaus 2016).

- A person can harbor more than one species of Borrelia, and finding several strains of Borrelia in one person is more the norm than the exception (Flores 2007).

- A recent study showed that half of US counties have ticks with Borrelia (Eisen 2016).

- Borrelia infection is a little bit different in every region and every person.

 - If you have ever been bitten by a tick, you may well have been exposed to Borrelia.

- The many different species and strains of Borrelia make diagnosing Borrelia infection very challenging.

OTHER BORRELIA-ASSOCIATED ILLNESSES

Borrelia infections are not limited to Lyme disease. Certain species of Borrelia are associated with illnesses that share many symptoms with Lyme disease, but also have unique features.

Even so, the basic mode of operation is still the same: infect by way of an insect bite, reproduce inside a susceptible host, and spread to other hosts via an insect. The twist is in how the unique species of Borrelia fools the host's immune system, resulting in odd symptoms.

STARI, standing for **Southern tick-associated rash illness**, is a Lyme-disease-like syndrome presently limited to the southeastern and south central United States (it may be spreading, but no one knows for sure). It is specifically associated with bites from the lone star tick (*Amblyomma americanum*).

The illness commonly presents with a bull's-eye rash (erythema migrans) and a flu-like syndrome that is like, but typically milder than classic Lyme disease. Though an absolute causative agent has not been defined, a species of Borrelia (no surprises here), called *Borrelia lonestari* has been isolated from some cases.

Relapsing fever is a form of Borrelia infection defined by abrupt onset of shaking chills, high fever, severe muscle aches, and headache. Associated enlargement of the spleen and liver is common. The acute phase resolves after 3 to 7 days, only to recur about a week later. Multiple recurrences are possible (varies with the species of Borrelia).

There are two types of relapsing fever, one transmitted by soft ticks[3] (tick-borne relapsing fever) and the other by lice[4] (louse-borne relapsing fever). Each is associated with different species of Borrelia, which are also different than those that cause Lyme disease.

Morgellons disease is a peculiar illness that is getting a lot of attention lately (though it is relatively rare). The illness is characterized by skin lesions containing filaments of varying colors (white, black, red, blue, purple, and green) and sensations of things crawling under the skin. Analysis of the filaments has shown that they are composed of abnormal keratin and collagen. Other symptoms include fatigue, neurological symptoms, and joint pain. Recently, an association has been made with spirochetes identified as Borrelia species (Middelveen 2015), though other tick-borne microbes may also be part of the syndrome.

BEYOND BORRELIA

To complicate matters even more, chronic Lyme disease is rarely Borrelia alone.

---

3 Soft ticks (as opposed to more common hard ticks) typically are found in rodent-infested cabins and feed at night. The bites are painless. About a half dozen species of Borrelia cause tick-borne relapsing fever worldwide, three of which are present in the United States (*B. hermsii, B. recurrentis,* and *B. miyamotoi*).

4 Louse-borne relapsing fever is mostly limited to poverty stricken areas of Africa (Ethiopia, Sudan) where lice infestations are endemic. *B. recurrentis* is the offending microbe. This louse-borne form of relapsing fever is associated with severe acute disease, but poor health status of those infected is likely a factor. With treatment, mortality is 1%, but antibiotics are often not available, and without treatment, mortality is 70%.

Ticks are nature's perfect vehicle for transmitting microbes (certainly as good as mosquitos, and possibly better because they feed longer), and many different types of microbes take advantage of this extraordinary opportunity.

A search on PubMed reveals citations for hundreds of different tick-borne microbes that have the potential to cause illness in humans and other animals. The list includes viruses, bacteria, protozoa, and even fungi.

In his 2015 book on Lyme disease, Stephen Buhner points out that "depth examination of Ixodes ticks has found they can carry up to 237 genera of microorganisms that are infectious to vertebrates" (and that's just one type of tick). A genus is a group of organisms with similar characteristics. For microbes, a genus can include many species. **Tallied up, the list of different species of tick-borne microbes adds up into the hundreds or even thousands.**

This shouldn't be surprising; all creatures harbor a wide variety of microbes. We humans are capable of harboring several thousand different microbe species. While we are a permanent host for these microbes, many microbes found in ticks are just using the tick as a vector to transfer from host to host.

Just like humans or any other creature, the spectrum of microbes present in different ticks is highly variable. Certain microbes are more prevalent in certain geographic regions. Certain microbes are also more prevalent in certain tick species or tick populations. But one thing is for sure: **all ticks carry a variety of microbes** (Moutailler 2016).

It is nature as intended. Microbes harbored by ticks are in the process of searching for a host. **Every tick bite is an opportunity for tick-borne microbes to infect and colonize a new host.** Microbes (usually more than one variety) always enter the host's bloodstream when a tick bite occurs.

If you have ever been bitten by a tick, tick-borne microbes have entered your bloodstream.

TICK-BORNE MICROBE SAMPLER

The most commonly described tick-borne microbes associated with Lyme disease include Borrelia, Mycoplasma, Bartonella, Babesia, Ehrlichia, Anaplasma, Rickettsia, and more recently, Chlamydia. Just like Borrelia, however, each one of these groups (genera) of microbes consists of many species and an almost unlimited number of different strains. And these are just the ones we know something about — who knows how many tick-borne microbes are still yet to be identified. Beyond bacterial species, research is also turning up a wide variety of viruses that can be carried by ticks (Estrada-Peña 2014).

Next to Borrelia, Mycoplasma is thought to be the most common microbe associated with chronic Lyme disease (about 75% of cases, but possibly even more, as Mycoplasma is also very hard to diagnose). It is also widespread in the general population. Virtually everyone has been exposed to Mycoplasma, and somewhere between 30 and 70% of different populations of people studied harbor it chronically without having symptoms (Razin 1998).

Mycoplasma is the smallest of all bacteria. There have been over 200 species of Mycoplasma classified, and at least 23 of them can infect humans (some are considered normal flora, but many can cause illness). Mycoplasma can be spread by ticks, but it also commonly occurs as respiratory and genital infections. Acute infections generally resolve without consequence in healthy individuals, but, like Borrelia, chronic infections can occur. The symptoms of chronic infection are nonspecific and very different from those of the acute infection.

Like most tick-borne microbes, Mycoplasma lives inside cells. They commonly infect white blood cells, which allow them to hitch a ride to every part of the body. The microbes must scavenge everything they need to survive; favorite sites include collagen-rich areas (joints, skin, brain) and myelin-covered nerves. To do this, they manipulate the immune system to generate inflammation to break down tissues. (Is this story starting to sound familiar?)

Chlamydia is extremely small bacteria with characteristics like Mycoplasma. Presently, there are nine recognized species of Chlamydia, but others will likely be uncovered. Chlamydia can be spread by ticks, but it is more commonly spread by respiratory infections (*C. pneumoniae*) and intimate contact with other people (*C. trachomatis*). More than half of people have been exposed to the more common species of Chlamydia, and chronic subclinical infection (chronic infection without overt symptoms) is very common. How often it occurs with chronic Lyme disease is currently unknown (but possibly very commonly).

Bartonella, the next most common chronic Lyme disease player, occurs widely in nature. All mammal populations harbor Bartonella (including whales and dolphins), and more than a dozen species of Bartonella can infect and cause illness in humans. As a Lyme disease coinfection, it occurs in an estimated 25 to 50% of cases. Like the other microbes discussed so far, most people have been exposed to some form of Bartonella, and a third of people carry it without having symptoms.

Bartonella is **spread by ticks, but also by other biting insects, especially fleas**. The most well-known acute Bartonella infection is cat-scratch fever (Bartonella henselae), but there are many other variations. It infects and reproduces inside specialized white blood cells that line blood vessels (slight variation on the theme). Symptoms arise from damage to small blood vessels (small vessel disease). Typical organs that can be affected include the liver, spleen, bone marrow, eyes, skin, and the entire vascular system, including the heart. This is important to note when vascular symptoms are part of the chronic Lyme disease complex.

While all of this sounds highly threatening, most people exposed to Bartonella do not get severely sick. After a brief flu-like illness, the person is back to full health; care from a doctor is rarely required, and a formal diagnosis of Bartonella is often never made. **Antibiotic therapy is rarely prescribed for an acute Bartonella infection.**

If immune function falters, however, chronic symptomatic infection can occur. Symptoms of chronic illness are nonspecific and very different than those of the acute illness. (This story should be sounding familiar by now — it is common to a wide variety of microbes, each microbe using a slightly different strategy for success).

Babesia, the next microbe on the list, is a protozoan. Protozoa are one-celled organisms with a nucleus surrounding their DNA (bacteria do not have a true nucleus). It is a distant cousin of malaria. **Though it is much less threatening than malaria, it is more threatening than other tick-borne microbes.** Fortunately, it is also less common than other tick-borne microbes and is associated with Lyme disease in only about 5 to 20% of cases.

There are more than a hundred-different species of Babesia, and at least a dozen are known to cause human illness. Babesia species, however, are more like groups of very similar organisms than distinct species; it has a near infinite ability to continually change its genotype (genetic presentation).

People bitten by a tick carrying Babesia may hardly get sick at all, or they may get very sick very suddenly. This may be a function of the strain or species of the microbe, the reaction of the person to the microbe, or both. In this way, it is very different than Borrelia and other tick-borne microbes. The one situation where infection with Babesia can be truly life-threatening is if the person has had a splenectomy. Anyone without a spleen suspected of having an infection with Babesia should be treated very aggressively with antimicrobial therapy.

Like malaria, it causes symptoms by infecting and destroying red blood cells (RBCs). It does this to scavenge essential nutrients from the cell. It can infect anything with RBCs (mammals, birds, reptiles, amphibians). It also infects white blood cells and can live inside different types of cells.

When people do get sick, they can get very sick. Common acute symptoms include high fever (105°° °F), severe fatigue and malaise, shaking chills and sweats, severe headache, muscle aches, joint pain, abdominal pain, jaundice, and a range of other symptoms. Severe infection can last weeks to months.

Also unlike Borrelia and previously mentioned tick-borne microbes, chronic illness with Babesia, when it occurs, is defined by relapses of acute symptoms (though some species may cause less severe recurrent symptoms).

The tick-borne microbes least commonly associated with Lyme disease include Ehrlichia, Anaplasma, and Rickettsia (5% or less of cases). The primary way these closely related microbes differ is by the cell type they infect. Ehrlichia and Anaplasma infect different types of white blood cells and are carried throughout the body (Ehrlichia causes more severe infections than Anaplasma). Rickettsia infects cells that line blood vessels.

Ehrlichia chaffeensis is the most common of seven known species of Ehrlichia. There are eight known species of Anaplasma with *A. phagocytophilum* being the most common. These microbes have been around for a long time, and as you might now expect, there are a huge number of possible strains of each species.

Like Babesia, infections with these microbes are either all or nothing: Two thirds of people will experience a mild illness that resolves without medical therapy, but some people will become very ill, very acutely. Acute symptoms include high fever, malaise, headache, confusion, joint pain, muscle aches, and a characteristic rash (more common with Ehrlichia and Rickettsia than Anaplasma).

Rickettsia rickettsii, **the microbe causing Rocky Mountain spotted fever, differs from the other two in that it infects cells lining blood vessels (endothelial cells).** This causes severe inflammation in blood vessels with obstruction. In addition to the symptoms above, it can cause loss of fingers and toes and organ failure. *R. rickettsii* is one of 26 known species of Rickettsia, most of which have potential to cause illness (Parola 2013).

These last three microbes are not ones to mess around with. When suspected, they should be treated aggressively with conventional antibiotics.

Diagnosis is based on clinical signs and symptoms and confirmed by labs after treatment is initiated. Labs are not helpful for the first 2 weeks when acute symptoms are most pronounced.

Chronic infection with these three microbes typically presents as recurrence of acute symptoms. Symptom-free phases can last months or even years.

Note that the above discussions are generalizations about the most well-understood species of tick-borne microbes; there are many different species and strains of each microbe. Each strain and species can have widely varying tendencies to cause illness. Milder species of Ehrlichia, Anaplasma, Rickettsia, and Babesia may be more commonly associated with chronic Lyme disease than once thought — making absolute conclusions about any microbe can be misleading.

ESSENTIAL LYME DISEASE FACTS

- Borrelia rarely travels alone; most cases of Lyme disease are associated with infections with other similar types of microbes (these other microbes are as much a part of Lyme disease as Borrelia).

- Because of other tick-borne microbes, Lyme-like illnesses can occur without the presence of Borrelia (and may be relatively common).

- Mycoplasma, Bartonella, and Chlamydia are much more common and much less threatening than Babesia, Ehrlichia, Anaplasma, and Rickettsia.

- High fever and lymph node swelling at initial infection are more typical of Babesia, Ehrlichia, Anaplasma, and Rickettsia.

- Like Borrelia, these microbes have been infecting humans for a very long time, and there are many species and strains of each microbe, each with a different potential to cause illness.

- This list may be just scratching the surface; who knows how many new species of tick-borne microbes exist.

4

Why Virulence Matters

All the microbes described so far have one thing in common — they are host dependent.

And host dependency is at the root of most problems caused by microbes.

Host-dependent microbes must, by necessity, scavenge resources and essential raw materials from the host's body. Though harm is not by intent (microbes cannot be defined as good or bad), a certain amount of harm is done by the process of extracting resources from a less-than-willing host. Illness occurs when harm is significant or accumulates.

Virulence is the potential for a microbe to cause harm or illness. All host-microbe relationships can be defined by virulence.

Throughout life, you are continually exposed to microbes seeking new host relationships. It is what microbes do. Spreading from one host to another is their purpose in life. Because environments are constantly fluctuating, adapting to new hosts helps ensure survival of that microbe's species. **The most successful microbes, such as Borrelia, quickly adapt to new environments and have adapted to a wide range of hosts.**

An infection from a microbe is simply a microbe attempting to use you as a host.

Each and every time you have ever gotten bitten by a tick, mosquito, flea, or some other biting insect; been nipped or scratched by a dog or cat; scraped or cut your skin; had sex with another person; kissed another person; even hugged another person; picked your nose; put your fingers in your mouth; given birth; been born; used a public toilet just after someone else had been there; taken a breath just after someone sneezed; been swimming in a natural pond, lake, or river; or consumed *any* food or beverage...you have encountered host-seeking microbes.

You are exposed to a wide variety of different microbes every day.

To access vital resources and nutrients, however, microbes must get past your immune system. Different microbes use different methods for manipulating the host's immune system to get what they want.

Fortunately, your immune system is extraordinarily sophisticated. It evolved because of repetitive exposure to an enormous number of different microbes over millions of years. For every new trick that different microbes have come up with to confound immune functions, the immune system has developed countermeasures to match it. **Every countermeasure has been permanently wired into your immune system.**

Therefore, most host-seeking microbes are immediately recognized and either dispatched or suppressed — so much so that most of the time you're not even aware that a confrontation has occurred. Rare is a confrontation that causes illness, and even rarer still, an illness that is truly life-threatening.

In other words, the **more familiar your immune system is with a microbe, the lower the chances of that microbe causing you harm** (lower virulence[1]). If the immune system knows a microbe (the human immune

---

1 Host-microbe familiarity is usually the most important factor that defines virulence, but other factors unique to the microbe can also affect virulence; there are exceptions to every rule.

system has confronted it before), then the natural aggressiveness of that microbe is curbed, and harm is minimized. **In some cases, the microbe and the host enter a well-balanced relationship in which the microbe persists and the host is not significantly harmed.**

This is the case with microbes referred to as normal flora. Your relationship with these microbes is so well balanced that the microbes gain benefit, but also provide benefit in return — the relationship is symbiotic. This type of mutual adaptation of one species to another **requires thousands upon thousands of years** of exposure between the host species and the microbe species. Our relationship with our normal flora likely dates back millions of years; we are extremely familiar with them.

At the other end of the spectrum, if the host's immune system has <u>no</u> familiarity with a microbe, then the immune system has <u>no</u> ability to inhibit the natural aggressiveness of the microbe.

This is what happens with an Ebola outbreak. Humans have rarely been exposed to the Ebola virus, and the human immune system has no familiarity with it. When a human host is infected with Ebola, the resulting host-microbe relationship is extremely unbalanced (and unnatural). The immune system of the infected person is completely blindsided, and the person quickly becomes severely ill. A wake of destruction spreads like wildfire until it eventually burns out.[2]

For humans, Ebola is possibly the most virulent microbe on the planet. On a 1 to 10 scale of virulence, Ebola would be a definite 10 (see figure 3).

---

2 Epidemics occur when a microbe skips from its established reservoir host to a naive host. (Virulence is increased when microbes skip to new hosts.) Strains of influenza virus that are well adapted to humans only cause mild-to-moderate illness. Every now and then, however, a strain of influenza jumps from another animal to humans (typically from birds), and the results are devastating. This is what happened with the 1918 flu epidemic that killed millions (Hoag, Study revives bird origin for 1918 flu pandemic, *Nature*, Feb 2014). Generally, epidemics of poorly adapted microbes are not sustainable; they run their course and eventually burn out.

Interestingly, microbe virulence is host specific; what is one host's pathogen is another host's normal flora. Every host-dependent microbe has a balanced relationship with at least one natural host (and some microbes, such as Borrelia, have many natural hosts). For the Ebola virus, the natural host is thought to be a spider that lives in Africa.[3] In that host, it exists without causing harm; the relationship is well balanced. On the spider's virulence scale, Ebola virus would be only a 1.

Similarly, on our virulence scale, our normal flora, the microbes that inhabit our intestinal tract, skin, and airway passages, would also be at 1. The potential for these microbes to cause illness is extremely low (but not zero[4]).

Everything on the human microbe virulence scale falls between 1 and 10. Microbes can be loosely separated into high virulence (5-10) and low virulence (1-5). The general traits and habits of high-virulence microbes are very different than those of low-virulence microbes.

High-virulence microbes are much more apt to cause acute life-threatening illness that requires acute medical intervention. Symptom profiles are typically indicative of the specific microbe causing the illness (most doctors would be able to identify AIDS, Ebola, or malaria from the symptoms alone). Chronic infections with higher virulence microbes, such as malaria, usually manifest as relapses of acute symptoms. In general, high-virulence microbes are best addressed with the potency of conventional therapies such as vaccines and synthetic antibiotics.

---

3 Sometimes the spider bites a bat, and the bat spreads the virus to other bats. Humans can become infected with the virus if they come in contact with the bat or the bat's excrement. When that happens, the results are devastating (Quammen 2015).

4 All microbes are greedy and aggressive; they will take as much as they can get. If immune function is disturbed, even normal flora can cause harm. This is best illustrated by the fact that when someone dies, it is normal flora, no longer constrained by the immune system, which rapidly break down tissues and cause a dead body to decompose.

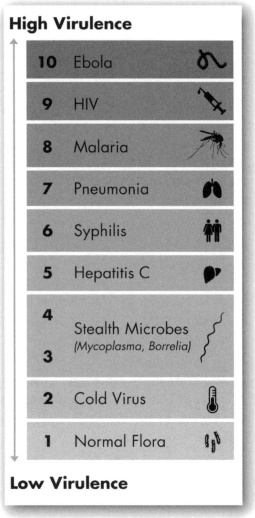

High Virulence

10	Ebola
9	HIV
8	Malaria
7	Pneumonia
6	Syphilis
5	Hepatitis C
4 3	Stealth Microbes *(Mycoplasma, Borrelia)*
2	Cold Virus
1	Normal Flora

Low Virulence

Figure 3 - Virulence Scale

Above 5 on the virulence scale, the rule of thumb is that one solitary microbe is the source of a symptomatic infection[5]. For microbes below

---

5 For a long time, science held to the assumption, defined by Robert Koch in 1884 (Koch's postulates) that microbial illnesses were caused by single specific microbes. While this still holds true for infections with high virulence microbes, it is much less true with low virulence microbes, in which multiple microbes together can cause illness (Peterson 2014).

5 on the scale, chronic infections generally involve multiple low-virulence microbes. Chronic Lyme disease is a typical example of a low virulence microbe illness. It is characterized by co-infections with Borrelia, Mycoplasma, Bartonella, and similar virulence stealth microbes.

Initial infections with lower virulence microbes (<5 on the scale) are typically mild and generally resolve without treatment (the immune system immediately makes recognition and takes countermeasures). **Resolution of symptoms, however, does not necessarily mean the microbe is gone.** Chronic infections can manifest with vague and nonspecific symptoms, such as those common to Lyme disease. Microbes at the lower end of the virulence scale are less likely to respond to conventional therapies, such as antibiotics and vaccines, and are often better addressed with natural therapies.

Note that the virulence scale can vary from person to person (we are all slightly different). One person's immune function against a microbe may be different from another person's. It depends on where one's great ancestors roamed the planet and what types of microbes they were exposed to. People from certain regions of Africa where malaria is endemic are much more resistant to malaria than all other people.

Similarly, some people are more apt to get sick from Borrelia than others. The same is true with Mycoplasma, Bartonella, Babesia, or any other microbe.

Virulence can also vary between different species of the same microbe. The different species of Borrelia that cause relapsing fever are more virulent than the species of Borrelia that cause Lyme disease. Similarly, there are some species of Rickettsia that are not as virulent as *Rickettsia rickettsii*, the microbe that causes Rocky Mountain spotted fever.

THE VIRULENCE PYRAMID

An interesting phenomenon that holds true for most microbes is that risk of exposure to a certain microbe is inversely related to its virulence.[6] In other words, **the more virulent a microbe is, the less likely you are to encounter it**. Most people on the planet will never be exposed to Ebola virus or HIV (even though these microbes notoriously get the most press attention). Everyone on the planet, however, has a balanced relationship with microbes that are considered normal flora.

Risk of exposure can be represented by stretching the virulence scale out into a pyramid shape (see figure 4). Highly virulent pathogens, such as Ebola virus and HIV, are represented at the very peak of the pyramid; risk of exposure is fortunately extremely low.

The broad base of the pyramid represents our normal flora. Every person on earth harbors benign microbes classified as normal flora; exposure is universal.

As you can see from the pyramid (see figure 4), there are a lot more microbes below the level of 5 than above it. This would be as expected. Over many thousands of years, humans have developed familiarity with most microbes that we will likely encounter. Because of host-microbe familiarity, they are less virulent.

This is especially true of tick-borne microbes. **Because ticks have been carrying microbes as long as there have been ticks, and ticks have been biting humans as long as there have been humans, humans are well acquainted with most microbes that ticks carry.**

---

6 This observation holds true for both developed and undeveloped countries. In developed countries, the total burden of potentially harmful microbes tends to be lower than developed countries, but risk of exposure is still proportional to the pyramid. In countries where living standards are poor, the microbial burden of *all* types of microbes is high, but it is proportioned with a greater preponderance of low-virulence microbes over high virulence.

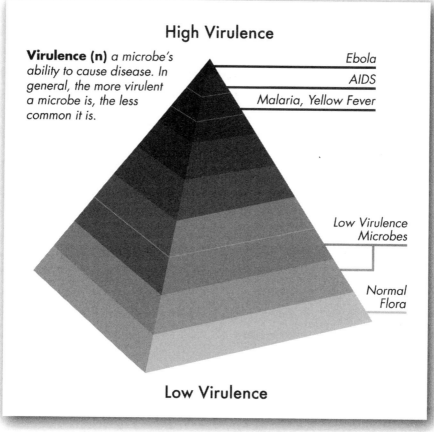

High Virulence

Virulence (n) *a microbe's ability to cause disease. In general, the more virulent a microbe is, the less common it is.*

Ebola

AIDS

Malaria, Yellow Fever

Low Virulence Microbes

Normal Flora

Low Virulence

Figure 4 - Virulence Pyramid

The tick-borne microbes most commonly associated with chronic Lyme disease all fall below 5 on the pyramid scale.[7] Mycoplasma, Bartonella, and Chlamydia are found in the 2-4 range. Borrelia is slightly more virulent (more apt to cause illness) and would fall in the 3-5 range.[8] In other

---

7 This, of course, is a generalization; there are many other potential species of microbes beyond these four that may be associated with chronic Lyme disease (both known and unknown). The list includes less virulent species of Rickettsia, Ehrlichia, and Anaplasma.

8 For the white-footed mouse, Borrelia would be a 1 on the virulence scale, the relationship is ancient. For a dog, Borrelia would be a 2; dogs can get mild arthritis from chronic infection with Borrelia, but generally are not severely affected. It implies that dogs have a longer and closer relationship with Borrelia than humans.

words, in humans, Borrelia is a persistent menace, but not a terrible monster like Ebola.

Ticks can carry higher virulence microbes, but they are rare. Powassan virus is the most virulent of all the tick-borne microbes. It is the only tick-borne microbe that might achieve a 10 on the virulence scale. If you even survived an infection with Powassan virus, it would likely leave you with permanent neurological damage. As you might predict, it is extremely rare (only 60 cases over the past 10 years). There is no cure, and because it is so rare, there probably never will be.

Rickettsia rickettsii, the microbe that causes Rocky Mountain spotted fever, is next on the list of higher virulence tick-borne microbes with a score of 7-8. As you might expect, infection with *R. rickettsii* is much less common than with Borrelia. Ehrlichia and Anaplasma are more common than *R. rickettsii*, but also less virulent (4-7 on the scale). Babesia, though it is a protozoan instead of bacteria, has similar potential to cause illness and would be found at 4-7 on the scale.

These microbes are more apt to cause severe acute disease and less likely to cause chronic illness.[9] Chronic illness, when it occurs, is generally associated with relapse of acute symptoms.

Interestingly, these microbes have been around just as long as Borrelia and the others, but human exposure may have been different through the course of time. There is some evidence that Borrelia is better at infecting than Rickettsia, so even though both microbes may be prevalent in ticks, human exposure may have been different (Buhner 2015).

---

9 Why some people get very sick and others do not get sick at all may be a function of the strain of the microbe, the variability of the host's virulence to that microbe, or possibly environmental or seasonal factors that are not yet evident. Less virulent species of Rickettsia, Ehrlichia, and Anaplasma may be more commonly associated with chronic Lyme disease than once thought.

THE VIRULENCE FACTOR

- Humans are constantly exposed to new microbes seeking to establish host-microbe relationships.

- Host-dependent microbes do harm by scavenging vital nutrients from the host and manipulating the host's immune system.

- Virulence is the potential for a host-dependent microbe to cause illness.

- The level of virulence is dependent on how familiar the host is with the microbe.

- The more virulent a microbe is, the less likely it is to be encountered.

- Microbe virulence can vary from person to person.

THE MICROBIOME AND STEALTH MICROBES

The total collection of all the microbes in the body is referred to as the microbiome. There are many thousands of different microbe species, totaling 100 trillion microbes that make up the human microbiome. A person's microbiome is as unique as his or her genes.

The microbiome consists predominantly of microbes considered to be normal flora, but it also contains microbes that would be considered "marginal". They are outliers...misfits...and we all have them. We collect them as we go through life. They enter the body at every opportunity by breaks in the skin or bug bites, consuming them in food or drink, breathing them in, or through sexual contact.

The human immune system is familiar with these microbes, but not enough to accept them as normal flora. They have higher potential to cause harm than normal flora, but they are still not high virulence (the many microbes between 2-5 on the virulence scale). Mycoplasma, Bartonella, Chlamydia, and Borrelia are certainly on the list, but there are many others.

They would like to join the normal mix of microbes in the body, but they haven't quite learned how to fit in — **they are *normal flora wannabes***. Instead, they live the life of a fugitive, always moving from host to host. Because of their questionable status, an invitation to stay around is never offered, and the immune system makes every effort to oust them.

Persisting is their specialty, however. They are experts at manipulating the immune system to stay one step ahead. It becomes a perpetual tug-of-war that neither party ever wins. The microbes are marginalized, and the potential for harm is minimized (their natural aggressiveness is kept in check), but they stubbornly prevail in the margins of the body.

Because of their fugitive status, they act very differently than normal flora. Normal flora microbes typically inhabit the skin, the gut, and other body cavities. Marginal microbes seek out immune-privileged sites in the body (brain tissue, joint cartilage, eyes, biofilms, and inside cells), where they are less apt to be targeted by immune functions.

For this reason, they are often called **stealth microbes** or **stealth pathogens**.

They are constantly pursued by the immune system and therefore typically occur in low concentrations in the body and grow very slowly (remember, that's all they need to do to complete their mission of moving to another host). This makes finding them extraordinarily challenging and getting rid of them even more challenging.

If healthy immune function is maintained, stealth microbes remain marginalized and do not cause overt illness.

Let immune function falter for even for an instant, however…

STEALTH MICROBE CHARACTERISTICS

- Strategies vary between microbes, but characteristics are similar.

- They are well adapted to human hosts, but not as well adapted as normal flora.

- Initial infection is generally mild; most infections resolve without treatment.

- Severe infection is unusual—stealth microbes rarely kill people directly.

- Multiple stealth microbes are typically present in the margins of the microbiome at one time.

- Everyone harbors stealth microbes, but people with chronic illness may harbor a wider spectrum of stealth microbes.

- Because of being constantly suppressed by immune function, they occur in low concentrations in the body and grow very slowly (even when intense symptoms are present).

- They can live inside cells, protected from immune function.

- Most stealth microbes can infect white blood cells and be spread throughout the body.

- Symptoms, when they occur, are related mostly to generation of inflammatory cytokines, and less to direct damage by the microbe.

5

Chronic Immune Dysfunction

The immune system has a big job. It's like being the officer in charge of a crew of misfits and ruffians on a sailing ship of days gone by.

Let your guard down for one moment and you will be overrun!

Microbes from the lower end of the virulence scale with stealthy character-istics are always present in the margins of the microbiome and always wait-ing for an opportunity — in everyone, but people who become chronically ill may be more apt to have a wider spectrum of marginal microbes. It's not one species of microbe, but many species of microbes all at once. Some, of course, have higher potential to cause illness than others.

In other words, chronic Lyme disease is not just an infection with a mi-crobe called *Borrelia burgdorferi*[1]. A person can harbor more than one species and several strains of Borrelia. At the same time, that person can harbor multiple strains and species of other microbes. Mycoplasma, Bartonella, and Chlamydia are common, but many others are possible (some known and others yet to be discovered).

If immune function falters for any reason, the natural aggressiveness of these microbes is no longer contained. The microbes are then able to

---

1 It's now becoming clear to scientists that many chronic illnesses are associated with disruptions in the balance of the entire microbiome (Peterson 2014).

manipulate immune messengers (called cytokines) in the body to generate inflammation. Inflammation breaks down tissues, allowing microbes to have access to the vital nutrients they need to survive.

Because each microbe has a slightly different strategy for manipulating the immune system, and each microbe may target different resources, symptoms are highly variable and seemingly unrelated to each other (chronic Lyme disease is a little bit different for every person).

Disruption of immune function sets up a vicious cycle. The lapse of immune function allows reactivation of herpes-type viruses, such as Epstein-Barr virus, cytomegalovirus, and others[2] that have been dormant in tissues (we all have these too). The lapse also affects gut microbes, allowing overgrowth of Candida (yeast) and other potentially harmful bacteria.

You can think of it as a covered pot boiling over on the stove. If immune function is healthy, stealth microbes remain restrained, and the pot stays at a low simmer. If immune function is disrupted, however, a low simmer gradually increases to a full boil, and then very suddenly everything pours over the side. Symptoms occur because the immune system can no longer keep a lid on things. The severity of symptoms depends on the degree of immune dysfunction, the types of stealth microbes present, and the burden they cause on the microbiome.

The kind of illness that occurs with a pot of stealth microbes boiling over is very different from that of a highly virulent microbe. In the case of infection with a highly virulent microbe (such as *Rickettsia rickettsii*), one

---

2 There are eight known herpes-type viruses that commonly infect humans: Epstein-Barr virus, CMV, HSV-1, HSV-2, herpes zoster virus, HHV-6a, HHV-6b, and HHV-7. Add that to the list of other viruses that can cause chronic illness including parvovirus B19 (most everyone is exposed), adenoviruses, and hepatitis B and C.

species of microbe acutely wreaks havoc on the body. The body either fails completely or recovers. Chronic infection is less likely.

Illness associated with stealthy opportunists is chronic and insidious. Multiple low-grade threats of different varieties (bacteria, viruses, fungi, or protozoa) are generally involved simultaneously. Once **chronic immune dysfunction** becomes established, the misery can last a lifetime.

"POT BOILING OVER" SYMPTOMS

Symptoms of illness associated with a stealth microbe infection are mostly caused by the tug-of-war that occurs between the microbes and the immune system. It amounts to a small war going on inside the body. Because the **small war typically involves multiple species of microbes, symptoms can be highly variable**.

Localized symptoms such as **joint pain**, **muscle pain**, **chest pain with heartbeat irregularities**, **eye pain**, **tooth pain**, **headaches**, and other neurological symptoms, such as **Bell's palsy** and **burning, tingling, and numbness**, are likely associated with the direct presence of microbes in tissues. The inflammation generated by microbes at those sites causes local damage.

Of all symptoms, **cardiac symptoms are the most concerning, and neurological symptoms are the most persistent**. Any person felt to have Lyme disease (with or without a positive test) who has chest pain, irregular heartbeats, or slow heart rate (<50), should receive immediate attention. Invasion of spirochetes into heart muscle can be life-threatening. Neurological symptoms can be just as disconcerting, but generally will gradually resolve as recovery progresses.

Most "pot boiling over" symptoms, however, are related to generalized inflammation resulting from circulation of inflammatory messengers (cytokines) throughout the whole body. These types of symptoms are non-localized and seemingly unrelated. Common non-localized symptoms include **fatigue, malaise, whole-body aches and pains, muscle weakness, intestinal symptoms, anxiety, depression, poor sleep, stress intolerance, brain fog, and flu-like symptoms.**

Fatigue is possibly the most universal symptom. It occurs anytime the body is chronically stressed in any way.

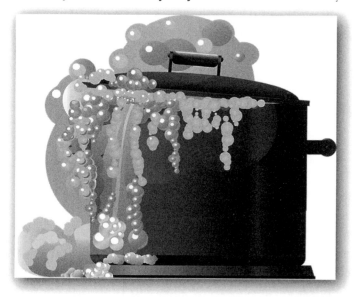

The stress of whole-body inflammation disrupts the natural balance of every system in the body (called homeostasis). Homeostasis is maintained by a small gland at the base of the brain called the hypothalamus. By way of the pituitary gland, the hypothalamus regulates the adrenal glands (stress glands), thyroid (metabolism), and ovaries/testes (reproduction). This central hormone system in the body is often referred to as the **HPA axis** (Hypothalamic-Pituitary-Adrenal axis).

The HPA axis is closely tied to the **autonomic nervous system**, which regulates functions in the body that occur automatically, such as breathing, heartbeat, and intestinal function. The autonomic system includes secretion of adrenaline from the adrenal gland and the sympathetic/ parasympathetic nervous system.

Disruption of the HPA axis and autonomic nervous system may be the cause of a wide range of symptoms including **cold intolerance, cold feet and hands, excessive thirst, sleep disturbances, anxiety, low blood pressure, sudden drop in blood pressure with dizziness (feeling faint), low/high heart rate, reduced sweating**, and **gastrointestinal dysfunction**. Symptoms associated with thyroid dysfunction and reproductive hormone imbalances (estrogen, testosterone) are also common.

Gastrointestinal dysfunction commonly includes "leaky gut". **Leaky gut** results from a combination of factors, including autonomic dysfunction, damage to the intestinal lining by microbes, such as Mycoplasma, and eating processed foods. Leaky gut allows food sensitivities to occur. (We'll cover leaky gut in **Chapter 24**, Digestive Dysfunction).

Similarly, toxins, chronic stress, and inflammation disrupt the blood brain barrier, resulting in "leaky brain." When the barrier is compromised, neurotoxins can pass into the brain. This contributes to a wide range of neurological symptoms including **brain fog, depression**, and **impaired mental functions**.

Endorphins, the chemicals in the body that promote feelings of well-being and act as natural pain relievers, are also secreted from the hypothalamus and pituitary gland. Disruption of hypothalamic function suppresses endorphin secretion, which **increases perception of pain and feeling low**. Endorphins are essential for supporting optimal immune function.

The ability of the body to rid itself of toxins is impaired, and toxins accumulate. Compromise of normal function extends all the way down to the cellular level; cells lose the ability to self-regulate and repair. The microbes also prevent abnormal cells that they have infected from self-destructing (this is called apoptosis), providing one possible link to cancer formation (Yandell 2016).

The fact that stealth microbes alter the cells they infect and widely manipulate the immune system may be a factor in the occurrence of autoimmunity. Autoimmunity is when the body attacks itself. All chronic Lyme sufferers likely have some degree of autoimmunity (Ghosh 2005), but some people will progress further to a destructive process defined as an autoimmune disease. Why this happens is unknown, but it may be a factor of different types of microbes coming together (bacteria and viruses) to disrupt immune functions (Steed 2014).

Some people with chronic Lyme disease experience **mast cell hypersensitization** (Talkington 1999). Mast cells (and some B cells) are associated with the immune pathway that deals with intestinal parasites (worms). Because Borrelia microbes have worm-like tails (flagella), these types of immune functions are sometimes directed at getting rid of the microbe. Because Borrelia is a bacteria and not a worm, however, it doesn't work very well, and overreaction occurs. Mast cells produce histamine. Excessive histamine is associated with **skin itching**, **rash**, **and allergic-type reactions**.

Of course, no symptom is absolute; every individual is different.

THE AGE OF CHRONIC IMMUNE DYSFUNCTION

The fact that many people who carry Borrelia and other stealth microbes never get sick suggests that there's more to it than just an infection with a microbe.

All humans have stealth microbes lurking in the margins of their microbiome (some more virulent than others; that part is the luck of the draw). If immune function is robust, the pot stays at a simmer, and overt illnesses does not occur.

If something chronically tips the balance toward immune dysfunction, however, the pot starts to boil.

Factors that tip the balance toward **chronic immune dysfunction** are more prevalent in the modern world than ever before in history. Slowly and insidiously, **the modern world has become saturated with toxic factors that disrupt immune function** (Bogdanos 2013). It is likely the reason why chronic Lyme disease, fibromyalgia, and many other similar illnesses have become so prevalent.

In other words, it's not more tick bites or increased prevalence of Borrelia and other stealth microbes that is causing more people to be ill. Instead, it is the result of a higher prevalence of factors causing **chronic immune dysfunction**.

We are complacent with these modern immune-disrupting factors because they are **connected to things that make life easier and more comfortable**.

In many respects, modern times are the best of times. Food is plentiful. Most people live and work inside comfortable temperature-controlled environments. Machines do all the back-breaking labor. Virtually anything can be made from plastic. It is possible to travel from one side of the planet to the other in less than a day. Artificial lighting has made the dark of night less restrictive.

Every coin has a flip side, however.

Food is plentiful, but most food that most people eat is artificially processed to satisfy taste buds, certainly not to benefit health. Over-farming with excessive use of pesticides and fertilizer has leached essential nutrients from soil. Oppressive stress has become synonymous with modern life. And the price of all the convenience is toxic byproducts from petroleum and coal.

It all adds up. Every system of the body is affected, but the immune system is especially hard hit. It shouldn't be surprising that illnesses, such as **chronic Lyme disease** and **fibromyalgia** have become so common.

A fitting name that I use for these immune-disrupting factors is **system disruptors**. System disruptors play a role in virtually all chronic illnesses. When I evaluate a patient, I spend more effort searching for system disruptors that are making the patient ill than trying to find a diagnosis.

System disruptors can be divided into **seven primary categories**:

- **Unnatural food.** The average diet for most people in the modern world is grain-based (processed grain products and grain-fed meat). Despite convenience and hitting all the right taste buds, modern processed food products are toxic to the intestinal system, disrupt immune functions, and cause hormone imbalances throughout the body. Beyond burdening the body with undesirable substances, the average American diet does not provide sufficient levels of vital nutrients and all-important antioxidants.

- **Toxin overload.** Over the past hundred years, **over 200,000 different manmade toxins have been released into the environment**. Most of them are from **petroleum, coal, or mining.** They are attached to things that make life easier and more comfortable. Because their presence is mostly hidden, we tend to ignore this insidious threat. Chemical toxins and heavy metals, however, accumulate in tissues and disrupt all systems in the body, including and especially the immune system. Toxins are not limited to those generated by humans. **Natural toxins, called biotoxins, are very present in every environment**. Most of the time, biotoxins do not occur in high enough concentrations to cause harm, but **mycotoxins produced by mold inside modern enclosed dwellings are potent immune disruptors.**

- **Chronic emotional stress.** Emotional stress is so pervasive that it has become accepted as part of modern life. The complexities of modern living cause a certain level of low-grade tension that is always present. The result is **increased susceptibility to anxiety and sleep problems, disruption of adrenal hormone balance, digestive dysfunction, and certainly immune dysfunction**.

- **Physical stress.** Beyond a hundred years ago, human physical stress would have been characterized by excessive physical labor (the iceman was worn down by carrying heavy loads for long distances). Today, we have the opposite problem. **Most people have sedentary jobs, and prolonged inactivity has become common to modern life**. Short bursts of intense activity in a gym are not enough to compensate (and sometimes can be harmful). Prolonged inactivity (especially sitting in front of a computer) is associated with decreased blood flow, retention of toxins, decreased endorphins, and, of course, immune dysfunction. This category also includes trauma and extremes in temperature or pressure.

- **Energy stress.** Artificial energy sources (computers, cell phones, electrical devices, microwave towers) very likely have **disruptive influence on the energy flow of the body**. How much this artificial force affects health is difficult to quantitate, but there is little doubt that disrupted energy flow in the body can adversely affect immune function.

- **Oxidative stress.** Everything is interrelated. All of the above factors increase production of damaging free radicals inside cells and in tissues. The damage caused by free radicals is called oxidative stress. Another form of oxidative stress, commonly called **inflammation**, results from excessive production of free radicals by overstimulated white blood cells. The average American diet is woefully deficient in protective antioxidants to curb the damage caused by oxidative stress and inflammation (and no, a one-a-day vitamin supplement is not enough to compensate).

- **Microbiome imbalance.** As we go through life, we continually add microbes to our microbiome — and some of them are not friendly. If chronic immune dysfunction becomes established, stealth microbes in the margins are no longer contained, and the pot boils over. Sometimes all it takes is a tick bite with introduction of yet another microbe (in addition to the ones inevitably already present) to tip the balance toward a boiling pot. In addition, infection with a higher virulence microbe, such as Rickettsia, Ehrlichia, Anaplasma, Babesia, or even a bad flu virus can initiate chronic immune dysfunction.

There's no getting around the role that system disruptors play in chronic Lyme disease. How different system disruptors come together influences how chronic Lyme disease will present.

THE MANY FACES OF CHRONIC LYME

The classic presentation of Lyme disease is onset of illness immediately after a tick bite. If some degree of immune dysfunction is already established when the tick bite occurs, the new infection with Borrelia becomes the tip of the balance that causes the pot to boil over. Though there are some people who can remember the tick bite that changed their lives, this presentation is less common than other presentations.

As mentioned in Chapter 2, the most common presentation of chronic Lyme disease is gradual onset. Most people are healthy when they first get infected and do not remember the tick bite or the initial infection. The microbe is present (along with other stealth microbes in the margins of the microbiome), but not causing harm. As cumulative stress from system disruptors adds up, immune function gradually deteriorates, and the pot starts boiling over with Borrelia in the middle of it all.

This scenario **brings up the question of how often mild arthritis or some other symptom attributed to aging might actually be a low-grade infection with Borrelia or other stealth microbes**. Mild symptoms are unlikely to be brought to the attention of a doctor. Even when they are, the doctor is unlikely to test for or become suspicious of a microbial illness.

Gradual onset, of course, is not the only presentation of chronic Lyme disease. Onset of chronic illness can be precipitated abruptly by an acutely stressful event (automobile accident, divorce, job loss, severe influenza, etc.). If Borrelia and other stealth microbes are present in a person's microbiome, acute disruption of immune function by the stressful event can tip the balance toward chronic illness.

It may be true that some people may be more genetically prone to develop chronic Lyme disease than others. Also, some microbes may be more virulent to some people than others. In addition, we all have genetic quirks that affect our susceptibility to certain diseases. For example, people who have the various methylation gene defects (5-MTHFR) may have more difficulty defending themselves against stealth microbes if nutrition is not up to par.

Simultaneous infection with multiple microbes by tick bite is yet another possibility. Acute infection with multiple species of microbes at once can be a real shock to the immune system. This is especially true if simultaneous infection occurs with Borrelia and a microbe of higher virulence, such as Babesia, Ehrlichia, Anaplasma, or Rickettsia. In this case, the pot rapidly reaches a full boil, and chronic debilitating illness becomes more likely. There are many less well-known (and usually not tested for) species of Ehrlichia, Anaplasma, and Rickettsia that may be involved.

This is where the story comes around full circle. When Dr. Willy Burgdorfer first analyzed the sera of patients infected in Lyme, Connecticut, many of them tested positive for a microbe he called the Swiss agent. He had discovered this microbe in ticks during a research trip to his native Switzerland in 1978 (but the specific type and species of the microbe had not been identified). At that time, the Swiss agent had not been associated with disease in humans. Because the spirochete, later named *Borrelia burgdorferi*, was more prominent in the analysis, it was given credit for causing the illness.

Years later, Dr. Burgdorfer played a role in identifying the Swiss agent as a species of Rickettsia, ultimately named *Rickettsia Helvetica* (Beati 1993). It became linked in Europe to a flu-like illness with symptoms including fever, headache, arthralgia (joint pain), myalgia (muscle pain) and occasionally a rash (similar to other spotted fevers caused by Rickettsia species). This species of Rickettsia is still not routinely tested for in the United States.

Simultaneous infection with both *Borrelia burgdorferi* <u>and</u> the Rickettsia microbe may explain why a cluster of people in Lyme, Connecticut became ill rather suddenly. Likely, both microbes had long been present in N. America, but coinfection with both together may have been unusual. The seventies era was also when people first started embracing fast food, fast cars, and a fast pace of life. It was the dawning of **the age of chronic immune dysfunction**.

BEYOND LYME

Though medical science would like to have everything fit into nice, neat boxes called diagnoses, the world of disease is mostly a big gray zone. Rarely does anything fit into a nice, neat box. The margins between different diagnoses are always blurred.

Not surprisingly, most anyone who ends up claiming a diagnosis of chronic Lyme disease has also entertained other possibilities before the test showed Lyme. The most common is fibromyalgia, but chronic fatigue syndrome, multiple sclerosis, and a range of other chronic illnesses also may have been considered. Some of those who ultimately pick the identity of chronic Lyme disease have testing absolutely indicating the presence of Borrelia, **but many do not**.

Conversely, many people who identify with fibromyalgia or chronic fatigue have suspected that they may have Lyme disease, but because testing for Borrelia was negative, they chose a different identification. Despite a negative test, however, some of those people harbor Borrelia.

Not surprisingly, there's a lot of overlap of symptoms.

If you overlay symptoms common to chronic Lyme disease with the classic symptoms of fibromyalgia and chronic fatigue syndrome, there is a lot of overlap. Continue with symptoms of early multiple sclerosis, Parkinson's, ALS, and most autoimmune diseases, and there is still a lot of overlap.

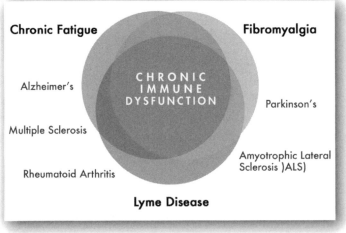

Figure 5 - Chronic Immune Dysfunction

This "pot-boiling-over" scenario not only explains many well-known diseases, but also accounts for all the "invisible" illnesses (Gulf War syndrome, adrenal fatigue, chronic fatigue and immune dysfunction syndrome, mixed connective tissue disorder, and myalgic encephalomyelitis — just to name a few) that fall between the margins of other diagnoses.

What type of illness a person ends up with depends on three primary factors:

- How different **system disruptors come together to initiate immune dysfunction**
- The **individual's genetic makeup**
- The **species and strains of microbes** that have been collected through life (some microbes or microbe combinations are more virulent than others — luck of the draw plays a role)

Borrelia is present in all confirmed cases of Lyme disease, but it is one of many microbes contributing to the illness. Fibromyalgia may or may not include Borrelia (many people diagnosed with fibromyalgia are carrying Borrelia, but do not know it), but other stealth microbes, such as Mycoplasma and Bartonella, may also be present. Chronic fatigue syndrome may include a different set of stealth microbes altogether.

Chronic Lyme disease, fibromyalgia, and chronic fatigue syndrome may be early stages of more advanced illnesses, such as multiple sclerosis, Parkinson's, and autoimmune diseases.

In other words, disease can be thought of as a continuum. It starts with mild symptoms. Early on, symptoms are not specific enough to define a diagnosis. This is the stage when many people end up being labeled as having fibromyalgia or chronic fatigue syndrome (disorders, not true diagnoses), or a not formally recognized diagnosis, such as chronic Lyme disease. With time, symptoms will progress and become more defined into a specific diagnosis, such as multiple sclerosis, Parkinson's, ALS, or an autoimmune disease.

The evidence supporting links between stealth microbes, microbiome imbalance, chronic immune dysfunction, and a variety of chronic illnesses is growing every year. Links have been made between Mycoplasma and rheumatoid arthritis, Chlamydia and multiple sclerosis, Alzheimer's and Borrelia (and other microbes), ALS and Borrelia (and other microbes), and autoimmune illnesses in general with a variety of stealth microbes. While medical science considers none of these links to be a smoking gun, the accumulated evidence is hard to ignore.

A CLOSING WORD ON PARASITES

The word *parasite* refers to any creature that requires a host to survive. So technically, all the microbes mentioned so far are parasites. To most people, however, the word *parasite* refers to intestinal worms. We may have these too, but rarely to the degree of causing symptoms and certainly not to the degree of people living in third-world countries.

Even so, many people seem to be intensely worried about them.

Intestinal parasites consist primarily of protozoa and worms. Protozoa are single-celled mobile creatures with the ability to reproduce by dividing like bacteria. They differ from bacteria in that their cells contain a nucleus separated by a membrane and contain mitochondria (called eukaryotic, the same as cells found in higher organisms). The most common intestinal protozoa are giardia (*Giardia lamblia*) and entamoeba (*Entamoeba histolytica*). Both are acquired from drinking contaminated water. In comparison, Babesia and malaria parasites are blood-borne protozoa transmitted by biting insects. Likely, there is a wider variety of blood-borne protozoa with stealth microbe characteristics that contribute to chronic illness than presently recognized.

One of them is *Toxoplasmosis gondii*. *T. gondii* is the most common protozoal infection in developed countries. Cat populations are the natural reservoir for the microbe. Humans become infected when they come in contact with feces from an infected cat. 30 to 50% of people have been infected with *T. gondii*. Symptoms of initial infection are generally mild, typical for a low virulence microbe. The microbe lives inside cells (obligate intracellular) and shares many characteristics with other stealth microbes. It is likely that most people infected become chronic carriers. Though most chronic carriers do not have symptoms, *T. gondii* has been associated with dementia, miscarriages, birth defects, blindness, and schizophrenia (Webster 2013).

The worms that everyone is worried about are multicellular higher organisms that can grow in size. Worms include roundworms and flatworms. They have very different life cycles than protozoa, bacteria, and viruses. The life cycle starts with eggs passed in some creatures' feces. The eggs hatch into larva, which can contaminate food, objects, or a drinking-water supply. The larva may infect another animal (cow, fish, pig), and if the undercooked meat is consumed by a person, infection can occur. Or, for some types of worms, unwary people consume the larvae in contaminated food or water. Some worm larvae can enter through the skin from contact with contaminated water or feces-contaminated objects.

Once consumed, the larvae carry on inside the host from larval to adult stage[3]. To survive, the organism scavenges resources directly from the host. If the burden of organisms on the host is low, the host doesn't suffer enough to notice. If infestation is large, symptoms include abdominal discomfort, loose stools, and bloody stools. Infestation is usually associated with immune compromise.

Once at the adult stage, the organism begins passing eggs. It will do so for the rest of its adult life. The eggs don't hatch inside the host's body (the infection is not self-maintaining), but are shed in feces (except in

---

3 For some types of multicellular parasites, the larvae enter the host through the skin when the host stands in contaminated water.

rare cases, hatched larvae can reinvade anal skin). The organism will then eventually die. Once the organism dies, the shedding stops, and the organism passes from the body. End of story...unless the host continues to consume new larvae.

To become infested with intestinal parasites, there must be large initial inoculation or continual re-inoculation. In other words, the person must consume or come in contact with a large dose of larvae or must be continually exposed to new larvae. Contaminated food or water is an essential part of the cycle. In third-world countries where sanitation is poor and fecal contamination of both food and water is common, much of the population carries a burden of multicellular parasites of different varieties (the degree of the burden is very dependent on immune function).

In developed countries where water sources are clean, people regularly wash their hands, and contaminated food is less common, harboring a significant burden of intestinal parasites is uncommon. We probably all pick up something occasionally on salads or undercooked meat, but it is just that — occasional and low grade. If you cook all your food thoroughly, the risk is even lower.

The biggest risk in developed countries is organic lettuce (but highly variable because of different methods of production). Manure can be sprayed on crops, but by law, it must not be applied after 120 days before harvest (Kaiser 2012). Other organic vegetables should be cooked, peeled, or washed thoroughly before consumption.

Unless you eat lots of undercooked meat, eat lots of uncooked, unpeeled organic vegetables or fruit, work in the agriculture or livestock industry where exposure to fecal contamination is high, or frequent third-world countries without being careful about what you eat and drink, intestinal parasites shouldn't be at the top of your list of concerns.

PART TWO
Gathering Information

6

A Holistic Approach to Evaluation

The process of figuring out why you're ill can be a roller-coaster ride that progresses from fear and desperation to hope, false hope, disappointment, restored hope, confusion, and finally to understanding, determination, and confidence in your own abilities.

QUEST FOR A DIAGNOSIS

When you're ill, the only thought on your mind is becoming well again. When wellness never comes and illness becomes chronic, fear paralyzes all rational thought. Ultimately, desperation leads to a trip to the doctor's office, where the **quest for a diagnosis** begins.

I know the process all too well. In medical school, I was taught the classic approach to diagnosis that most doctors use today.

It starts with a history focused on cataloging symptoms of illness. Next, a physical exam is performed to search for any physical signs of illness. From this information, possible diagnoses are considered. Labs and other diagnostic tests are ordered to confirm or dismiss different possibilities.

For most acute illnesses, such as acute pneumonia, a broken leg, or even something such as Ebola virus, this method works well. The symptoms are specific for a very limited number of possibilities, and targeted diagnostic tests quickly reveal the diagnosis. Treatment is immediate and specific.

With chronic illnesses, however, things get complicated. **The symptoms of many, if not most, chronic illnesses are nonspecific**. In other words, the symptoms that occur are common to many illnesses, but do not point to any one specific illness. Abnormal physical signs often do not show up until someone is very sick.

Without symptoms or signs to guide the next step, ordering labs is a shot in the dark. By default, most doctors end up taking the shotgun approach: pull the trigger, and see what falls. There are thousands of labs that can be ordered, but none of them are quite as specific or reliable as you might think. Most lab results end up being filed away as unremarkable.

Certain symptoms, such as neurological, cardiac, or intestinal symptoms, may trigger referral to a specialist. This, of course, incurs more lab tests and diagnostic procedures that add expense and waiting time. Often as not, these tests too are unremarkable. The most you can expect is reassurance that you don't have MS, cancer, an impending heart attack, or some terrible autoimmune disease (yet).

All the while, you, the patient, end up entombed in the perpetual wait for a diagnosis — for without a diagnosis, treatment cannot begin. When a diagnosis never comes because all the labs and procedures are unremarkable, you ultimately get pinned with fibromyalgia or chronic fatigue syndrome — **because nothing else fits**.

And those labels won't get you very far because they are **classified as disorders, not true diagnoses**. A true diagnosis can be defined by tests, and potential cures are available. A disorder is simply a name applied to a collection of symptoms for which the cause is unknown (at least by medical science), and "cure" simply doesn't apply. Your doctor may offer prescriptions to alleviate symptoms, but little more.

Without a *real* diagnosis, you often end up being treated like a second-class citizen.

I know how it feels because I've been on both sides of the fence. As a physician, it's frustrating not to be able to find anything, and it's all too easy to focus that frustration back on the patient (it's not my fault...it's all in the patient's head). As a patient, I've felt the heat of that frustration, but at the same time, felt helpless and desperate to find answers — ultimately it can erode the doctor-patient relationship.

THE LYME TEST
The one test that people often turn to in hopes of changing that situation is the test for Lyme disease. A positive test means you have a *real* diagnosis and a potential cure. Hope is often pinned on that test being positive.

Most doctors, however, will not routinely order a test for Lyme disease unless you report a tick bite. Considering that most people with chronic Lyme disease don't remember a tick bite, it is usually not part of the initial evaluation (unless you happen to ask for it).

Sooner or later, however, Lyme disease will come up as a possibility.

When it does, your doctor will likely order the screening test for Lyme disease (ELISA). If you have been sick for a while, this test may well be negative (even if you do have Lyme disease). With a negative test, your provider may refuse to go any further...in which case, you will probably end up searching for another provider.

If your medical provider happens to be a bit savvier, he or she will also order a Western blot for Lyme. The standard Western blot for Lyme that is run by many conventional labs, however, is missing several key bands (they were excluded years ago when a vaccine that ultimately didn't work was being developed, but the bands were never put back in the test), so correct results are about 50/50 at best.

Also, microbial testing is **geared toward diagnosing acute infection.** If you've been sick for a while, your chances of a getting a positive test are even lower.

If the test is negative, you continue with a label of chronic fatigue or fibromyalgia (even though you may have Lyme disease). At that point, you become a real thorn in your medical provider's side — a chronic complainer who never gets well.

If the test is positive, you may receive a short course of antibiotics lasting several weeks. While this may provide some benefit, it is unlikely to make you well. Few providers are willing to write for repeated or prolonged courses of antibiotics (they may be right on this one; there is no evidence that prolonged antibiotic therapy has any benefit for chronic Lyme disease).

Hope turns into false hope and disappointment.

LYME SPECIALISTS

At this point, you may give up on the conventional medical community entirely and seek out someone with specialized knowledge. Hope for a treatable diagnosis is restored, whether you had a positive Lyme test or not, and the quest takes on a new direction.

Prepare to be overwhelmed, however. If your situation is disparate, your new medical provider will likely order a wide assortment of different tests to determine why you are ill. Often these tests provide useful information, but sometimes they just make things more confusing; the body is extremely complex and we still don't understand everything about how it works.

Also, be prepared to pull out your checkbook. Many of these tests are not recognized by the conventional medical community. Therefore, they are not covered by health insurance, and you will likely pay for them out of pocket. The bill can run into many thousands of dollars.

If you had a negative Lyme test before, but still feel you have chronic Lyme disease, a blood sample sent to IGeneX labs may be able to prove you right (for a cost of about $600). The test, however, is only 70% good at best and is specific for *Borrelia burgdorferi*; it does not test for other species of Borrelia.

If that test is positive, you may also decide to test for "coinfections" (for an additional cost). Whatever microbes the testing turns up, however, may just be scratching the surface — there are many more unknowns than knowns, and all forms of testing are far from being absolute. You may still have the microbe being tested for, even if testing is negative.

By the end of it all, you will have accumulated a huge amount of information about different functions in your body and different microbes that may be present, but unless you have a provider who truly understands a holistic approach to recovery, you may end up more confused than anything else.

Use caution as you proceed further. The common practice of independently treating each lab abnormality and each microbe that turns up is painstakingly difficult — it can work, but it's very complicated and expensive.

To get your life back, you must address the whole as well as the individual parts.

DIAGNOSIS FROM A HOLISTIC PERSPECTIVE
Stop...take a deep breath...let it out slowly.

It is possible to overcome chronic Lyme disease without spending thousands of dollars on testing and flying across the country to see a specialist.

The process of gathering information needn't be complicated or frustrating. It's just a matter of putting things in perspective.

Certain types of testing can be important, but the success of your recovery does not hinge on any one test. In fact, you could bypass lab testing altogether and your recovery would likely progress just fine.

This is especially true of microbe testing. The current state of microbe testing, especially for chronic infections with stealth microbes, is limited at best. It is not uncommon for someone to be infected with Borrelia, have all the symptoms of chronic Lyme disease, but test negative for Borrelia. It's just as possible to have all the symptoms of chronic Lyme disease, but not have Borrelia at all — many stealth microbes have characteristics like Borrelia.

There's always more to it than just an infection with a microbe, however. It's not uncommon for people to harbor Borrelia (and/or other stealth microbes) and not be sick at all. Something else must be present for chronic illness to occur.

That something is **chronic immune dysfunction**. It results from a combination of factors, both natural and unnatural. These factors are the **system disruptors** mentioned in Chapter 5. Sometimes the effects of system disruptors have been adding up for a while, and an infection from a tick bite tips the balance. Other times, Borrelia and/or other stealth microbes have been long present, but immune dysfunction and chronic illness doesn't occur until the negative effects of system disruptors add up. Symptoms gradually appear and worsen over time.

With a holistic approach to diagnosis, the effects of system disruptors are considered just as much as any formal test results. Therefore, a holistic evaluation begins with an assessment of your health habits. The next chapter, **Chapter 7**, begins with a survey of your present health habits. It's a reflection of the impact that system disruptors are having on the healing systems of your body. Other methods of self-assessment are also included in the chapter.

During your recovery, you will need to establish a relationship with one or more healthcare providers (if you haven't already). A conventional healthcare provider can order labs and other tests to rule out the possibility of something other than Lyme disease. A doctor can also prescribe medications if needed. Medications are sometimes beneficial for controlling symptoms early in your recovery. You also need access to the medical system if you have an emergency. The guidelines in **Chapter 8** will help you maintain positive relationship with the medical system. A description of different types of providers and specialists is also included.

There are literally thousands of different types of lab tests, most of which are not important for your recovery. You will need the basics, however. **Chapter 9** provides guidelines on which labs offer the most benefit. A list of labs for defining immune dysfunction is also provided, along with explanations of specialized labs that a Lyme specialist may order. This type of testing is rarely essential for your recovery, however. Plenty of people have gotten well using a holistic approach to recovery without it.

You may not be able to resist the urge to test for microbes (we all want to know as much as we can), but please read the beginning of **Chapter 10** thoroughly before jumping down that rabbit hole. Most people don't require extensive microbe testing to get well (or any microbe testing, for that matter), but the current state of microbe testing is provided in the chapter for those who are interested.

Time to move forward with your recovery!

7

Self-Assessment

Some of the most important information for your recovery is information that you can gather yourself. This type of information is different from that provided by lab tests, but it is just as valuable.

Your self-assessment begins with a simple health survey. The better your health habits, the faster your recovery will progress. The survey evaluates the impact that various system disruptors are having on your body. Curtailing system disruptors is a key part of your recovery.

How do your present health habits stack up? Have they improved since you started struggling with chronic illness? Repeat the survey at 3 months and 6 months to track your improvement.

Assign yourself 0 for answers on the left, 1 for answers in the middle, and 2 for answers on the right. Be honest. Add up all the numbers at the end. A low number score reflects poor health habits. The higher the number, the better your health habits. The lowest possible score is, of course, zero, and the highest possible score for the survey is 60.

Diet

Serving of Fresh Vegetables Daily:	0-1	2-4	>5
Serving of Fresh Fruit Daily:	0-1	2-4	>5
% of Food Wrapped or Packaged: (processed food)	>70%	30-70%	<30%
Bean Products (proportion of diet):	large	moderate	small
Nuts (including peanuts):	large	moderate	small
Fish/Seafood Consumption:	rarely	1-2x/wk	3x+/wk
Meat Consumption (chicken):	daily	4x/wk	1-4/wk
Egg Consumption:	daily	4-6 eggs/wk	1-4 eggs/wk
Meat Consumption (pork, beef):	often	1-3x/wk	1-3x/wk
Dairy (milk, cheese):	often	occasionally	light use
Cakes, Cookies, Pastries:	often	occasionally	rarely
Bread & Similar Products:	often	occasionally	rarely

Toxins and Hazardous Substances

Cigarette Smoking:	still smoking	quit for > 1 year	never
Alcohol Consumption:	> 2 drinks/day	1-2 drinks/day	1 or less/day
Visible Mold in Living Space:	present	possible	absent
Stale Smell in House:	strong	mild	absent
Computer/Cell Phone Use:	> 6 hrs/day	2-4 hrs/day	< 2 hrs/day
Drink Purified Water	rarely	occasionally	often
Eat Organic Food	rarely	occasionally	often
Known Toxin Exposure:	high	moderate	low

Lifestyle

Exercise:	rarely	occasionally	often/daily
Exercise Intensity:	intense	light	moderate
Practice Relaxing:	rarely	occasionally	often
Avg. Hours of Sleep/Night:	< 4	4-6	> 7
Take an Afternoon Nap:	rarely	occasionally	often/daily
My General Energy Level is:	low	comes & goes	normal
Feel Stressed:	often	moderately	occasionally
Manage Stress:	poorly	okay	well
Work:	> 8hrs/day	avg 8 hrs/day	< 8hrs/day
I Enjoy My Work:	rarely	occasionally	mostly

MEASURING WELLNESS

Wellness is the absence of illness. Wellness can also be defined as the absence of symptoms. Therefore, not having symptoms is certainly an indicator of wellness. Monitoring symptoms, however, is very subjective. It's easy to become complacent about symptoms and accept their presence over time. It's also easy to forget how bad it was in the past.

Even so, keeping track of symptoms is an effective way to measure present health status and progress forward. The more objectively you catalog symptoms, the more useful the information will be.

Journaling. Jotting your thoughts down is a great way to monitor your recovery. It doesn't have to be an actual journal; a file on your computer works just fine. You don't have to be a master at writing to gain benefit from journaling.

A symptom log is a very important part of your journal. Objectively measuring and logging symptoms helps you see progress...or the lack thereof. A symptom log can be created in a notebook or in an Excel file.

Pick 5 to 10 of your most prominent symptoms, and list them on a chart. Create columns on the chart adjacent to the symptoms, allowing for multiple entries. Rate each symptom on a 1-to-10 scale in terms of intensity, with 10 being the most intense. Each month, repeat the assessment, and enter a rating. This will help you monitor improvement from month to month. Seeing progress is important in your recovery.

Pain as a symptom. Pain is very commonly associated with chronic illness and is a hallmark feature of fibromyalgia. Pain is generally associated with inflammation and is generally limited to the area of the body that is inflamed, but this is not always the case; pain can be referred from another area. Pain associated with other symptoms (fever, vomiting, etc.) is generally more concerning than isolated pain. Any unexplained

Symptom	Month 1	Month 2	Month 3	Month 4
Fatigue	10	8	6	4
Joint Pain	9	7	4	3
Insomnia	9	6	5	4
Brain Fog	10	8	7	4
Body Aches	8	7	3	1

Figure 6 - Sample symptom survey

pain, severe pain, worsening pain, or pain associated with other symptoms should immediately be brought to the attention of a healthcare provider. Resolution of pain is one of the most positive (and desirable) indications of getting well.

MONITORING BODY FUNCTIONS

Tongue. The Chinese have been studying tongues for thousands of years, and whole encyclopedias are devoted to diagnosing disease by tongue analysis. The tongue is a barometer for the rest of the body. While in-depth analysis in rarely indicated, an examination in the mirror can provide valuable information.

The surface of a normal tongue is wet, pink, and mildly grooved. Dryness with white or yellow plaque across the surface and associated burning is a sign of poor digestion, immune compromise, and intestinal bacterial imbalance. It can also represent a yeast infection (thrush), which generally only occurs under the above conditions. Improvement in tongue health generally follows improved health in general, but thrush must be diagnosed and treated by a healthcare provider.

Throat. The back of the throat is a great barometer for airborne toxins. A scratchy throat in the absence of a viral infection often indicates the presence of threatening toxins in the environment and a debilitated state of health. As your health improves, you should become less sensitive to toxic threats.

Abdomen. A distended abdomen can be a sign of trapped gas in the small intestine. The abdomen will be tense like a drum. Sometimes you can even thump it and make a drum-like sound. Trapped gas in the small intestine results from excessive concentrations of bacteria and/or Candida (yeast) in the small intestine (normally, concentrations of bacteria in the small intestine are low). It often results from poor digestion and low stomach acid. It can also result from excessive consumption of starches and sugar.

Getting rid of trapped gas is a matter of starving out the microbes by cutting out starches and sugar and improving digestion. Digestive enzymes and apple cider vinegar with meals (1-2 tbsp. with 8 oz. of water with each meal) often helps improve digestion. Probiotics sometimes help and sometimes make it worse. In this situation, avoid probiotics containing lactobacilli. Use probiotics containing only Bifidobacterium.

Stools. Although a taboo topic in daily conversation, stools can provide a wealth of information about the digestive tract. Digestive dysfunction is common in all types of chronic illness, including chronic Lyme disease.

- *Frequency.* Normal bowel movements consist of soft, but formed stools that occur spontaneously 1-2 times daily. Gas and bloating are minimal.
  - o Constipation is defined as the absence of spontaneous bowel movements associated with impaired colonic activity. It is often closely associated with consumption of processed

food products. Stools are generally hard. Flatulence is common. Frequency is anything less than once daily, but going several days to even weeks is not uncommon. Some individuals are more prone to constipation than others.

- o Loose stools in the form of poorly formed or liquid stools, typically occurring more than once daily, are a sign of impaired digestion and gut inflammation. When accompanied by gas and bloating (usually present), loose stools are a sign of abnormal bacterial overgrowth.

- *Undigested food.* Nuts, such as sunflower seeds and pumpkin seeds, and corn typically come through undigested, but other food substances should not be identifiable. Loose stools containing undigested food are a strong sign of low acid production in the stomach and low digestive enzymes. In this case, digestive enzyme supplements and vinegar with meals can be very beneficial (2 tbsp. apple cider vinegar in 6-8 oz. water).

- *Color.* The normal color of stool is reddish brown. The color represents bile in stool, which is necessary for digesting fat. Light grey stools suggest stagnant bile production from the liver and gallbladder. Tar-like stools can represent bleeding in the stomach, and a significant amount of bright red blood is never a good sign.

- *Float or not.* Normal stools sink. Floating stools, especially if loose and light grey, indicate poor digestion of fat. It is a sign of insufficient enzyme production from the pancreas and stagnant bile production.

- *Odor.* Normal stools have odor, but odor strong enough to run you out of the bathroom is a strong sign of extreme bacterial imbalance. Foul-smelling flatulence is just as indicative.

Urine. Adequate urine flow indicates normal hydration. If you are drinking the right amount, urine will be the color of lemonade. Normal voiding should occur several times daily and 1-2 times at night. If your urine is as clear as water, you are probably over-hydrating. Urine the color of apple juice indicates dehydration.

Urine should not have a foul odor (unless asparagus have been consumed) or be cloudy. These are indications of infection or bacterial contamination.

Everyone always wants to know exactly how much to drink, but the answer is very dependent on physical activity and sweating. Color of urine is the best guide. Don't forget: vegetables and fruit contain high quantities of water compared to processed food, which generally contains little moisture.

Urinating large amounts frequently is generally a result of drinking lots of liquids, but it can also be a sign of an underlying problem. The way to know for sure is by doing a liquid fast for 6 to 12 hours. If the flow slows down and urine concentrates, then you don't have a problem.

MEASURING YOUR VITAL SIGNS
Pulse. Average pulse is 72 beats per minute. To find your pulse, turn your wrist so it's facing up, then place your index and middle finger just on the other side of the largest tendon until you feel your heartbeat. Check for consistency; beats should occur very regularly. Count each beat for 30 seconds, then multiply the number of beats by two.

- Consistently low pulse rate (less than 60 beats per minute) can be an indication of hypothyroidism, Chronic Immune Dysfunction, and/or compromised adrenal function.

- Low pulse rate (less than 60 beats per minute) associated with exercise intolerance, and persistent low rate with exercise, can be a sign of heart block (can occur in Lyme disease). This needs the direct attention of a doctor.

- Irregular pulse with skipped beats can be a sign of microbial infection of the heart, especially if accompanied by chest pain (heart involvement is somewhat common in Lyme disease). This also needs attention from a doctor.

- Persistent elevated pulse during rest (over 100 beats per minute) should also be brought to the attention of your healthcare provider.

Heart Rate Variability Monitoring (HRV). Cell phones are useful for a multitude of functions, including monitoring stress tolerance and wellness. Most smartphones have a built-in app for measuring heart rate. You simply engage the app and place your finger over the light by the camera. Heart rate is measured along with the change in rate between beats. This information can be used to define stress tolerance.

In healthy individuals, normal heart rate varies very slightly from beat to beat. The random up-and-down changes of beat-to-beat variability reflect a healthy autonomic system. The autonomic system of the body regulates breathing, heartbeat, and digestive processes. It is deeply connected to all functions in the body. When the body is stressed, autonomic functions are affected, and beat-to-beat heart rate variability (HRV) is lost.

The Chinese have been aware of this phenomenon for thousands of years. Pulse diagnosis is an important part of traditional Chinese medicine. Skilled practitioners used changes in pulse to diagnose different conditions and ascertain overall wellness.

In the West, HRV has been used to measure fetal well-being in laboring mothers for over 40 years. Having practiced obstetrics for 20 years of my life, I am very familiar with the technology. When an unborn infant becomes stressed in labor, the fetal heart rate tracing loses variability and becomes flat. With continued stress, the flat heart rate gradually increases, and with acute stress (contractions), drops subtly, a sign designated as late decelerations. As such, it is a reasonable guide for intervention in cases of assisted delivery or cesarean section.

Over the past 20 years, heart rate variability has also been found to be a strong predictor of death from heart attack or the presence of cardio-vascular disease in healthy adults. Most recently, it has been used for monitoring exercise tolerance and general well-being.

There are numerous apps that measure HRV that are available for smart-phones. Check the app marketplace for your brand of phone to see what's available.

While HRV is not yet good enough to diagnose specific illnesses, it is a great way to monitor stress tolerance. If your heart rate shows good variability at rest, but decreases with the addition of any sort of stress (physical, emotional, toxins, radiation), it indicates that your reserves are low. In that case, you need to let up on the stress.

Body temperature. Average temperature is 98.6 degrees Fahrenheit, but variations are normal. Temperature is generally lowest first thing in the morning and higher during the day. Exercise can raise body temper-ature. Temperature varies during different times in the menstrual cycle and increases with pregnancy. Basal body temperature (BBT) is taken by oral thermometer (digital preferred) first thing in the morning, before your feet hit the floor. Consistent BBT under 97.5 degrees is a possible indication of low metabolism, which could indicate hypothyroidism. High temperature (over 99 degrees) could indicate an active infection.

Winter can be a miserable time of year for people with chronic Lyme disease. Cold hands, cold feet and feeling chilled to the bone are a normal state much of the time. The metabolic fires are just not burning hot enough to keep everything warm. See **Chapter 21**, for advice on staying warm.

Blood glucose. Abnormally elevated insulin levels and elevated blood glucose levels are major system disruptors. Considering that most people in the developed world consume excessive amounts of processed carbohydrates, it is a significant concern.

Monitoring blood glucose levels several times a day can help you gain control. An inexpensive device for measuring blood glucose, called a glucometer, can be obtained from any pharmacy. Obtaining a measurement does require sticking your finger with a lance, but it's not that bad, and you can get used to it. Use an automatic lance, and stick on the side of your finger instead of on the pad where the nerves are.

Measure fasting blood glucose in the morning before eating and post-prandial (after eating) blood glucose 2 hours after a main meal. Testing can reveal the effect of different kinds of foods. Test regularly while you are making dietary modifications and intermittently once your diet is improved. Your target is blood glucose of less than 90 mg/dl fasting and less than 110 mg/dl postprandial.

8

Making Best Use of the Medical System

You will need to work with other people to get well, and having positive relationships with medical providers is important. Many Lyme disease and fibromyalgia sufferers often become frustrated with the medical system. Generally, it is a result of asking the system for something it is not designed to deliver. Getting best use of the system is a matter of respecting its limitations.

The conventional medical system is specifically designed to deliver acute medical care. Your doctor is trained to treat acute medical conditions. Drugs and surgery act acutely. In other words, the medical system and your doctor are equipped to offer primarily acute, symptomatic support for Lyme disease, fibromyalgia, chronic fatigue, chronic aspects of autoimmune disease, and most other chronic illnesses. **If you ask your doctor to do more, both you and your doctor will come away frustrated.**

The medical system is very procedure driven. All services are defined by the coding system as being procedures, even a basic office visit. Of all procedures, basic office visits providing counseling are reimbursed at the very lowest level — **so you can see why your provider is very motivated to order procedures and much less apt to spend time talking with you.**

Medical providers should be viewed not as potential saviors, but as part of a team for helping you get well. You are the head of that team. You are ultimately responsible for any decisions that are made. Do your homework.

If you follow the simple guidelines in this chapter, you are likely to have a positive relationship with most healthcare providers you encounter.

WHAT YOU NEED FROM YOUR GENERAL PROVIDER

Rule out acute, life-threatening illness. Don't expect your doctor to cure chronic conditions such as chronic Lyme disease and fibromyalgia. These conditions are the great mimickers, however, and you do want to make sure that your symptoms are not masking an acute, life-threatening condition such as cancer or heart disease. Your doctor can help you with this. It will require lab tests and possibly diagnostic procedures, which will hopefully all be negative (fingers crossed), but just the same, you need to have them done for peace of mind.

Order labs. Any doctor can order basic labs covered by health insurance. Basic lab tests are often unremarkable in chronic Lyme disease and fibromyalgia patients (except for vitamin D levels), but can be helpful for defining general health status or ruling out some other treatable condition. Some doctors also can order testing for food sensitivities and heavy-metal toxicity, which can be important if you are not getting well. (Specific tests are covered in the next chapter.)

Your doctor can also order basic tests for Lyme disease. The ELISA for Lyme disease is specific for *Borrelia burgdorferi* and is **only valuable for diagnosing acute Lyme disease**; it has little value for people who have been sick for a long time. The Western blot for Lyme is more reliable for diagnosing chronic Lyme disease, but still has a low predictive value. In other words, it is not uncommon to have symptoms of chronic Lyme and be harboring Borrelia, but have a negative Western blot. (This is covered in more detail in **Chapter 10**, under Testing for Microbes.)

Provide prescription medications. Relief of symptoms such as pain, anxiety, and insomnia, even if only temporary, can be helpful for recovery. Use of medications for this purpose, however, must be approached cautiously. These types of medications can be quite habit-forming. Symptoms associated with habituation can inhibit and prolong recovery. Well-meaning physicians often do not understand drug habituation and write prescriptions for narcotics and benzodiazepines (Valium, Xanax, Ativan, Klonopin) much too liberally.

If you decide to use drugs to treat symptoms, especially narcotics and benzodiazepines, use them carefully and intermittently. Learn about what the drug can do to your body (any drug can be researched on the Internet) and the potential for habituation before taking the drug. If you do this, you will probably know more about the drug than your doctor (and you should; it's your body that it's affecting!).

In certain situations, such as an acute tick bite, antibiotics are indicated. The standard for symptomatic acute tick bite is doxycycline 100 mg twice daily for 14 to 30 days or until most acute symptoms resolve. Doxycycline covers all the coinfections except for Babesia (see Babesia blog).

ESTABLISHING A GOOD RELATIONSHIP WITH YOUR GENERAL PROVIDER

There are several guidelines you should follow to have a more positive, productive relationship with your general healthcare provider:

1. Never walk into your provider's office with a list of 20 concerns that you want addressed during that visit. Be very specific about the goal you want to accomplish during that visit, and make it reasonable.

2. Be respectful of your provider's time. The system is designed around strict time limitations. Your provider only has about 15 minutes (30 minutes at the most) to spend with you.

3. Be organized. Have information readily available, such as previous lab results and/or personal observations, which may be helpful in achieving the goal of the visit.

4. Accept that your provider will likely offer only drugs and possibly surgical procedures. Your provider's knowledge and training generally does not extend beyond conventional therapies.

5. Don't be afraid to ask questions. If something isn't clear, make sure it is clear before you move forward.

6. You may know more about Lyme disease than your doctor, but never try to "one-up" your doctor in knowledge. It will get you nowhere.

7. Remember, you always have the last say. You can research information about any drug or lab test on the Internet. Many doctors know less about the long-term side effects of the drugs they prescribe than they should. Also, many doctors take a "shotgun" approach to ordering labs with little regard to cost or whether results will influence outcome. Be smart about your choices.

WHEN TO CONSIDER A MEDICAL SPECIALIST

If you have significant cardiac, neurological, or gastrointestinal symptoms, your general provider will likely refer you to a specialist in those areas. A specialist will order or perform specialized tests to evaluate the possibility of a treatable diagnosis.

Most of the time, you do need to undergo any recommended diagnostic procedure, sometimes for nothing more than the peace of mind, especially if the procedure carries little risk and is covered by insurance (do your research, however, as the potential for benefit should always be balanced by the risk). Fortunately, most often, specialized testing is negative or equivocal. This is a good thing because it indicates that illness has not progressed beyond the point where restoration of normal health is possible.

WHEN TO CONSIDER A LYME OR ALTERNATIVE SPECIALIST

Specialists who focus on treating chronic Lyme disease and fibromyalgia include Lyme-literate medical doctors, integrative doctors, and functional medicine doctors (see descriptions below). In general, if you have mild to moderate illness that is responding well to the recommendations provided in this book, you do not need to seek out a Lyme specialist. If your illness is severe, however, a specialist in this field can help you get your life back. Alternative providers are more sensitive to the needs of chronic Lyme and fibromyalgia than conventional doctors. They can order advanced lab testing and provide alternative therapies. Be aware, however, that **services offered by alternative providers are often not covered by health insurance**. You, the patient, should always be in control. Ask about the cost for every service and the potential for benefit that might be gained from every service.

TYPES OF PROVIDERS

Conventional Medical Doctor. Everyone needs a general medical provider (family physician or internist) for ruling out life-threatening conditions, providing medical therapy for symptoms when indicated, and dealing with acute situations. In certain situations, you may need to see a specialist (cardiologist, neurologist, rheumatologist, gastroenterologist). Most doctors undergo specialty training for 3-5 years beyond medical school. Primary care providers do additional training in family medicine, pediatrics, internal medicine, obstetrics/gynecology, or emergency medicine. Specialists do additional training in a medical or surgical specialty.

Doctor of Osteopathy (DO). DOs are the equivalent of MDs. They go through similar training and have similar skills. Some DOs are more apt to understand natural approaches to healing.

Nurse Practitioner/Physician's Assistant. NPs and PAs work under the license of a Medical Doctor. Generally, they work in the same office as the doctor who sponsors them, but they can work in free-standing offices. In general, NPs and PAs will take more time with you than a doctor. They can tap into the knowledge of the doctor when necessary. They tend to be more knowledgeable about nutrition and other aspects of healing than a physician (and are generally more willing to take the time to help in this regard).

Lyme-Literate Medical Doctor. Medical doctors who specialize in treatment of Lyme disease are much more aware of the complexities of the disease process than their conventional colleagues, but many LLMDs still limit their practices to drug therapies. As such, they tend to be strong advocates of long-term IV antibiotic therapy. Some, however, are starting to accept alternative therapy options like integrative or functional medical doctors (see below).

Integrative Medical Doctor. Integrative physicians are defined by use of alternative therapies or alternative applications of drugs therapies. They do much more extensive laboratory evaluations than conventional doctors, with the hope of picking up subtle abnormalities that can be corrected with nutrients, vitamin-like substances, or drugs. If your body is in a total tailspin, this approach may be necessary to restore stability. It can, however, become quite complicated. Like their conventional colleagues, integrative physicians tend to be procedure driven. Procedures commonly offered include IV nutrient therapy, IV chelation, IV ozone therapy, and hyperbaric oxygen. Integrative doctors, in general, take more time with patients than conventional doctors, and procedures often can improve well-being acutely, but it all comes with a hefty price tag. Both lab evaluations and office procedures are often not covered by insurance. If you decide to work with an integrative physician, know up front the purpose of each lab and procedure, along with the overall cost to you.

Functional Medical Doctor. Providers trained in functional medicine are much more apt to take a holistic approach to therapy. They look for underlying causes that can be reversed with diet, lifestyle changes, and supplements. They typically spend much more time with you and are less likely to do unnecessary procedures. They are much more apt to consider herbal therapies. It can be a best-of-all-worlds situation. The only drawback is that the healthcare system does not pay them to practice this way. Therefore, most functional medicine providers are only found in large cities, typically do not take insurance, and are very, very pricey.

Naturopathic Doctor. Naturopathic doctors are very much like functional or integrative medical doctors, except they are more likely to use natural herbal therapy. In states where they are licensed, naturopaths can write prescriptions for drugs. They are only licensed in some states.

Chiropractor. Most chiropractors rely on realignment of the musculoskeletal system to reduce symptoms of pain and discomfort. A chiropractor can be very valuable for relieving musculoskeletal symptoms without the use of drug therapy. Some chiropractors also offer care very much like functional medical doctors, but they cannot write prescriptions. A few chiropractors specialize in Lyme disease and fibromyalgia and are more knowledgeable about natural therapy options than conventional physicians.

Acupuncturist. An acupuncturist uses specialized needles or pressure at specific points on the body to restore balance in the energy fields of the body. Studies have documented benefit for many types of conditions. Achieving benefit generally requires multiple sessions, and benefit fades when sessions are discontinued. Many acupuncturists are also trained in Traditional Chinese Medicine with Chinese herbs.

Massage Therapist. Massage therapists are not trained to diagnose and offer treatment for medical conditions, but a skilled massage therapist can do wonders for body aches and pains.

Energy Medicine. There are many different forms of energy medicine and just as many different types of practitioners. All of them use personal energy or energy conducted through their body to balance and restore the energy of the patient. Some people respond to energy medicine very favorably; others do not. It all depends on the chemistry between the provider and the recipient.

Health Coach. This type of provider is an authority on wellness who motivates individuals to be proactive about improving health habits. A health coach can help you with setbacks and keep you moving in a positive direction with your recovery.

Laboratory Evaluation

The human body is an immensely complex biological machine with millions of different biochemical functions happening simultaneously. Lab tests provide an ever so small glimpse at certain key functions. From those indicators, determinations can be made about how well the body is functioning and whether illness is present.

Laboratory assessment, however, is far from absolute. Because the human body is so complex, the ability of lab testing to predict a specific chronic illness is often limited. All labs are subject to variability and different interpretations.

For this reason, it's important not to get too wrapped up in lab results alone. The problem of chronic Lyme disease cannot be solved exclusively by looking at lab results. If fact, getting too obsessed with lab results can hold back your recovery.

There are literally thousands of different lab tests that can be performed, but only a fraction of them are well understood. Many should be left for research purposes only. Problems arise when doctors order obscure tests that are still poorly understood.

Before you have labs drawn, ask your doctor to explain the purpose of each test.

The information provided by labs is only valuable if it is put to good use. Millions of dollars are wasted yearly on labs that were obtained, but the information was never used. Before you have labs drawn, ask yourself and your doctor: **"Will the information provided by this lab (or any other diagnostic test) influence my approach to getting well?"** If the answer is no, then you may want to reconsider having that test performed.

For chronic illnesses such as chronic Lyme disease and fibromyalgia, general lab evaluations are often unremarkable. The greatest value of labs is ruling out the possibility of a more threatening condition. Lab values that are mildly abnormal generally return to normal as wellness is restored.

The following is a guide to the labs that I find to be most valuable in evaluating chronic illnesses such as chronic Lyme disease and fibromyalgia. It is, by no means, an absolute or exclusive list.

BASIC TESTING THAT EVERYONE NEEDS
There are certain basic tests and a few specialized tests that have great value. These are the tests that everyone should consider getting. The following list of labs can be ordered by any healthcare provider. Typically, these tests are covered by health insurance.

Complete blood count (CBC with diff). Measures cellular components of blood.

- *White Blood Cell count (WBC).* Low WBC (<4000) can indicate chronic infection with virus or low-virulence bacteria such as Mycoplasma, but it can occur in healthy people. Elevated WBC (>11,500) can indicate an active infection.

- *Differential (diff).* Measures different types and ratios of white blood cells present. Sometimes it can be helpful for defining an infection (bacteria vs. viral vs. parasite), but it is not always absolute.

- *Hemoglobin (Hb).* Anemia is indicated by Hb < 12.0. Anemia can be caused by blood loss (heavy periods), inadequate production of RBCs (chemotherapy), and increased destruction of RBCs (infection: malaria, Babesia, Bartonella). Hb levels > 16.0 can be associated with smoking, living at altitude, and excessive iron stores in the body (hemochromatosis).

Blood chemistries. Measure of common chemical components of the body.

- *Electrolytes.* Sodium, potassium, chloride, CO_2— these are generally normal, unless you are really sick.

- *Liver function.* Abnormal values suggest an elevated rate of liver compromise, possibly from toxins or viruses such as hepatitis. Elevated bilirubin suggests increased breakdown and turnover of RBCs (Babesia, Bartonella). Certain low-virulence microbes (Bartonella) destroy RBCs.

- *Kidney function.* BUN and creatinine screen for kidney disease. Unrecognized kidney disease can be a factor causing fatigue.

Glucose metabolism. Excessive carbohydrate consumption is a major system disrupter that must be controlled before recovery is possible. Three primary tests: fasting blood glucose, hemoglobin A1c, and fasting insulin define insulin resistance and abnormal glucose metabolism.

- *Fasting blood glucose.* Levels >100 mg/dl suggest pre-diabetes. Levels >126 mg/dl suggest overt diabetes.

- *Fasting insulin.* Levels defined as elevated suggest insulin resistance (normal range varies depending on the lab). Insulin resistance is a factor contributing to immune dysfunction and hormone imbalances.

- *Hemoglobin A1c (HbA1c).* HbA1c measures the cumulative damage done by excessive carbohydrate consumption. It is one of the most important tests on the list. Excessive carbohydrate consumption disrupts hormone pathways and immune function. Your target for optimal recovery is 4.8-5.2%. Anything higher will hold you back. Levels > 5.6% indicate pre-diabetes. Levels > 6.4% indicate overt diabetes.

Minerals. Magnesium and calcium are the primary minerals measured.

- *Magnesium.* Magnesium levels are often low during chronic illness. Supplementation is indicated if levels are low, but over-aggressive use of magnesium supplements can often worsen Lyme symptoms.

- *Calcium.* Persistently elevated calcium levels can indicate the presence of a small benign tumor producing excessive parathyroid hormone (PTH). Symptoms can mimic fibromyalgia and chronic Lyme disease. Follow-up testing should include PTH levels.

Thyroid function. Complete thyroid function should include Thyroid Stimulating Hormone (TSH), free T_4, free T_3, reverse T_3, and thyroid antibodies. Illnesses associated with chronic immune dysfunction are commonly associated with abnormal thyroid function. Correcting abnormal thyroid function can accelerate recovery. Testing for thyroid antibodies (TPO and thyroglobulin) is important to identify Hashimoto's disease, a form of autoimmune thyroid dysfunction.

Lipid panel. Basic evaluation for cardiovascular risk. Cholesterol commonly increases with age and decline in liver function. The nutrition guidelines in this book help maintain normal cholesterol levels. Significantly elevated cholesterol, however, should be addressed by your healthcare provider.

Autoimmune Testing. Chronic Immune Dysfunction and stealth microbes play a major role in autoimmunity. The type of autoimmune illness that occurs is related to the factors that disrupt immune function, the person's genetics, and the spectrum of stealth microbes. Though diagnosis of specific autoimmune illnesses is complex and requires extensive testing, basic screening for autoimmunity can be done with two tests.

- *Rheumatoid factor.* A standard test if severe arthritis is present.
- *ANA titer.* Positive in many types of autoimmune disease.

C-reactive protein (CRP). CRP is a measure of inflammation. It is probably more valuable for monitoring health habits than anything else. High levels (>10) correlate with poor health habits and increased risk of disease. Normal CRP levels, however, are often present in individuals who follow good dietary habits, despite suffering from a chronic illness. It is not a specific marker for Lyme disease, fibromyalgia, or chronic fatigue.

Vitamin D. Vitamin D is not only important for healthy bones, but also very important for normal immune function. There are several forms of vitamin D — calcidiol (25 OH vitamin D) is the most commonly measured form in blood tests. Normal ranges for blood levels of Vitamin D and indications for supplementation are both controversial. The official Institute of Medicine defines calcidiol levels >20 ng/ml as normal and >50 ng/ml as too high. Their recommendations for daily vitamin D include sun exposure or 600-1000 IU of vitamin D3 daily. The Vitamin D Council, however, recommends 40-100 as the normal range, generally requiring much higher doses of supplementation. Levels of >40 ng/ml have been associated with reduced risk of many cancers and chronic disease in general. Achieving consistent vitamin D levels >40 ng/ml is important for recovery. Ideally, have your levels checked every 6 months.

Vitamin B12. Low B12 levels (normal ranges vary between labs) can be a sign of low intake (vegetarians), but more commonly a sign of inadequate absorption and gastric dysfunction. Vitamin B12 generally increases spontaneously with improved health habits, but in the short term, B12 injections or sublingual (under the tongue) supplements can improve energy levels. Activated forms of B12 are better absorbed orally than the more common inactive forms used in most multivitamin products.

Ferritin. Ferritin measures iron stores. Low ferritin levels can indicate low stores of iron in the body, which can be associated with fatigue and restless legs syndrome. High ferritin levels indicate abnormal retention of iron in the body (called hemochromatosis), which can be associated with liver damage and nonspecific symptoms. High levels can also be associated with autoimmunity and chronic infection (Zandman-Goddard 2009).

Urinalysis. Test strips for urine testing can be obtained over the Internet without a prescription.

- *pH.* Urine pH should be consistently alkaline, reflecting high consumption of vegetables and fruit.

- *WBCs, nitrites.* These tests show evidence of a urinary tract infection.

- *Protein.* Elevated levels can indicate kidney disease.

- *Bilirubin.* Elevated levels show increased turnover or destruction of RBCs.

- *Trace blood.* Can indicate the presence of a kidney stone or other kidney disease.

Mold and mycotoxins. Evaluation for mold is indicated anytime there is any suspicion of mold. Mycotoxins (mold toxins) are potent immune disruptors and cause a wide spectrum of nonspecific symptoms including neurological symptoms and persistent insomnia. Testing for mold in your environment can be important for your recovery (see **Chapter 27**, Mold and Mycotoxins for more information).

TB skin test. The skin test for tuberculosis should be performed if there is a history of recent exposure or chronic pulmonary symptoms.

Omega-3/omega-6 ratio. The ratio of omega-3 fatty acids to omega-6 fatty acids is a marker for balance of inflammatory factors in the body. Optimal omega-3/omega-6 ratio balances inflammation in the body. The vast majority of people do not get adequate intake of omega-3 fatty acids. Testing can guide optimal supplementation.

ADVANCED TESTING

If you have all the symptoms of chronic Lyme disease (or fibromyalgia or chronic fatigue), then immune dysfunction, the presence of stealth microbes, adrenal dysfunction, hormone imbalances, and mitochondrial dysfunction can all be assumed — you don't necessarily need labs to prove it. And, if you are going about recovery in the right way and all the symptoms are resolving, you don't necessarily need specialized labs to prove that you are getting well.

If your illness is severe or you are not getting well, however, specialized lab testing can sometimes help direct your recovery efforts. Most Lyme specialists or integrative doctors will require you to get a large battery of tests as part of the evaluation. The following discussion is provided to help you understand what the different tests mean and the value they may offer.

Testing for Immune Dysfunction and Disrupted Homeostasis

Chronic immune dysfunction is a given in chronic Lyme disease, fibro-myalgia, and chronic fatigue syndrome, but sometimes defining the level of dysfunction can help guide recovery.

Th1/Th2 Pathways

Immune function pathways can be defined by types of lymphocytes (white blood cells) and chemical messengers (cytokines) that are used to direct immune functions. T lymphocytes (because they originate from the thymus gland) are important for cell-mediated immunity (direct neutralization of threats by white blood cells). Neutrophils and natural killer cells (NK cells) are an important part of cell-mediated immunity. B lymphocytes (originate from bone marrow) produce antibodies against threats. Specialized lymphocytes, called T helper lymphocytes (Th), direct the immune response by secreting cytokines. Though there are a variety of different T helper subsets, for chronic illnesses associated with stealth microbes, Th1 and Th2 pathways are most important.

- **Th1 pathway.** Associated with cell-mediated immunity, activation of NK cells, and conversion of IgM to prolonged IgG response against intracellular pathogens. When overactive, it is associated with inflammation. Primary cytokines are IL-12, **IFN-gamma**, and TNF-alpha.

- **Th2 pathway.** Associated with antibody-mediated immunity and extracellular parasites. A polarized Th2 response is associated with asthma, allergies, and certain types of autoimmune diseases. Cytokines **IL-4**, IL-5, IL-6, **IL-10**, and IL-13.

In the early stages of Lyme disease (or infection with any intracellular stealth microbe), the immune system mounts an aggressive Th1 response. Stealth pathogens upregulate IL-10 to suppress the Th1 response and shift it to Th2. Shifting to a Th2 response allows the pathogens to maintain a low grade chronic infection. This happens over months to years. Herbs that aggressively stimulate Th1 functions (astragalus, echinacea) are beneficial in acute Lyme disease, but should be avoided in chronic Lyme disease. Other herbs for modulating immune function are discussed in **Chapter 14**. Though measurement of key cytokines can sometimes be useful, the cytokine dynamics of chronic stealth microbe illness can be quite strange; cytokines are not always as expected.

Lymphocyte Activity

Testing can be done for specific types of WBC activity, including natural killer cell activity (NK cell: CD 16 and 56), T lymphocytes (CD 3), and T helper cells (CD 4).

CD 57 markers are a subset of mature natural killer cells that have more deadly killer-cell activity. CD 57 markers are sometimes low in Lyme disease, but are not always reliable or specific (see Borrelia testing in **Chapter 10**).

Coagulation Factors

Microbial infections commonly cause activation of coagulation as part of the body's defense mechanisms. How much coagulation is activated depends on the degree of illness. In a severely ill patient, fibrin, one of the chief components of scar formation, can coat the inner lining of blood vessels. This can block absorption of nutrients and hormones such as thyroid (hypothyroid symptoms occur even with normal thyroid hormones). Labs for monitoring coagulation function include D-dimer, prothrombin fragment 1+2, thrombin-antithrombin complex, and SFM. Testing is only indicated with severe illness.

ATP profile

ATP is the energy molecule of metabolic functions. The ATP profile is an indirect measure of ATP activity in neutrophil mitochondria. It has value in analyzing mitochondrial activity in the body and also the presence of acute infection. Individuals with chronic fatigue often display low ATP function, suggesting decreased mitochondrial function and reduced neutrophil capacity (which is a fundamental problem associated with any fatigue-related disorders, so testing for it isn't usually necessary).

IGF-1 (insulin-like growth factor-1)
IGF-1 affects tissue and bone growth by regulating growth hormone. IGF-1 secretion mirrors growth hormone secretion, but unlike growth hormone, which fluctuates, IGF-1 is stable throughout the day, making it useful for monitoring secretion of growth hormone. Low IGF-1 is associated with aging, chronic illness, and decreased immune function.

Summary of Indicators
Because chronic immune dysfunction is different for every person (different microbes, different genes, different system disruptors), defining immune dysfunction with labs is rarely straightforward. None of following markers are always abnormal.

- *Low NK cell function*

- *Low CD 57 cell function*

- *Low ATP function*

- *Low IGF-1*

- *Elevated coagulation factors*

Hormone testing

- *Adrenal function.* Adrenal dysfunction is a given in any chronic illness. Elevated cortisol levels, associated with increased physical and emotional stress contribute to sleeplessness, stress intolerance, agitation, and anxiety. Prolonged adrenal stress can result in inadequate cortisol secretion, with symptoms of extreme fatigue, total stress intolerance, and excessive sleeping (but sleep is dysfunctional and not restful). Adrenal dysfunction generally resolves (gradually) with herbal therapy, stress management, and adequate sleep. Testing is only indicated if symptoms do not resolve with appropriate restorative therapy. Routine testing is not necessary.

- o Salivary cortisol, measured 4 times over 24 hours — measure of adrenal function.

- o DHEA-S — adrenal precursor to male and female hormones; peaks at age 30 and steadily declines thereafter. Abnormally low levels of DHEA-S for age can be associated with inadequate adrenal function.

- o Some doctors also order pregnenolone, another adrenal hormone, and ACTH, the pituitary hormone that regulates adrenal function.

- *Reproductive hormones.* Menopause can exacerbate symptoms of any chronic illness. Though usually obvious, with the absence of periods, menopause can be confirmed by elevated levels of a pituitary hormone called FSH. Levels >25 indicate menopause. Other hormone levels, including estrogen and progesterone, are generally not necessary to measure, but may be recommended by your healthcare provider. In men with fatigue, total and free testosterone is sometimes indicated if severe fatigue and loss of vitality are present.

  - o Female — salivary or blood E_1, E_2, E_3, free testosterone, progesterone, FSH, (screening FSH, estradiol levels)

  - o Male — free testosterone, total testosterone

Management of stress and menopause will be addressed in **Chapter 28**.

Testing for Toxins

- *Heavy metals.* Build-up of heavy metals and other toxins can be a hidden factor in chronic illness. People suffering from chronic illness have a harder time getting rid of heavy metals from the body and heavy metals build up in tissues. Every person living on the planet today, however, is carrying some heavy metals, and no one knows how much is too much. The biggest sources of concern are amalgam dental fillings, contaminated water sources, and food, such as large fish.

The recovery protocol in this book will address mild to moderate accumulation of heavy metals. Testing is only indicated if you are severely ill or not getting well.

- ○ Hair samples — the least reliable method of testing for heavy metals.

- ○ Blood test — valuable only for testing for acute exposure.

- ○ 24-hour urine after DMSA — most accurate assessment. Urine is collected for 24 hours after use of DMSA 100 mg to pull heavy metals out of tissues. DMSA (dimercaptosuccinic acid) is an organosulfur compound that binds heavy metals.

- *Organic toxins.* The presence of organic toxins (pesticides, plastic residues) is almost a given and can be addressed with dietary and lifestyle modifications. Chlorella is excellent for pulling organic toxins out of the body (use of chlorella will be discussed in Chapter 25).

What to do about heavy metals and organic toxins will be discussed more thoroughly in **Chapter 26**, Curbing Toxic Threats.

Gastrointestinal Function
Food sensitivities. Chronic gastrointestinal dysfunction is often associated with sensitivities to commonly consumed foods (not the same as food allergies, such as peanut allergy). Symptoms associated with food sensitivities are commonly delayed for 1-2 days after the food is consumed. Typical symptoms include fatigue, joint pain, muscle pain, and general achiness—in fact, food sensitivities alone can be the root of many symptoms. Food sensitivities will be discussed more thoroughly in **Chapter 24**, Digestive Dysfunction.

- Food sensitivities are best defined by an elimination diet—a diet designed to selectively identify and eliminate problem foods (covered in **Chapter 25**, Gut Restoration Protocol).

- Problem foods can also be delineated with specific IgG and IgA testing. A basic food-sensitivity panel can be obtained for about $120. This shows general categories of foods to be avoided.

Breath testing. Testing the breath for hydrogen and methane after taking a dose of glucose or lactulose is used to define the presence of Small Intestine Bacterial Overgrowth (SIBO). SIBO is commonly associated with symptoms of gas, bloating, nausea, and diarrhea. It can also be associated with fatigue, joint pain, and depression. Generally, symptoms alone are satisfactory for diagnosing SIBO, but in severe cases, breath testing can be valuable. SIBO is discussed in **Chapter 24.**

Comprehensive stool analysis. Stool analysis is valuable for defining gastrointestinal dysfunction and diagnosing parasites and yeast overgrowth. This expensive test is generally reserved for extreme cases when dietary modifications and supplements are not enough to overcome gastrointestinal problems. It is rarely necessary.

Folate and methylation

MTHFR is a gene that codes for an enzyme called **methylenetetrahydrofolate reductase**. This enzyme is vital for creating 5-methyltetrahydrofolate, an essential substance for **converting the amino acid homocysteine into the amino acid methionine**. Methionine is essential for amino acid synthesis, formation of glutathione (important intracellular antioxidant), formation of DNA, and detoxification. Methionine is important for formation of SAMe, which plays a key role in metabolism of dopamine, serotonin, and melatonin.

There are about 40 different genetic mutations that can affect MTHFR. About 40% of the population has one affected gene. About 12% of the population has two affected genes. It is important to note that mutations cause variations in the enzymes, not defective enzymes. The enzymes are still functional, but to varying degrees. It is also important to note that because methylation is so important, the body has many redundant pathways for methylation; it is not solely dependent on MTHFR.

Problems that have been weakly associated to MTHFR mutations include elevated risk of stroke and heart attack; increased cancer risk; defects in embryo development (spinal tube defects); and neurological symptoms including insomnia, irritability, depression, brain fog, neuropathy (burning/tingling feet and hands), restless legs syndrome, fibromyalgia, and chronic Lyme disease. How much of a factor it is in these illnesses is still controversial.

For five years of my medical practice, I had the fortune of being associated with a lab that did MTHFR mutation testing for free. Therefore, virtually every one of my patients had MTHFR testing. This amounted to a couple thousand people. Surprisingly, I found it played less of a role in recovery than I expected. I had chronic Lyme sufferers who were severely symptomatic who had no mutations and perfectly healthy people who had double mutations. It may be a factor in chronic illness, but is probably minor compared to other things.

TESTING
MTHFR problems can be detected indirectly by checking for elevations of homocysteine and deficiencies of RBC folate in the blood. MTHFR mutations can also be detected directly by specialized labs. Avoid DIY home labs because testing may be inaccurate. Avoid practitioners who suggest that all your problems are related to MTHFR mutations.

SOLUTIONS
The best solution is getting plenty of natural 5-methyltetrahydrofolate (methylfolate for short). Leafy greens are a great source, but if know you

have a mutation, supplementing is a good idea. Folic acid, found in most multivitamin products, will not work because it must be converted by the deficient enzyme.

You must supplement with 5-methyltetrahydrofolate. 5-methyltetrahydrofolate 400-800 micrograms daily is generally adequate for anyone with a single mutation (especially if you eat plenty of leafy greens). If you have a double mutation, it is a good idea to take an extra 400-800 micrograms daily. For additional benefit, you can add SAMe 400-800 mg daily. SAMe supports detoxification and can improve sleep (by taking it in the evening).

Chemical components called "methyl groups" that are essential for proper detoxification can also be supplied by vitamin B6 and vitamin B12. It is, however, important to get the activated forms of these important vitamins. The activated form of vitamin B6 is pyridoxal 5-phosphate, and the active form of vitamin B12 is methylcobalamin. You can also take SAMe (400-800 mg daily), especially if poor sleep and depression are an issue.

Healthful diet and adequate supplementation of substances that provide methyl groups is generally adequate for recovery. MTHFR testing is only necessary if recovery is not progressing.

TESTING BEYOND THE LABORATORY
Certain types of symptoms require evaluation by diagnostic procedures conducted by specialists in their respective field.

Neurological symptoms - Severe neurological symptoms are evaluated with a nerve conduction test and MRI of the brain. The purpose is ruling out multiple sclerosis.

Cardiac symptoms - Chest pain and irregular heartbeat are evaluated by EKG and Holter monitor. Findings may lead to cardiac catheterization.

GI symptoms - Stomach pain and symptoms are often evaluated by upper endoscopy. Lower intestinal and colon symptoms are evaluated by colonoscopy. Routine colon cancer screening with colonoscopy is recommended every 10 years for everyone over 50.

10

Testing for Microbes

"B. burgdorferi doesn't like to come out in the open, so checking Blood, CSF, and SF is like looking for cockroaches in the middle of a busy highway."

- MIKE D. MADDOX, DC, LYME SPECIALIST

We'd all like to know as much as possible about which microbes may be present...but you don't want to hold your recovery back because of the lack of information either.

Frankly, the present state of technology for microbial testing is somewhat limited. It's a lot better than it was in 1981, but the microbes that are being routinely tested for account for a small fraction of many possibilities. There are at least a dozen species of Borrelia that can cause Lyme disease, but most labs test only for one species, *Borrelia burgdorferi*. Beyond Borrelia, there are literally hundreds of possible species of stealth microbes that could be present, but current testing is only available for a handful of species.

And that's just the ones we know about. New stealth microbe species are discovered every year.

Testing that is available is **mostly geared toward diagnosing acute infections**. Most people who want to be tested, however, have chronic illness...and testing for chronic infections is poor at best.

The long and the short of it is, all ticks carry potentially pathogenic microbes. If you have ever been bitten by a tick, you have been exposed to stealth microbes. **If you have all the symptoms of chronic Lyme disease, then the chances that you are carrying some species of Borrelia (and other stealth microbes as well) is very high** — no matter what testing shows.

It ultimately begs the question: why test for microbes at all?

If you choose a conventional route of therapy, you may not have much choice in the matter; many doctors will not consider writing a prescription until testing is done and results are available. Considering the extreme limitations of the present state of testing for stealth microbes, it is just one of the extreme drawbacks of pursuing a purely conventional route of therapy.

If you choose a natural route of therapy, testing is much less mandatory. A comprehensive herbal protocol accounts for Borrelia and most other possibilities; it is assumed that they are there. When your goal is restoring immune function and suppressing stealth microbes in general, knowing exactly which microbes are present becomes less relevant. Many people have gotten well without doing any testing at all.

The biggest reason to test is if you are not improving. Sometimes testing can uncover the presence of a more virulent microbe (Babesia, Ehrlichia, Rickettsia, Anaplasma) or reactivation of a herpes-type virus for which a prescription antimicrobial might provide benefit.

If you decide to do microbe testing, the place to start is with tests covered by your medical insurance. Insurance policies are highly variable, however, and **it is up to you (not your doctor) to find out what is and isn't covered.**

Most health care insurance policies will cover testing for Borrelia and possible coinfections with in-network labs. Most in-network labs, however, only provide a basic level of testing, which often carries a low probability of diagnosing an offending microbe (in chronic illness especially).

Testing for *Borrelia burgdorferi* alone may not be sufficient. If you decide to do any testing at all, you should probably test for as many possibilities as there are available. Considering the many species of Borrelia that can cause Lyme and all the other possible stealth microbes that may be present, plan on spending hundreds of dollars — all for tests that may have very little actual impact on your recovery.

SPECIALTY LABS

Because of demand, there is a proliferation of specialty labs doing testing. The oldest and possibly the most well-known is IGeneX, but there are many new and innovative testing labs coming on the scene. Blood can be drawn at the doctor's office and sent to a specialty lab, but you will be responsible for the bill.

Specialty labs do more advanced and sophisticated lab testing, but the **testing is mostly focused on diagnosing acute infection, not chronic.** If you suffer from chronic illness, the probability that any testing will provide useful information is more limited than you might think. Tests from specialty labs are generally not covered by insurance — each test can run anywhere from $200 to $900. If your budget is limited, your money may be better spent on other aspects of your recovery.

Conventional labs have little incentive for bias in reporting results. Tests are ordered by doctors and paid for by health insurance. It does not matter to them whether the test is positive or negative.

Specialty labs, in comparison, do have strong incentives to deliver positive tests. People pay higher costs out of pocket because they expect a better result than that offered by a conventional lab. The incentive to deliver a positive test motivates specialty labs to be more innovative and often offer higher accuracy testing, but it also pushes them to lower standards to allow for more positive tests. This potentially increases the number of false positive tests (the test is positive, but the person doesn't have the microbe).

REASONS TO TEST

- You need to know...that burning curiosity that we all share as humans.

- Testing for a specific microbe is primarily valuable for acute symptoms after a tick bite.

- Some stealth microbes are more virulent than others and respond better to antibiotic therapy; a positive test can help direct therapy.

- Obtaining lab tests for microbes supports research in discovering new microbes.

- Testing offers financial support for labs and institutions doing testing.

- Testing for Epstein-Barr virus (EBV), cytomegalovirus (CMV), and other herpes-type viruses (there are 8 that commonly infect and are carried by humans) can be valuable because high titers associated with reactivation of these viruses may respond to antiviral therapy.

LIMITATIONS OF TESTING

- **Most testing is geared toward diagnosing acute infection, not chronic** (testing for chronic infections with stealth microbes is a relatively new concept).

- During chronic infection, stealth microbes occur in very low concentrations in isolated areas of the body and live inside cells, thus decreasing chances of detection.

- Testing is very dependent on adequate antibody production; in chronic infection with stealth microbes, production of antibodies is often depressed.

- **A positive test for a specific microbe can provide false peace of mind,** because other threatening microbes are often present that were not tested for.

- **A negative test does not exclude the possibility of that microbe being present** (especially during chronic illness).

- **Cross-reactivity with other bacteria is common,** including normal flora.

- Most **testing is species specific;** many species of each type (genera) of microbe are possible; testing is only available for a limited number of species.

- **Symptoms of chronic Lyme disease can occur without the presence of Borrelia** and can be caused by other stealth microbes (though Borrelia may be present, but the test is falsely negative).

- **Everyone harbors stealth microbes**; the microbiome is extremely complex.

- Testing for the many possibilities **can run into many thousands of dollars**, often not covered by insurance.

- **Testing may not affect your chances of successful recovery.**

The following is a detailed discussion of the current state of microbial testing. It is not mandatory reading for progressing forward with a holistic approach to recovery.

TYPES OF TESTING FOR MICROBES

Testing is getting better, and there are a variety of different ways to test, but none of them are anywhere near 100% accurate. **Testing is mostly useful for diagnosing acute illness.** This is especially true when symptoms of illness suggest infection with a higher virulence microbe that might respond to acute treatment with antibiotics. New innovations may gradually improve testing for chronic illness associated with stealth microbes, but right now, testing for chronic infection is very limited.

Direct testing includes visualizing the microbe directly in tissue or blood samples or growing the microbe out of tissue or blood samples in media that is specific for that microbe. Direct testing is not species specific, so any species of the microbe can be diagnosed. Polymerase chain reaction (PCR) tests directly for the microbe's DNA. It is species specific (uncommon species may be present but will not be diagnosed).

These forms of testing are most useful for diagnosing acute infections. Because stealth microbes occur in such low concentrations in the body during chronic infection, are not present in the blood in high numbers, can occur in dormant or cyst forms, live inside cells, and gravitate toward isolated recesses of the body, direct methods of testing are not reliable for chronic infections.

Indirect testing relies on antibody production to the microbe (serology). Evidence of acute infection is best evaluated with IgM antibodies and late acute or chronic infection with IgG antibodies. Some testing regimens require serial titers (testing at different time intervals) to distinguish between acute and chronic infections. Different types of serology are available for different microbes. Accuracy for testing chronic illness associated with stealth microbes is greatly limited by low concentrations of the microbe in the body and corresponding low levels of antibody production.

Common Types of Testing for Microbes

- Direct

  o *Tissue/blood* — direct visualization

  o *Tissue/blood culture* — uses culture media specific for the microbe to grow the microbe in culture

  o *Polymerase Chain Reaction (PCR)* — direct detection of microbe DNA

- Indirect (serology)

  o *Enzyme-linked Immunoassay (EIA) or Enzyme-Linked Immunosorbent Assay (ELISA)* — measures antibodies in the patient's serum that is specific to microbial antigens (part of the microbe) by using labeled enzymes to bind the antibody for measurement

  o *Enzyme-Linked Fluorescent Assay (ELFA) or Immunofluorescence Assay (IFA)* — utilizes fluorescent dyes to identify the presence of microbe-specific antibodies in the patient's serum. Newer and faster than ELISA.

  o *Western Blot* — detects antibodies to multiple different microbial antigens by measuring different protein bands. Collectively, the presence of multiple bands allows diagnosis of infection with a specific microbe; more sensitive than ELISA for Borrelia

ACCURACY OF TESTING

To determine accuracy (sensitivity), a test must be compared to a known standard. To standardize a microbe test, the test is used on a population of people (or lab animals) proven to have the microbe by some other means (usually culture). If a test is stated to be 96% sensitive for a microbe, then it was found to be positive 96% of the time in that proven population. These people (or lab animals) are generally acutely infected and have high concentrations of microbes in their bloodstream.

This makes statements of test accuracy somewhat misleading. When that same test is used for people with chronic infection, the sensitivity can be dramatically lower that the stated 96%. This is especially true with chronic infections with stealth microbes, which typically occur in very low concentrations in the body.

DIAGNOSING BORRELIA

The stealth nature of *Borrelia burgdorferi* makes it very difficult to diagnose. Because it stays deep in tissues, can live inside cells (intracellular), has elaborate ways of tricking the immune system, changes its genetic signature readily, and doesn't require high concentrations of microbes to cause illness, developing testing is a real challenge.

Most testing is specific for *Borrelia burgdorferi*, but presently there are 12 species of Borrelia that can cause Lyme disease. In Europe, two other species of Borrelia, *Borrelia afzelii* and *Borrelia garinii*, are more common than *Borrelia burgdorferi* as a cause of Lyme disease. Because of mobility of people (and ticks carried by birds), different species are constantly being circulated around the world. It is gradually becoming evident that other species of Borrelia are much more common than once thought.

Posted on the FDA website:

FDA public health advisory: "**FDA is advising you about the potential for misdiagnosis of Lyme disease. The results of commonly marketed assays for detecting antibody to *Borrelia burgdorferi* (anti-*Bb*), the organism that causes Lyme disease, may be easily misinterpreted. It is important that clinicians understand the limitations of these tests. A positive result does not necessarily indicate current infection with *B. burgdorferi*, and patients with active Lyme disease may have a negative test** result." "*Assays for anti-Bb should be used only to support a clinical diagnosis of Lyme disease.*"

Bull's-eye rash (erythema migrans). The classic bull's-eye rash, redness extending outward from the tick-bite site with an outer, more prominent red ring. Symptoms of Lyme disease associated with a history of tick bite and bull's-eye rash are the most reliable way to diagnose infection with Borrelia, but even that is far from being absolute. There are likely other types of microbes that can cause a bull's-eye rash. Only one third of people with Lyme disease will have a bull's-eye rash, and only 10% of bull's-eye rashes are associated with the presence of Borrelia in the blood.

Blood/Tissue culture. The most definitive test for proving the presence of a microbe is growing it in the lab from a tissue or blood sample. Because Borrelia exists in such low concentrations in blood and tissues, and because Borrelia is so difficult to grow under artificial conditions, cultures have very limited usefulness for diagnosing Lyme disease.

ELISA. Tests for host's antibodies produced against Borrelia. It is recommended as a screening test for Lyme disease. The CDC (Centers for Disease Control) defines this test as an important screening test for Lyme disease, but in clinical practice, most healthcare providers who treat Lyme disease find that the test has poor predictive value and limited usefulness. The rate of false-negative testing in chronic illness is high, but it is also possible to have a positive ELISA and negative Western blot in someone who is carrying Borrelia chronically. **It has some value for diagnosing acute Lyme disease, but limited value for chronic Lyme disease.**

PCR for *B. burgdorferi*. Tests directly for Borrelia DNA in the host's blood. Because the microbe clears from the blood quickly, the value of PCR testing is limited to only acute infection. **PCR tests should be**

limited to only acute tick-bite exposure, but even then, a negative test does not rule out the possibility of an acute Borrelia infection. The test is specific for *B. burgdorferi* and does not test for other species of Borrelia.

Western blot. The Western blot for *Borrelia burgdorferi* relies on production of antibodies by the host's immune system for different parts (antigens) of the bacteria. Antibody production does not occur until the body's secondary defense kicks in and is dependent on the host's ability to mount an immune response. The Western blot test may provide a more accurate diagnosis of Lyme disease than most of the other available tests, but testing is more valuable for the late acute than chronic illness. In addition, the test is oriented toward diagnosis of *Borrelia burgdorferi* and no other species of Borrelia that may cause Lyme disease.

Because Borrelia shares antigens with other bacteria, multiple positive antibodies (called bands) are required for a true positive test. Western blot is performed for both IgM and IgG antibodies in an effort to separate acute from chronic illness.

IgM antibodies are indicative of acute Borrelia infection. Testing can be positive as early as 1 week after infection remains positive for 6-8 weeks after initial exposure, but then typically declines. CDC guidelines require two positive bands out of three (23-25, 39, 41). IGeneX labs adds three extra bands (31, 34, 83-93), the first two of which were removed from the CDC criteria during development of an unsuccessful vaccine and never replaced.

The IgG antibody is typically present a few months following initial infection. **IgG antibodies are more indicative of chronic infection** (but may not be present in longstanding illness). CDC guidelines require five positive bands out of ten (18, 23-25, 28, 30, 39, 41, 45, 58, 66, 83-93). The IGeneX criteria is two bands out of ten (18, 23-25, 28, 30, 39, 41, 45, 58, 66, 83-93).

Band 41 is specific for the flagella (tail) of spirochetes (corkscrew bacteria), but is not absolutely specific for Borrelia. Recently reported data from IGeneX supports that some Lyme patients may only have a restricted IgM response to *B. burgdorferi*. **Because Lyme patients have different immune systems, only approximately 70% of those with Lyme disease will generate a positive Western blot.** Patients who test positive for rheumatoid factor or Epstein-Barr virus may have false-negative tests. Acute viral infections can cause false-positive results. IGeneX Western blot costs about $600.

IGeneX Western blot may also detect *B. afezelii* and B. *garnii*. *IGeneX is now offering PCR testing for Borrelia miyamotoi (associated with relapsing fever) for $245. IGeneX is also offering immunofluorescence testing (FISH) for Babesia, Anaplasma, Ehrlichia, and Rickettsia.*

I-spot Lyme test. This is a new test as of March 2013. It is an enhanced form of enzyme-linked immunospot assay (ELISPOT) that tests T-cell response to *Borrelia burgdorferi* antigens. It allows earlier detection than the Western blot. It can also be used to monitor treatment.

The test has been evaluated by only one study that included 25 individuals fitting strict criteria for Lyme disease or with proven *Bb* infection and 23 controls. The test showed 84% sensitivity (was positive in individuals with *Bb*) and 94% specificity (specific for *Bb*). While this sounds promising, it is a very small study in a distinct population of people. This would suggest the test **has value primarily for diagnosing acute Lyme disease**. Whether it will pick up Borrelia in chronic illness is completely unknown.

The test is specific for *Borrelia burgdorferi* and **will not pick up other Borrelia species** that cause Lyme disease. The cost is $375-$400, presently not covered by insurance. At the time of this writing, the test is waiting for FDA approval. The test is available through Neuroscience, Inc.

Ceres Nanotrap. This test, performed on a urine sample, captures the outer surface protein from Borrelia bacteria. The company claims high specificity for Borrelia bacteria and high sensitivity for picking up acute infection. The biggest advantage of the test is that it is not species specific; it will pick up a variety of different species of Borrelia. At this time, the value of the test for diagnosing chronic Lyme disease is unknown. Expect to pay $400 for this test.

Advanced Laboratory Services improved culture. After enhanced culture, Borrelia microbes are identified by immunostaining, PCR, and DNA sequencing. This test has the advantage of being less species specific. A study published in 2013 showed 94% serum/blood positive at 16 weeks' growth in a group of 72 patients who met all CDC criteria for Lyme disease as compared with 48 negative controls. Time will tell how promising this test really is. Expect to pay up to $900.

CD 57 natural killer cells. Natural killer cells are WBCs that destroy cancer cells, viruses, and bacteria. CD 57 cells are best described as a subpopulation of NK cells that are more mature and cytotoxic than other killer cells. CD 57 cells are commonly increased in cancer and viral infections, but often low in autoimmune disease (it is speculated that CD 57 cells have a regulatory role, and unsatisfactory levels of CD 57 may allow autoimmunity). Infection with Borrelia has been associated with decreased CD 57 counts (which may be a link between stealth microbe infections and autoimmunity).

Though low CD 57 counts have been proposed as a marker for chronic Lyme disease, other microbes, such as Babesia, also cause low CD 57 counts. In addition, one study found that there was no difference in CD 57 levels in post-treatment Lyme disease individuals, symptomatic chronic Lyme disease individuals, and healthy controls (Marques 2009). This suggests that monitoring CD 57 levels for chronic Lyme disease is neither specific for Borrelia nor sensitive enough to provide reliable information.

Direct tick testing. If you actually kept the tick that bit you, it is possible to have the tick checked for certain microbes. The testing, however, does not check for all possibilities. Tic-Kit will check the tick for only certain species of Borrelia, Bartonella, Babesia, and Ehrlichia (tic-kit.com).

STARI. Bite of the lone star tick is associated with a Lyme-like illness named **STARI (Southern Tick-Associated Rash Illness).**[1] It can be associated with a bull's-eye rash and all the symptoms of Lyme disease, but tests for Borrelia are always negative. The cause of STARI is presently unknown, but another form of Borrelia (possibly *B. lonestari*) is suspected.

DIAGNOSING COINFECTIONS AND RELATED MICROBES
There are quite a few microbes spread by blood-sucking insects (ticks, mosquitoes, fleas, lice, chiggers, biting flies, scabies) that have similar stealth microbe characteristics to *Borrelia burgdorferi*; some we know about, and others are still waiting to be discovered.

They all have stealth characteristics and have the ability to infect and thrive inside cells. They are masters of evading the immune system and can be even harder to diagnose than Borrelia. Symptom profiles are similar to Borrelia and related mostly to stimulation of cytokine cascades, not concentrations of microbes. Though they each have slightly different strategies, their motive is the same: complete a life cycle stage within the host and move on.

The primary known players in chronic Lyme disease include Mycoplasma, Bartonella, and Chlamydia species. Higher virulence microbes, including the more well-known species of Babesia, Anaplasma, Ehrlichia, and Rickettsia, are more apt to cause acute illness and less apt to be

---

1 http://www.cdc.gov/stari/disease/

associated with chronic illness, but research is discovering lesser known and lesser virulent species of these microbes that are associated with chronic Lyme. Reactivation of herpes-type viruses is common in chronic Lyme.

Though testing is possible for some species of these microbes, when a natural route of recovery is chosen, extensive testing is not necessary and can actually be very misleading.

MYCOPLASMA

Diagnosis of Mycoplasma is challenging, especially chronic infections. Most commonly, amplified PCR tests for DNA specific for the microbe in a blood sample are used for diagnosis. PCR is species specific and focused on diagnosing acute respiratory or genital Mycoplasma infections. When testing for Mycoplasma, ask to be tested for all the possible species (*M. fermentans, M. genitalium, M. penetrans, M. hominis, M. pneumoniae, M. synoviae, Ureaplasma urealyticum*). 75% of acute infections show cold agglutinins (clumping of RBCs).

Serial titers testing for antibodies with enzyme-linked immunosorbent assays can be used to test for acute infection. Persistent, elevated titer may indicate chronic infection or asymptomatic carrier, but in general, chronic infection with Mycoplasma is difficult to diagnose. 25% of chronic infections show low WBC count.

The University of Alabama School of Medicine runs a research lab specializing in Mycoplasma. The lab utilizes culture, nucleic acid amplification technology and serology, and performance of in vitro susceptibility testing for detection and identification of human Mycoplasmas. Testing is reasonable, with an average of $100-$150 per test. The <u>website posts no information</u> about sensitivity or specificity of testing (how accurate it is). www.uab.edu/medicine/pathology/Mycoplasma-Home.

BARTONELLA

The best test for Bartonella is an amplified version of PCR called ePCR by Galaxy Diagnostics (Research Triangle, NC; www.galaxydx.com). The company offers both ePCR and serology testing for Bartonella. Standard PCR for Bartonella costs $220, and ePCR costs $480. Testing is species specific; the most common species are including in the testing protocol. The company also offers standard PCR for Anaplasma, Babesia, Ehrlichia, and Rickettsia (most common species) for $220 each (or $590 for a total tick panel).

Galaxy Diagnostics says, "Even the most sensitive DNA detection methods can produce false negatives due to extremely low levels of DNA in a given sample. We overcome this testing limitation by enriching samples for one week in a patented enrichment media called BAPGM (Bartonella Alpha Proteobacteria Growth Medium), which increases the bacterial load in patient samples up to detectable levels for PCR testing." According to their website, they "sequence verify all positive PCR results to identify the species of infection, ensuring the highest level of specificity achievable. Sequence identification is an important step for Bartonella detection, as virulence and treatment resistance may vary across species."

BABESIA

Indirect Immunofluorescent Assay (IFA) tests for IgG and IgM antibodies against Babesia. Diagnosis relies on a fourfold rise in antibody titer over several weeks. The first sample should be taken as early in the disease process as possible, and the second sample taken 2-4 weeks later. PCR detects microbial DNA in a blood sample. IGeneX uses an amplified version of PCR and FISH together for improved accuracy of testing for *B. microti* and *B. ducani*.

EHRLICHIA/ANAPLASMA/RICKETTSIA

These microbes have the potential to cause severe illness; therapy should not await laboratory diagnosis if acute infection with any of

these microbes is suspected. Blood can be drawn when therapy is initiated to confirm the infection. The most accurate test is serial serology using IFA. Diagnosis depends on a fourfold rise in titer from the first sample taken as early in the disease process as possible, to the second sample taken 2-4 weeks later. PCR is 60-85% effective for diagnosing Ehrlichia and 70-90% effective for diagnosing Anaplasma, but less valuable for diagnosing Rocky Mountain spotted fever. Accuracy for diagnosing chronic infection is unknown. There are many new species of these microbes being discovered for which routine testing is not yet available.

CHLAMYDIA

Pelvic infection associated with *C. trachomatis* is diagnosed by vaginal swab in females (either patient or clinician collected) and urine sample in males. Nucleic acid amplification tests (NAATs) are the most sensitive. Yearly screening for females < aged 25 is recommended by the CDC. Testing for *C. pneumoniae* (respiratory infection) is performed with PCR specific for *C. pneumoniae* DNA from a blood sample. Present testing includes only the two most common species out of nine known species.

VIRUSES

The list of viruses that can cause chronic infection with chronic reactions in the human body is long. A partial list includes Epstein-Barr virus, cytomegalovirus (CMV), HSV-1, HSV-2, herpes zoster virus, HHV-6a, HHV-6b, HHV-7, parvovirus B-19, adenoviruses, and hepatitis B and C. Reactivation of dormant viruses is commonly associated with immune dysfunction that occurs with fibromyalgia, Lyme disease, and similar chronic illnesses. Testing for specific viral reactivation is generally not necessary, but if you are interested, the best source of information about testing is www.labtestsonline.org.

The two most common reactivated viruses associated with chronic flu-like symptoms are Epstein-Barr virus and cytomegalovirus.

Epstein-Barr virus (EBV)

To evaluate acute and chronic infection for EBV, four antibodies commonly tested are viral capsid antigen (VCA) IgG, VCA IgM, D early antigen (EA-D), and Epstein-Barr nuclear antigen (EBNA).

- The presence of VCA IgG antibodies indicates recent or past EBV infection.

- The presence of VCA IgM antibodies and the absence of antibodies to EBNA indicates recent infection.

- The presence of antibodies to EBNA indicates infection sometime in the past. Antibodies to EBNA develop 6 to 8 weeks after the time of infection and are present for life.

- The presence of VCA IgG, EA-D, and EBNA may indicate reactivation of the virus.

Cytomegalovirus (CMV)

To evaluate acute and chronic CMV infection, a blood sample is tested for IgG and IgM antibodies to CMV.

- The presence of CMV IgM indicates a recent active infection.

- The presence of both CMV IgM and CMV IgG can indicate active primary infection or reactivation of dormant virus.

- The presence of CMV IgG only indicates past exposure.

INTESTINAL PARASITES

Intestinal parasites are common in third-world countries where sanitation and waste disposal systems are poor, but much less common in developed countries. Parasite eggs are consumed with contaminated food, hatch inside the body, go through a life cycle, lay eggs, and then die. The eggs do not hatch inside the body, but are shed in feces. Chronic parasite re-infestation requires continual consumption of contaminated food.

People in developed countries do occasionally consume parasite eggs from eating raw foods and can occasionally harbor very low levels of parasites, but rarely enough to cause symptoms of infestation. Infections are always self-limited unless contaminated food is again consumed. Testing is rarely indicated. Testing stool for eggs and parasites is not very sensitive and is most always negative unless infestation is large.

TRANSMISSION VECTORS

Different stealth microbes have different transmission routes. Knowing the mode of transmission can sometimes be helpful in diagnosis. Many of the stealth microbes can be transmitted by ticks. For Borrelia, STARI, Babesia, Ehrlichia, and Anaplasma, this is a major route of transmission. If the type of tick is known, sometimes it can be helpful in defining types of microbes that are present. **This is not absolute, however**. Most tick-borne microbes can be spread by a variety of ticks.

In addition, many stealth microbes are also spread by other biting in-sects (mosquitoes, fleas, lice, biting flies, chiggers), sexual contact, blood transfusions, and air droplets. Mycoplasma and Bartonella are more commonly spread by other means and can already be present, but silent at the time of infection with a different tick-borne microbe. Mycoplasma and Bartonella are probably more common in individuals diagnosed with fibromyalgia and chronic fatigue (along with other stealth microbes).

Borrelia: Black-legged deer tick (*Ixodes scapularis*), most common in the northeastern, mid-Atlantic, north-central US, and western black-legged tick (*Ixodes pacificus*) on the US Pacific coast.

STARI: Lone star tick (*Amblyomma americanum*), most common in the southern US extending out to Oklahoma and Texas, and mid-Atlantic extending up into northeastern US.

Mycoplasma: Mostly respiratory and sexual transmission, but can be spread by biting insects, including ticks, probably numerous species.

Numerous species of Mycoplasma are widely distributed worldwide. Mycoplasma may be primary factor in fibromyalgia, chronic fatigue syndrome, and autoimmune disease.

Bartonella: Most commonly associated with a scratch of an infected animal (cat, dog), but also can be spread by fleas and lice. Ticks are a vector, but specific tick species have not been specified. Bartonella may be a primary factor in fibromyalgia and chronic fatigue.

Babesia: Black-legged deer ticks (Ixodes scapularis), most common in New England, New York, New Jersey, Wisconsin, Minnesota, but spreading southward; southeastern US with Georgia as the epicenter.

Ehrlichia: Most common in mideast and southeast US, most concentrated in a band stretching from North Carolina to Oklahoma (South, South-central, Southeast), the distribution of the lone star tick (*Amblyomma americanum*). Ehrlichia is also transmitted by black-legged (Ixodes scapularis) and western black-legged (Ixodes pacificus) ticks, along with other tick species worldwide.

Anaplasma: Black-legged tick (*Ixodes scapularis*; NE and upper Midwest) and western black-legged tick (*Ixodes pacificus*) in northern California.

Rickettsia (Rocky Mountain spotted fever): American dog tick (*Dermacentor variabilis*) most common distribution in mid-states east of the Rockies, Rocky Mountain wood tick (*Dermacentor andersoni*), and brown dog tick (*Rhipicephalus sanguineus*, Arizona); Rocky Mountain spotted fever is widely distributed across the US and can occur in any state.

HALLMARK SYMPTOMS

Chronic infection with any stealth microbe is associated with nonspecific symptoms (it is their very nature). Even the symptoms that are considered classic for a particular microbe do not always occur. There are numerous species and strains of each of the different microbes, each of which have slightly different characteristics. If a classic symptom is present, however, it may help with diagnosis.

Borrelia: Microbes bore into areas of the body with collagen (skin, joints, brain) → bull's-eye rash (⅓ of cases), migrating arthritis, brain fog.

STARI: Probably another species of Borrelia with same characteristics as Lyme → bull's-eye rash (⅓ of cases), migrating arthritis.

Mycoplasma: Infect tissues lining areas in the body → initial respiratory or pelvic symptoms (depending on infection site), fatigue, intestinal issues. Systemic symptoms are typically different from initial symptoms. Arthritis is common.

Bartonella: Infect WBCs and cells lining blood vessels, scavenges RBCs for food → bone pain from infection in bone marrow, pain in soles of feet (from damage to blood vessels when walking). Damage to blood vessels can also cause stretch marks on legs.

Babesia: Infect RBCs, liver, spleen → relapsing high fevers with drenching sweats, liver/spleen enlargement.

Ehrlichia/Anaplasma: Infect specific types of WBCs → high fever, headache, muscle pain. Acute illness is most common. Chronic infection presents as relapses of acute symptoms.

Rickettsia (Rocky Mountain spotted fever): Infect cells lining blood vessels causing severe vasculitis → high fever, spotted rash (90%), severe swelling in extremities. Acute illness is most common. Chronic infection, when it occurs, generally presents as relapses of acute symptoms.

Chlamydia: *Chlamydia trachomatis* can be spread by ticks, but is more commonly spread by sexual contact or respiratory infection. It can, however, be present at the time of infection of other microbes by tick bite. It is a common stealth microbe associated with chronic fatigue. It also has possible links to MS. Chlamydia is spread as a sexually transmitted disease and has been associated with chronic pelvic pain in women, infertility, and chronic fatigue. *Chlamydia pneumoniae*, which is associated with acute respiratory infection, has also been associated with chronic fatigue.

PART THREE
Therapies for Getting Well

11

A Holistic Approach to Recovery

Controlling symptoms and killing or suppressing microbes are important for overcoming chronic Lyme, but if that's the limit of your efforts, the chances of success are greatly diminished. To accomplish your ultimate mission of wellness, you must also reduce inflammation generated by the microbes, restore the normal ability of the immune system to control marginal microbes, restore the natural healing capacity of the body, and support repair of damage in the body. That requires a holistic approach to recovery.

Essential Components of Overcoming Chronic Lyme Disease:

- Control symptoms

- Suppress stealth microbes (not just Borrelia)

- Control inflammation

- Restore normal immune function

- Restore healing and repair damage

- Restore homeostasis (hormonal balance)

The method you use to overcome illness is defined as therapy. Therapies can be divided into three main types: **restorative**, **symptomatic**, and **heroic**. Each type is important. A holistic approach to recovery from chronic illness generally utilizes all three.

RESTORATIVE THERAPY

Of the three, **restorative therapy** provides the most comprehensive benefit. Restorative therapy focuses on reducing stress caused by system disruptors, which allows the healing systems of the body to flourish. It includes suppressing microbes, but the primary (and all important) goal is restoring normal immune function. As long as immune function is disrupted, you will not get well — no matter how hard you hit the microbes.

Embracing a healthful diet and lifestyle is an essential part of this approach, but that alone is rarely enough to restore wellness — **medicinal herbs are the cornerstone of the restorative therapy**.

Medicinal herbs come from plants selected for their remarkable healing properties. Of all therapeutic modalities, herbs offer the highest potential for healing (no drug on earth comes close). The biochemical substances present in herbs (called phytochemicals) suppress a wide range of microbial threats, neutralize free radicals and mutagens (cancer-causing substances), reduce inflammation, modulate immune functions, and restore homeostasis (hormonal and metabolic balance) to all systems in the body.

Because the phytochemicals present in herbs mesh naturally well with human biochemistry, most herbs are associated with very low toxicity. This allows herbs to be used for extended periods without concern.

Herbs with antimicrobial properties are ideal for reining in unstrained stealth microbes. Because stealth microbes grow slowly, can live inside cells, and favor isolated areas of the body, constant suppression must be applied for months or even years to get ahead. Because antimicrobial herbs have such low potential for toxicity and do not disrupt normal flora like synthetic antibiotics, they can be used for long durations.

The biggest limitation of restorative therapy is that healing takes time. Symptoms are not treated directly, but only gradually resolve as healing occurs. Pronounced symptoms, however, can be a real impediment to progress. Symptoms of pain and poor sleep are especially aggravating. For this reason, therapy directed primarily at relieving symptoms can be beneficial.

SYMPTOMATIC THERAPY

Symptomatic therapy, as you might expect, is therapy that is specifically directed at controlling symptoms. Sometimes treating specific symptoms directly and aggressively can expedite recovery. It mostly comes in the form of drugs, but there are some natural and alternative options that fit into this category.

The benefits of symptomatic therapies are generally limited to acute relief of symptoms. The contribution to healing and wellness is generally minimal. Suppression of symptoms is transient and only lasts as long as the therapy is administered. Over time, symptomatic therapies lose effectiveness. Dependence and habituation can be a problem with some drugs in this category. Use of symptomatic therapy becomes less necessary as healing occurs.

HEROIC THERAPY

Heroic therapy is listed last, but heroic solutions are the solutions most people turn to first. When you're sick, you want to be well immediately — and you want any and all heroic measures available to be directed at that goal. What works for acute or life-threatening situations, however, is not necessarily a good fit for chronic illnesses such as chronic Lyme disease.

Heroic therapies are designed to acutely and directly inhibit processes of disease. In the Middle Ages, heroic therapies consisted of mercury and leeches. In the 21st century, the concept of heroic therapy has been modernized with the advent of synthetic antibiotics, vaccines, pharmaceuticals, and modern surgery.

Heroic therapies are best reserved for when something truly heroic is needed: a broken leg, an acute pneumonia, or a heart attack. In such cases, when all the marvels of modern medicine are focused on fixing one thing, remarkable outcomes can occur. Today, the best heroic therapies include life-saving interventions for acute trauma, heart attack and stroke, cancer, and surgical procedures for restoring lost functions.

In chronic illness, however, the role of heroic therapies is less well defined. Because the entire body is in the process of breaking down in multiple ways, use of heroic therapies in chronic illness is like plugging leaks in a failing dam — without rebuilding the entire structure, collapse is inevitable. The greatest value of heroic therapies in chronic illness is when the holes and cracks are so bad and so deep that something heroic must be done immediately. Once the structure is stabilized, restorative therapy can take over to heal the entire structure.

Heroic therapies commonly used in Lyme disease include synthetic antibiotics, steroids, and anti-inflammatory drugs of various types. Alternative forms of heroic therapies use oxidation, electricity, and various types of radiation. Heroic therapies focus primarily on killing specific microbes or shocking systems in the body back into working order. The price of any heroic therapy is toxicity to tissues with the risk of disrupting systems in the body even further — generally the more potent a heroic therapy is, the greater the potential for harm.

A holistic approach to recovery uses restorative therapies as a foundation, symptomatic therapies in early stages as necessary, and heroic therapies only when specific indications are present. Often wellness can be achieved with restorative therapy alone.

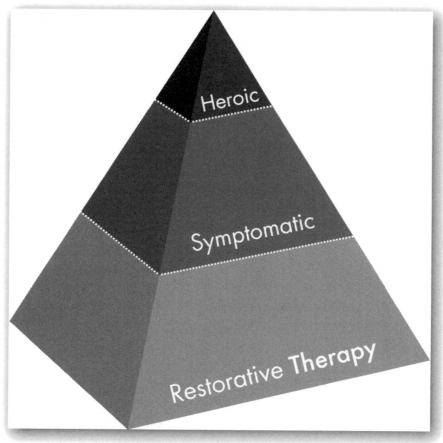

Figure 7 – Therapies in Perspective

LOOKING AHEAD

The next chapter, **Chapter 12**, will review the **indications for synthetic antibiotics in Lyme disease**. Antibiotics have a place in acute Lyme disease treatment, but use in chronic Lyme is controversial. The reasons why will be discussed in detail.

The three chapters following that are devoted to **understanding herbal therapy** and why it is such a good fit for chronic Lyme. In **Chapter 13**, you will learn about the wide range of beneficial properties offered by herbs and different herbal preparations. **Chapter 14** is a discussion about specific herbs useful for chronic Lyme disease. **Chapter 15** summarizes the **core herbal protocol** and provides tips for taking herbal supplements and establishing a supplement routine.

Inflammation is the source of many symptoms. The core supplements will gradually reduce inflammation, but in the short term, severe inflammation can slow your recovery. Symptoms associated with brain and joint inflammation are particularly disturbing. **Chapter 16** goes into more detail about inflammation and discusses both **drugs and natural substances that are useful for curbing inflammation acutely**. Specific guidelines for **reducing joint inflammation and brain inflammation** are discussed.

Lack of **sleep and pain are common roadblocks to recovery. Chapters 17 and 18** provide advice on dealing with these disrupting symptoms, both acutely and chronically. Both medications and natural options are discussed.

Chapter 19 reviews some of the more **common heroic therapies being utilized for Lyme disease**, both conventional and alternative.

Recovery from Lyme disease is an up and down process. **Chapter 20** provides advice for dealing with different types of **setbacks and relapses**.

Chapter 21 discusses **far infrared sauna and other ways to use heat to enhance your recovery**.

This block of chapters ends with a complete discussion of everything you need to know about **biofilm**.

The next block of chapters after that moves on to guiding you through the process of **establishing a healing environment in the body**. This is the ultimate key to staying well and living a normal life!

12

Antibiotics and Lyme Disease

There is a place for antibiotic use in chronic Lyme disease, and certainly there are people who get well with use of synthetic antibiotics alone, but if most people, or even a large portion of people with chronic Lyme got well using antibiotics, there wouldn't be hordes of people searching for other solutions. Many people either don't tolerate antibiotic therapy or don't get well with antibiotics.

The best use of antibiotics in Lyme occurs when something truly heroic is indicated — early-stage Lyme disease, chronic Lyme disease with severe involvement of heart or brain, when there is suspicion of a highly virulent microbe such as Rickettsia, or when nothing else works. The usefulness of antibiotics is limited by their inherent toxicity. Often, antibiotics must be discontinued because toxicity builds up, sometimes even within a few weeks.

Whenever you decide to use synthetic antibiotics, you enter a race — can you kill off all the pathogens before the toxic effects of the antibiotics catch up with you? You're much more likely to win the race against a highly virulent pathogen, which typically responds well to synthetic antibiotics, than you are with stealth pathogens, which typically respond very slowly to synthetic antibiotics.

Selective killing is the reason why synthetic antibiotics have *any* use for treating *any* bacterial infection. Antibiotics kill pathogens and, with short-term use, are less destructive to the trillions of normal flora in your body. With continued or chronic use, however, the harm inflicted on normal flora also adds up.

One of the keys to selective killing is bacterial growth rate. The microbes that make up your normal flora reproduce very slowly and maintain stable concentrations in the body. **Synthetic antibiotics rely on the rapid growth rate of pathogens for killing.** Aggressive pathogens, such as those that cause pneumonia, divide very rapidly and concentrate at specific sites in the body (in the case of pneumonia, congestion of lobes of lungs). This type of infection is very susceptible to synthetic antibiotic therapy.

The survival strategy used by stealth microbes makes them very resistant to antibiotic therapy. Like normal flora, stealth microbes such as Borrelia grow very slowly. *Streptococcus pneumoniae*, a common pneumonia-causing pathogen turns over a generation every 20 minutes. In contrast, it takes Borrelia 12 hours to turn over a generation — they win by persistence, not aggression. This factor alone makes a stealth microbe such as Borrelia much less susceptible to antibiotic therapy.

Stealth microbes do not concentrate at specific sites. They disperse throughout tissues in the body and occur at very low concentrations. They have an uncanny ability to penetrate the most isolated recesses of the body where they are protected from immune functions and antibiotics. Stealth microbes can live inside cells where they are protected from many types of antibiotics. They also have the ability to exist inside biofilms, though this is likely only a minor survival strategy for stealth microbes (See **Chapter 22**, Understanding Biofilm).

Borrelia (and others) have the ability to wrap themselves into protective cysts when a hostile environment is encountered. When antibiotics are administered, Borrelia microbes rapidly encyst and become dormant (note that a healthy immune system is well equipped to mop up cysts). The harder you hit them with antibiotics, the more they encyst until all Borrelia microbes in the body are present in antibiotic-resistant cyst forms. **When the antibiotics are discontinued, they return to normal form and go about life.**

In general, the less virulent a microbe is, the worse its response to synthetic antibiotics. In other words, Rickettsia will respond to doxycycline much better than Borrelia. Of all the stealth microbes, Mycoplasma is probably the most resistant to synthetic antibiotics.

To kill off stealth microbes with synthetic antibiotics, antibiotics must be used in high concentrations (sometimes several antibiotics at a time) for very long periods of time (months). This makes winning the race problematic on multiple levels.

Normal flora microbes are less susceptible to antibiotics, but prolonged use of high concentrations of antibiotics does have an adverse effect. **Disruption of normal flora allows for emergence of pathogens.** There are always potential pathogens present in the mix of microbes in the body, but they are suppressed by normal flora. When normal flora microbes are inhibited by antibiotics, pathogens are able to flourish. Overgrowth of pathogens, such as *Clostridium difficile* (*C. diff*) in the gut, has become commonplace with overuse of antibiotics.

It's only a matter of time before a pathogen develops antibiotic resistance. When an antibiotic is used against a pathogen, most of the bacteria are killed, but a few of the microbes develop resistance to the antibiotic and survive. With each new generation, antibiotic-resistant survivors accumulate until all of them are resistant to the antibiotic[1]. If healthy immune function is not present to mop up the resistant survivors as they develop, the antibiotic becomes useless.

Chronic immune dysfunction allows antibiotic-resistant survivors to flourish and displace normal flora. This disrupts immune function even further. With time, a vicious cycle develops that is hard to overcome.

Excessive use of antibiotics in both human and animal populations (antibiotics are heavily used in the livestock industry) **creates resistance and enhances virulence in nonpathogenic bacteria**. Antibiotic-resistant strains of bacteria that were once every day normal flora have now become quite aggressive. Methicillin-resistant *Staphylococcus aureus* (MRSA) on the skin, and pathogenic strains of *E. coli* and other microbes in the gut, have become a worldwide health hazard. These new pathogens are much more destructive than stealth microbes.

Long-term antibiotic use breaks down beneficial biofilms in the large bowel. Friendly microbes create biofilm in the mucous lining of the distal small intestine and the large colon. This type of biofilm is protective and essential for a healthy colon. Long-term use of antibiotics can disrupt this very important protective barrier. Studies show that loss of bifidobacteria in this layer with replacement with pathogenic bacteria is associated with gut illnesses such as ulcerative colitis and colon cancer (Macfarlane 2005, 2007, 2011).

If all that wasn't enough, **synthetic antibiotics have been found to destroy mitochondria in normal cells** (Morgun 2015, Kalghatgis 2013). There is evidence that mitochondria, the powerhouses within every cell

---

1 The faster a microbe grows, the quicker it can become antibiotic resistant. Aggressive pathogens would be expected to become antibiotic resistant much faster than stealth microbes, which would become resistant faster than normal flora. Viruses are very fast growing and can become resistant to antivirals very rapidly.

in the body, were once primitive bacteria. A billion years ago, when higher life was evolving, primitive bacteria with high-energy capacity were hijacked by cells of higher living creatures to produce energy. Eventually, they became part of cells of all higher life forms, but they still retain bacteria-like characteristics.

Having bacteria-like characteristics makes mitochondria susceptible to damage by many types of antibiotics. This may be why many people experience fatigue with antibiotic use. Antibiotics are especially damaging to cells lining the intestines.

In summary, usefulness of **prolonged antibiotics for chronic stealth microbe infections is limited** because:

- Stealth microbes typically **grow very slowly** (most antibiotics depend on rapid growth)

- Stealth microbes **occur in very low concentrations** in isolated areas of the body

- Stealth microbes are able to **live inside cells** and areas of the body shielded from antibiotics

- Certain stealth microbes, such as Borrelia, are able to **form antibiotic-resistant cysts**

- Prolonged antibiotic use results in the **emergence of antibiotic-resistant pathogens**

- Use of antibiotics commonly **causes yeast overgrowth in the gut**

- Prolonged antibiotic **use kills normal flora in the gut and allows overgrowth of pathogens**

- Antibiotics **damage mitochondria** inside cells, especially cells lining the intestines

- Antibiotics may **disrupt microbial biofilms that protect the lining of the intestines and colon**

- Chronic antibiotic use **disrupts immune function** — normal immune function is essential for getting well

People suffering from chronic Lyme disease do report getting well with long-term antibiotic therapy, but it may be the exception rather than the rule.

CURRENT RECOMMENDATIONS FOR ANTIBIOTICS IN LYME DISEASE

There is a place for use of antibiotics for treatment of Lyme disease, but when and how to administer antibiotics, however, remains controversial.

Current recommendations for the treatment of Lyme disease, per the Centers for Disease Control and Prevention (CDC) are defined in a scientific article published in the journal, *Clinical Infectious Diseases*, in 2006. The article has not been updated in the intervening years and is criticized by many experts who treat Lyme disease.

The current recommendations for treatment of "adult patients with early localized or early disseminated Lyme disease associated with erythema migrans or positive serologic testing, in the absence of specific neurologic manifestations or advanced atrioventricular heart block" is **"doxycycline (100 mg twice per day), amoxicillin (500 mg 3 times per day), or cefuroxime axetil (500 mg twice per day) for 14 days** (range, 10–21 days for doxycycline and 14–21 days for amoxicillin or cefuroxime axetil)". However, many doctors prescribe 30 days of treatment.

Routine use of antimicrobial prophylaxis or serologic testing is not recommended by the CDC for prevention of Lyme disease after a recognized tick bite. "**A single dose of doxycycline may be offered to adult patients (200-mg dose)** when the tick can be identified as an adult or nymphal *I. scapularis* tick that is estimated to have been attached for >36 hours." Antibiotics must be administered within 72 hours of attachment.

The article goes on to recommend ceftriaxone, 2 g once per day intravenously for 14 days (range, 10–28 days) for acute neurological symptoms and similar treatment for acute cardiac manifestations of Lyme disease. This brief treatment is considered curative by the CDC.

For symptomatic late-stage Lyme disease, the article recommends 14 days of oral or intravenous antibiotics (depending on the type of symptoms) and suggests that this is also curative.

The article does not recognize "chronic Lyme disease", but does recognize "Post Treatment Lyme Disease Syndrome (PTLDS)". The authors strongly suggest, however, that the symptoms are not related to persistent Borrelia bacteria in the body: "The notion that symptomatic, chronic *B. burgdorferi* infection can exist despite recommended treatment courses of antibiotics in the absence of objective clinical signs of disease, is highly implausible as evidenced by the lack of antibiotic resistance in this genus." They go on to imply an emotional link: "Delayed convalescence can be related to the emotional state of the patient before onset of the illness."

Studies cited in the article strongly supported use of antibiotics in early-stage Lyme disease, but not use of prolonged antibiotic therapy in late-stage or post-treatment Lyme disease.

Many doctors in the Lyme community disagree very strongly with this seemingly outdated and narrow-minded summation of Lyme disease treatment. For persistent Lyme disease symptoms, many doctors prescribe 6-9 months of either oral or intravenous antibiotics. To date, however, there are no studies supporting this practice either (Berende 2016).

In fact, **one recently published study challenges everything accepted about Lyme disease by both the conventional medical community and the Lyme community** (Rudenko 2015).

In the study, published in March 2016, researchers tested people from around the country who had atypical symptoms of Lyme disease (typical presentations are not the norm), had a *negative* Western blot for Lyme disease, and were treated for 6-9 months with antibiotics, but continued having symptoms.

In several of these people, using special techniques to culture and isolate the microbe (not practical for routine use), they were able to isolate *two* species of Borrelia from blood samples: *Borrelia burgdorferi* and *Borrelia bissettii.*

Negative Western blot, atypical Lyme symptoms, aggressive prolonged antibiotic therapy, persistent Lyme symptoms despite therapy, followed by positive culture for two species of Borrelia are **direct evidence that Borrelia is very hard to diagnose and responds poorly to any level of antibiotic therapy**, especially with chronic illness. (The study also provides hope and verification to all the patients who have had a negative Western blot, but still feel they have Lyme disease.)

In summary, scientific evidence does support use of antibiotic therapy in early-stage Lyme disease. This makes sense because bacteria are migrating through the bloodstream and have not disseminated deeply into tissues. It is unlikely that antibiotics alone eliminate all Borrelia microbes, but it may give the immune system the upper hand enough to gain control. It does not, however, completely eliminate the possibility of chronic infection.

In contrast, treating chronic Lyme disease for months on end continually with synthetic antibiotics is highly controversial. There is no good science to back it up, and the potential for toxicity is quite high.

Some physicians have started **pulsing antibiotics** for several weeks to a month on and several weeks to a month off to reduce potential toxicity, but there are no studies supporting this practice. It may be worth considering, however, especially in conjunction with herbal therapy in a person who is not making progress with herbal therapy alone. Short courses of antibiotics during relapses or setbacks may enhance recovery without accumulating the toxic effects of long-term antibiotic use.

ANTIBIOTICS FOR OTHER TICK-BORNE INFECTIONS

Use of antibiotics for treatment of low-virulence stealth microbes, including Mycoplasma, Bartonella, and Chlamydia should be mostly reserved for acute infections. When infection by these microbes occurs by tick bite, however, the initial acute infection is often not recognized.

Synthetic antibiotics are most useful for acute infections with more virulent bacteria that grow rapidly. For tick-borne microbes, this mostly includes acute infections with Rickettsia, Ehrlichia, Anaplasma, and Babesia species.

The potential for acute severe illness with these microbes is high, especially with Rickettsia. For this reason, **anyone presenting with a history of tick bite, high fever, and severe flu-like illness should receive 30 days of antibiotic therapy.** Antibiotics should be started empirically without waiting for test results.

Rickettsia, Ehrlichia, and Anaplasma respond well to tetracyclines, such as doxycycline. The **standard treatment protocol is doxycycline, 100 mg twice daily for 30 days or 3 days after symptoms subside completely**. The course of antibiotics can be repeated if symptoms are persistent. Alternative antibiotics for acute infection are posted on the CDC website (www.cdc.gov).

Equally concerning is an acute infection with Babesia. Babesia is a protozoan, which does not respond to doxycycline. The current CDC

Guidelines for Babesia recommend treatment for 7-10 days with two antibiotics: **atovaquone 750 mg twice daily** and **azithromycin 500-1000 mg initially followed by 250-1000 mg daily** or **clindamycin 600 mg 3 times daily** or **600 mg IV 4 times daily** and **quinine 650 mg 3 times daily.**

Aggressive therapy for Babesia is especially indicated in someone who has had a splenectomy. Individuals who have had the spleen removed are especially at risk of severe life-threatening infection with Babesia.

Atovaquone is associated with high incidence of side effects; some people are very sensitive to it. The clindamycin/quinine combination is an older regimen also associated with a high incidence of side effects. **Clindamycin should never be used orally** because it can stimulate overgrowth of *Clostridium difficile* in the gut. *Clostridium difficile* (*C. diff*) is a notorious pathogen associated with severe bloody diarrhea.

As a less toxic alternative, some physicians are prescribing **metronidazole 500 mg twice daily for 14 days** (metronidazole should never be used for more than 2 weeks because of toxicity) or **tinidazole 500 mg twice daily for 14 days** (less toxic, but more expensive). This is not a standard protocol, however.

Chronic Babesia infection is characterized by relapsing high fever or positive test for Babesia. A relapse of Babesia should be treated just like an acute infection.

It should be noted that Babesia is actually harder to kill than malaria because it grows slowly and occurs in low concentrations in the body (a characteristic in common with lower virulence stealth microbes; Babesia is on the fence between low virulence and high virulence). Limiting duration of therapy to 7-10 days is associated with a high relapse rate of 40-50%. Longer therapy of 6-8 weeks, especially in immunocompromised individuals, is recommended by most experts who regularly treat Babesia. Longer treatments with any of the antimicrobials used for Babesia, however, are associated with high rates of side effects and toxicity. Natural therapies discussed later in the book provide a potentially safer long-term solution.

Symptoms associated with Babesia infection are related to clumping of blood cells and blockage of small blood vessels. This process impedes recovery. There is evidence that heparin, a commonly used anticoagulant administered by subcutaneous or IV injection, has value for treating severe Babesia. Heparin inhibits blood coagulation, reduces cerebral impacts (brain blood clots), and suppresses replication of organisms.

GENERAL GUIDELINES FOR ANTIBIOTIC USE IN LYME DISEASE

- Doxycycline covers for Borrelia and all known coinfections except Babesia. Other antibiotics can be added at the discretion of the healthcare provider.

- If acute infection is suspected, follow CDC guidelines for antibiotic choices.

- For alternative recommendations on antibiotic use in Lyme disease, reference the International Lyme and Associated Diseases Society at: www.ilads.org/lyme/treatment-guidelines.php.

- Whether a single antibiotic or combination antibiotics are used, therapy **should only extend for 30 days or until symptoms resolve**. Detrimental effects accumulate the longer antibiotics are used.

- **A break of at least 30 days** should be taken before repeating antibiotic therapy to allow the immune system and intestinal tract to recover.

- **Pulsing antibiotics with continuous herbal therapy** may have value (but has not been studied). For someone having a severe or persistent setback, short courses of antibiotic therapy (2-4 weeks) with continuous herbal therapy provide a way to increase pressure on microbes without the cumulative toxicity associated with continuous antibiotics.

- Probiotics including Lactobacillus, Bifidobacterium, and a friendly strain of yeast called *Saccharomyces boulardii* (inhibits *C. diff.*) should be taken daily (hours apart from antibiotics). Dosage: 20-50 billion cfu daily.

- Yeast overgrowth in the gut can be partially controlled by strictly limiting dietary sugar and starch. Many herbs have antifungal properties. If yeast overgrowth requires use of antifungals, such as Diflucan, the drug should only be used long enough to control the problem. Long-term use (6 weeks) creates drug-resistant yeast.

- **Synthetic antibiotic therapy is best accompanied by herbal therapy**. Herbs support immune function and reduce inflammation. Herbs may reduce the time period required for antibiotics to work. Herbal therapy can be continued indefinitely.

- A gut-friendly diet should be followed while taking antibiotics.

- **Clindamycin, an antibiotic commonly prescribed for Lyme disease coinfections, should never be used orally**. Clindamycin is commonly associated with overgrowth of *Clostridium difficile* in the gut. Overgrowth of *C diff.* causes severe bloody diarrhea often requiring hospitalization.

13

With synthetic antibiotics, you can indiscriminately kill bacteria...but that's about all.

With herbs, you can do so much more. In fact, if you consider chronic Lyme disease as a total body dysfunction related to a pot of stealth microbes no longer constrained by a dysfunctional immune system, herbs couldn't be a more perfect solution.

Plants are exposed to the same stress factors as any other living thing on earth. Plants deal with these stress factors by producing a complex spectrum of biochemical substances (phytochemicals) that provide protection against a wide range of threats, including a huge variety of microbes, free radicals, toxins, and radiation. Because different plants evolved in different environments under different stress factors, the phytochemicals in plants are highly variable. Plant biochemistry also generates food for the plant from the sun, carries oxygen, rids the plant of toxic waste, and repairs damage.

Plants and animals have been intimately linked since the beginning of life on earth. **When animals consume plants, they gain more than just food.** Animals also benefit from the protective properties found in those plants.

Humans knew this instinctively. While some plants were consumed primarily for food, others, now known as medicinal herbs, were selected primarily for their healing properties — different plants were chosen for different healing properties. The medicinal herbs were naturally chosen over more toxic plants because their biochemistry meshed particularly well with human biochemistry. Therefore, the potential for benefit was high, and the potential for harm was extremely low.

Herbal therapy has been a part of human civilization for thousands of years. The herbal traditions of the world predate science and were based on observations. The effects of illness on the human body were observed, and specific herbs were applied to counteract those observations and return the body to a normal state of health. These observations were passed from generation to generation by oral and written traditions. All the world's healing traditions, including traditional Chinese medicine and Ayurvedic medicine, were founded around this concept.

MODERN HERBOLOGY
Herbal medicine is gradually evolving beyond those traditions. Because of science, it is now possible to evaluate the medicinal effects of specific biochemical substances found in herbs. When both tradition and science are considered, we know more about herbs than any other source of healing on the planet.

The wide range of benefits provided by plant biochemistry includes:

- Broad-spectrum antimicrobial properties (against bacteria, viruses, protozoa, and harmful fungi)
- Anti-inflammatory properties
- Immune modulation (balances immune functions)
- Anti-mutagenic properties (anti-cancer)

- Antioxidant properties

- Hormone-balancing properties

- Anti-fatigue and enhanced stress resistance

- Enhanced detoxification and cellular functions

- Protection against harmful radiation

These properties, common to all herbs, provide benefit by directly counteracting system disruptors. The seven categories of system disruptors discussed in Chapter 5 are the primary root causes of all illnesses. The phytochemicals found in herbs counteract all of the negative aspects of system disruptors. When the effects of system disruptors are minimized, healing systems of the body flourish. This makes herbs a perfect choice for restoring wellness.

Because different plants evolved in different environments under different stress factors, the spectrum of phytochemicals present in plants is highly variable. Therefore, different herbs provide different healing properties. Different herbs can be combined to broaden the spectrum of healing potential.

Herbal therapy is remarkably different from drug therapy. Head-to-head, it's like comparing apples to oranges. Drugs are single chemical substances specifically designed to affect or block specific pathways in the body to inhibit disease. Because the effect is artificial and the biochemistry of the body is so complex, there is a high potential for side effects and toxicity with use of any drug. **All drugs have the potential to be poisonous.**

These profound differences are no more evident than when comparing synthetic antibiotics to herbal therapy.

ANTIMICROBIAL PROPERTIES OF HERBS

Synthetic antibiotics are single chemical agents selected to interfere with some key aspect of bacterial survival. **Antibiotics are potent, but subject to bacterial resistance with continued use.** Synthetic antibiotics indiscriminately kill normal flora and disrupt the entire microbiome, often with far-reaching negative effects to health.

The antimicrobial properties of herbs are quite different than synthetic antibiotics. In many respects, herbs are much more sophisticated than synthetic antibiotics. **Medicinal plants contain a spectrum of hundreds or even thousands of chemicals designed to suppress microbial function in different ways.** The evolution of plant chemistry is the result of millions of years of exposure to every variety of microbes. Not surprisingly, resistance to herbal therapy is much less common.

The antimicrobial properties of herbs are not limited to bacteria, but also include viruses, protozoa, and threatening fungal species. Plants, however, figured out the friend-versus-foe problem a long time ago. Herbs are less apt to kill normal flora or disrupt the microbiome. **In fact, many herbs support intestinal health by suppressing harmful microbes in the gut and allowing normal flora to flourish.**

Herbs with antimicrobial properties are not as potent as synthetic antibiotics, but one of the advantages of herbal therapy is being able to apply constant pressure against stealth microbes without disrupting other functions in the body. Because herbs are associated with such inherently low toxicity, they can be used continually for long durations (years or even a lifetime) without any negative effects.[1] In fact, long-term use of

---

1 Some plants that can be used as medicines do have drug-like effects. Examples include St. John's wort, cannabis, valerian, and kava. Of course, these herbs have a higher potential for toxicity. They are the exceptions. As such, they should be used with more caution than most other herbs.

herbal therapy is associated with a wide range of benefits, including support of immune function.

All herbs contain antimicrobial properties, with some better suited for one given purpose or another. The list of advantages provided by herbal therapy for stealth microbe infections includes:

- Very low potential for herb toxicity, which means **herbs can be safely used** for extended periods of time
- Unlike antibiotics, many herbs are effective for **suppressing stealthy opportunists** and can affect intracellular microbes (microbes existing inside cells)
- Multiple herbs can be used safely to create **synergy against different types of microbes**
- Herbs **support normal flora** (friendly bacteria) in the gut and on the skin
- The range of coverage with herbs extends to **viruses, protozoa, and harmful yeasts**
- Herbs enhance **immune function** and support healing in the body
- **Bacterial resistance is rare** (This can happen with use of an herb, but it takes a very long time!)

HERBAL PREPARATIONS

Herbal medicines can come from different parts of the plant, including the leaves, bark, stems, roots, rhizomes, flowers, and fruit. Which part of the herb to use has been decided by thousands of years of traditional use with each plant (though modern science is finding that other, less traditional parts of certain plants are also valuable, in some cases).

For herbs to work, you have to get them inside of you. There are a variety of ways to do that.

One way to gain the benefits of herbs is by eating them with food. This is how prehistoric people used herbs and how certain herbs are currently used today. Culinary herbs (basil, oregano, thyme, rosemary, turmeric, cinnamon, cardamom, ginger, and many others) not only add spice to food, but also provide potent medicinal value. Gram for gram (or ounce for ounce), turmeric, cinnamon, ginger, and oregano have ten times the antioxidant power of blueberries (Halvorsen 2006). Culinary herbs also provide antimicrobial and other healing properties. **Making use of culinary herbs is a great way to get started with herbal medicine!**

Another common traditional method of enjoying herbs is by brewing fresh or dried herbs in hot water as a tea. Tea brewed from the leaves of *Camellia sinensis* is the most commonly consumed beverage in the world. Green tea, prepared from fresh leaves that are steamed and dried, is the most popular way to consume tea in the East. The black tea preferred in the West is crushed and allowed to oxidize before drying. Both forms of tea come from the leaves of the *Camellia sinensis* plant.

Both types of tea have about the same amount of caffeine, but **green tea contains an amino acid called l-theanine, which counteracts the stimulating effects of caffeine**. Both also provide potent antioxidants (but black less than green because the leaves have been oxidized) and other important medicinal properties. The biggest limitation of drinking tea regularly (green or black) is the presence of tannins. **Tannins dry tissues (think leather tanning) and can damage the lining of the stomach and intestines with regular use (something to keep in mind if you are taking powdered supplements regularly).**

Tea from *Camellia sinensis*, of course, is not the only herbal tea. There are many other teas that can be prepared from fresh or dried herbs. **One of the limitations with any herbal tea, however, is getting enough of the medicinal ingredients to provide benefit.**

To extract more of the beneficial phytochemicals, herbs can also be prepared as a decoction. To make a decoction, the herb is simmered in water until the brew is very concentrated. While a few herbs, such as ginger, work well as a decoction, **most herbal decoctions can be too bitter to drink.** Another limitation of a decoction is that the high heat destroys some of the beneficial phytochemicals.

Possibly the most popular way to prepare herbs is by extraction. There are different types of extractions, but the most popular (and historically the most available) is with water and alcohol. To make an **extract**, the whole dried herb is soaked in a mixture of water and alcohol (usually 20-70% alcohol). The alcohol pulls both water-soluble and some oil-soluble chemicals out of the herb without using heat.

Extractions are very concentrated, so only a small amount of liquid needs to be consumed to provide full benefit (usually in the range of 15-30 drops). This is a good thing because many medicinal herbs are very bitter.

You could grow, harvest, and prepare your own herbs, but gaining the variety and quantities of different herbs for a comprehensive regimen for treating Lyme disease would be a real challenge. Fortunately, high-quality herbal products are readily available commercially. Commercial preparations of herbs include powdered dry whole herb, water/alcohol extractions, powdered extractions, essential oils, and supercritical CO_2 extractions. Knowing the differences is important.

Powdered dry whole herb involves taking the whole herb (whatever part, leaves, stems, or roots, is indicated), drying it, and then grinding it into a powder. It is then encapsulated, formed into tablets, or sold as loose powder. **Whole-herb powders are generally not standardized, so it is hard to judge quality and potency.** Because whole-herb powders contain inert fiber from the plant, they are by far the least potent way to take herbs, but also the least expensive (you get what you pay for). The biggest advantage of whole-herb powders is that you get the full spectrum of chemicals present in the herb.

Water/alcohol extractions (tinctures) are a very popular way to market herbs commercially. Extracts are potent and good value for the money. **The biggest disadvantage of water/alcohol extractions is all the alcohol.** If you were taking a full dose of 8-12 different herbs, 30 drops of each herb several times a day, you would be consuming a lot of alcohol. Alcohol is a toxin that can hold back your recovery. Also, many herbs are quite bitter and unpleasant tasting.

The remedy for this is **dried powdered extract**. To make a dried powdered extract, a water/alcohol extraction is sprayed on a surface, and the water and alcohol are evaporated off, leaving a concentrated powder of the plant phytochemicals. Typically, some of the powdered whole herb is added back in to make the powder more usable. The powder is then encapsulated or made into tablets (less common). **It is by far the most potent herbal preparation.** Capsules of powdered extract are easy to take and travel well.

The only disadvantage of powdered extracts is that the powder is very dry. Taking powdered extracts several times a day can dry tissues lining the stomach and intestines, eventually causing problems. **For this reason, it is best to take powdered extracts with a fatty substance, such as coconut or almond milk, which helps protect tissues.** (Some critics of powdered extracts would also say that you miss the full experience of tasting the herb…if you really want that experience.)

Both water/alcohol and dried powder extracts can be standardized. Standardization is a way to measure potency and consistency between batches of herbs and different herbal products. An extract is standardized by measuring a key chemical substance in the herb. This substance may be one of the more active phytochemicals in the herb, but not the only active chemical. It is simply a marker. The only problem with standardization is that un-reputable product suppliers sometimes spike marker substances into low quality extracts to beef them up — reputable supplement companies are very aware of these issues and know how to avoid substandard extracts.

Fat-soluble chemical substances (oils) can also be extracted from herbs using steam distillation. Steam distillation removes the oil-based chemicals from the plant. Oils are stored in specialized vesicles in leaves, stems, bark, roots, and flowers (varies per plant). Called **essential oils**, these herb extractions are extremely potent and generally dosed a few drops at a time. Because concentrated essential oils have higher potential for toxicity to mucous membranes, they are most commonly administered by aromatherapy, though certain essential oils can be diluted and used topically or internally in capsules. (See the end of **Appendix A** for more information about essential oils.)

Some herbs are most commonly found as water/alcohol extractions, and some are most commonly found as essential oils. A few can be found both ways. Though the oil extractions and water/alcohol extractions from the same herb are different sets of chemicals, the benefits are often similar (both lavender essential oil and lavender herb are calming).

The most modern way to prepare herbs is by CO_2 extraction. Supercritical CO_2 extraction utilizes carbon dioxide held at liquid state by temperature and pressure as a solvent. Both oil and water solvent components of the herb are extracted at once. The biggest disadvantage of supercritical extracts is high cost and a final product that can be harsh on tissues. It is the most popular method of preparing medicinal cannabis.

Liposomal preparations of herbs are made by blending herbal powder with some type of fat such that the herb particles become surrounded by a layer of fat. This is purported to enhance absorption of the herb. While there are studies showing increased absorption with single-agent drugs, liposomal herbal preparations have not been well studied. Most liposomal herbal preparations are overpriced and often underdosed. There is no evidence that having an herbal product made this way justifies the extra expense of creating the product. Besides...all you really have to do to achieve this effect is take your herb capsules with coconut milk. The stomach will blend the herbs and coconut fat into liposomes.

EVIDENCE FOR HERBAL THERAPY

If the only information available about using herbs was from history of traditional use, there would still be enough information to safely use and gain benefit from herbal therapy. Thousands of years of observation and recorded use have great value.

But historical information is far from being the limit; science has been applied to the study of herbal medicine much more intensely than most people realize. Over the past 50 years, hundreds of independent scientific studies have been done on commonly used herbs. Studies include laboratory studies, animal studies, and a surprising number of human clinical trials.

Human clinical trials are the studies most accepted by medical science. Clinical trials evaluate how a group of people with an illness respond to a particular type of therapy. This type of study is great for evaluating drugs, which act rapidly and specifically, but less so for evaluating herbs. Herbs induce healing, do not treat symptoms directly, and take time to work. Therefore, short-term clinical trials targeting a specific effect often do not reveal the full benefit of an herb. Though many herbs have shown benefit under this type of scrutiny, it is still not the best method for evaluating herbal therapy.

Clinical trials are far from being the only type of scientific study. Modern science has the ability to study the biological activity of individual phytochemicals, such as reducing inflammation or affecting inflammatory messengers. In addition, the effects that standardized herb preparations have on different systems of the body, such as the immune system, can be studied in animal and human models. When it comes to studying herbs, this is the most valuable type of science.

To sum up, science supports most traditional uses of herbal therapy. It also strongly supports the notion that herbs are profoundly safe and well tolerated by the human body.

ANTIMICROBIAL HERBS AND LYME DISEASE

When choosing herbs for antimicrobial properties, both history and science are important. Even before humans readily understood and accepted germ therapy (that certain illnesses are caused by microbes), herbs were often effectively used for illnesses that were caused by microbes. Once a microbe causing an illness is identified, it can be assumed that the herb historically used to treat that illness has activity against that microbe.

The antimicrobial value of herbs can also be evaluated by test-tube studies (in vitro) and in living models (in vivo). In test-tube studies, an herb is placed in a tube or on a plate growing a particular microbe. If the microbe dies, it is assumed the herb has activity against it. In a living model, some type of laboratory animal is infected with a microbe. Observation is then made about how the animal responds to treatment (with an herb or a drug). In vivo studies are much more valuable than in vitro studies[2] because intestinal absorption of the herbal components and activity in a living model is considered.

---

2 The best recent example of misinterpretations caused by in vitro studies has to do with stevia. An in vitro study showed that when the natural sugar alternative, stevia, was placed in a petri dish with live Borrelia, the stevia inhibited growth of the microbe. The reasoning is flawed, however, because the compounds found in stevia are not absorbed through the intestines; that's why it works as a no caloric sweetener. If the stevia compounds are not absorbed into the bloodstream, they can have no activity against Borrelia in the body.

Accumulating specific information about herbs through scientific methods, however, is tedious and slow. It comes in bits and pieces and is sometimes limited in scope. Using clinical science to answer the specific question of whether herbal medicine is effective for Lyme disease could take decades, if it happens at all.

Interestingly, some of the most valuable evidence supporting herbal therapy, especially for antimicrobial purposes, doesn't come directly from the scientific community. It comes from experiences of people using herbs reported on the Internet.

The Internet provides a way for people to share experiences, both positive and negative. And people do readily and willingly share experiences. Billions of people worldwide use herbs, and millions of them have posted their experiences online. That information becomes public domain. If a topic is one that many people care about or are struggling with, the magnitude of experiences reflected on the Internet can be profound.

Before the Internet, answering the question of whether herbs were effective for Lyme disease would have been nearly impossible. But over the past 20 years, many people have used herbal therapy for Lyme disease. And many of those people have posted their experiences on the Internet. In fact, there are thousands of online reports suggesting positive benefit of herbal therapy for Lyme disease.

The consensus of prevailing information is not only powerful enough to **strongly support the possible effectiveness of herbal therapy for chronic Lyme disease**, but also the **low potential for toxicity as compared to other options**. As such, this information is becoming common knowledge. Common knowledge is information held to be true by a majority of people.

One particular selection of herbs, called the Buhner protocol, has recently gotten a lot of attention. The Buhner protocol was introduced in

2005 by an herbalist named Stephen Buhner. The herbs used in the protocol were very well researched by Buhner, and thousands of people, by way of the Internet, have reported significant benefit from following the protocol. Though no formal studies have been done on the protocol, it is becoming common knowledge that the Buhner protocol is safe and effective for overcoming Lyme disease.

Though there are many herbs that likely have value for Lyme disease, the Buhner protocol has become a standard to follow. The herbal protocol that I have used in my clinical practice for the past 10 years is based on the Buhner protocol. My experience with these same herbs suggests they are safe and effective for chronic Lyme.

Again, these are not the only herbs that work for chronic Lyme. The Buhner protocol can be replaced with other herbs that would be just as effective, but there is value in standardization. **Right now, the Buhner protocol is the best standard to follow.**

BEYOND HERBS — NATURAL BIOIDENTICALS
Herbs are not the only substances used for natural supplements. Vitamins, vitamin-life substances, organic mineral compounds, amino acids, and a host of other active chemicals in the body are commonly found in natural supplement products. Because these substances are the same (or nearly the same) as biochemical substances in the body, they can be classified as **bioidenticals**. Medicinally, they are used to replace or enhance normal levels of the same compound in the human body. This can have a therapeutic effect.

Bioidenticals can be subdivided into essential and nonessential substances. Essential refers to substances that must be obtained from dietary sources to support human life. This brief list includes vitamins, minerals, essential fatty acids, and nine essential amino acids. With aging and disease, however, certain nonessentials can become essential. Coenzyme Q-10 and the antioxidant, glutathione, are readily synthesized by the body, but synthesis declines with age; replacement in certain individuals can be life enhancing. Certain bioidenticals, such as insulin for diabetics and thyroid hormone, are controlled by prescription.

Because the body is so complex, using bioidenticals for therapy is extremely tricky — much more so than herbs (which are inherently safe). Bioidenticals have been around for less than a hundred years and have been studied less than any other medicinal approach. The safety of many bioidenticals has not been well defined. Only a handful have been defined as safe and effective for use.

14

Core Herbal Protocol

Herbal therapy can be thought of as an orchestra of healing. In a symphony, no single instrument matters; rather, it's the entire orchestra playing in perfect harmony that makes beautiful music and creates a larger-than-life experience. The sound produced by each instrument is replaced by a unique sound created by the sum of all the instruments.

Similarly, in herbal medicine, **the sum of all the herbs is more powerful than each herb individually** (a concept called **synergy**).[1] This is especially true of medicinal herbs that each contain a broad spectrum of antimicrobials, antivirals, and antioxidants. When different herbs are taken together, suppression of a variety of microbes hidden in your system is enhanced, and the healing systems of your body are stimulated.

Finding herbs with antimicrobial activity that might be valuable for Lyme disease is not difficult; virtually all plants display at least some antimicrobial activity — with some providing stronger antimicrobial properties than others. Typically, cultivated food plants[2] have the least antimicro-

---

1 Using multiple herbs to gain synergy is practical because the inherent toxicity of herbs is so low. When multiple drugs are used together, it's often the toxicity of the drugs that synergizes and becomes amplified, instead of the benefits.

2 The trade-off in cultivating plants to primarily produce food is that the foods lose natural protective qualities, such as antimicrobial properties. This is why food plants require the application of pesticides. Medicinal herbs have been cultivated for medicinal properties and have retained the natural antimicrobial properties inherent to the plant.

erties, and medicinal herbs have the most. Certain herbs, of course, will have more potent antimicrobial properties than others.

Standardization is important. Therefore, the herbal selection for my protocol is based on the protocol for Lyme disease introduced by Stephen Buhner in *Healing Lyme* (2005). Over the course of 10 plus years since it has been in print, thousands of people have reported benefit from following Buhner's basic core protocol. **I used it personally and began recommending it in my medical practice, all with extraordinary responses.**

Over the years, as my knowledge has grown, I expanded the core protocol to provide coverage against other stealth microbes and provide other medicinal benefits. In late 2015, Stephen Buhner made similar additions in the new edition of *Healing Lyme*, released in late 2015.

Because fibromyalgia, chronic fatigue syndrome, autoimmune diseases, and many other chronic illnesses likely have roots in **chronic immune dysfunction** and chronic infections with stealth microbes, I suspected the protocol might work well for these illnesses also. As expected, many such patients have achieved great benefit from following the protocol. Because the protocol addresses most all of the factors associated with chronic illness, its use is not dependent on having a formal diagnosis. People with chronic Lyme symptoms, but without a formal diagnosis of Lyme disease, have achieved benefit.

In 2014, I had the ingredients for my protocol combined into four multi-ingredient supplements using high-grade standardized powdered extracts. One downside of the Buhner protocol is that the herbs have to be sourced from multiple places. **I wanted to make herbal supplements easy to obtain and easy to take.** My protocol specifies taking three capsules of each of the four formulas twice daily (though taking lower or higher doses more than twice a day is certainly allowed).

The protocol is supported by daily emails providing guidance on how to take the supplements, along with encouragement and education about diet and other supportive practices. The daily email series lasts for 6 months. Surveys occur at monthly intervals to track participant progress.

So far, the surveys indicate 75% of people report some improvement and 50% report significant improvement. Most everyone has been very satisfied with the program (see **Resources**).

I strongly agree with Stephen Buhner that there is no "one size fits all" for chronic Lyme disease. Every person is a unique individual, and Lyme disease (or fibromyalgia or chronic fatigue or any other chronic illness) is different in every person. **This protocol is a starting point, not an ending point.**

I hope those who use this protocol or similar protocols will go on to try other herbs and embrace the power of herbal therapy. We live in a world where high-quality herbal products are more available than ever before in the history of mankind. Once you understand what to look for, it's relatively easy to find good herbal products. **Appendix A provides an extensive list of other herbs, bioidenticals, and essential oils that have value for chronic Lyme disease and general health.**

When adding a new herb, it's nice to know the science and history behind the herb, but sometimes the best way to find out whether it works for you is simply by trying it. While you would never do this with a drug because of the potential for toxicity, it's quite reasonable with most herbs.

PRIMARY SUPPLEMENTS

The natural supplements listed in this chapter should be considered essential for supporting the healing processes in the body. **These supplements provide properties that restore energy to the body, reduce**

inflammation, restore normal immune function, and suppress stealth microbes.

Optimal benefit comes from taking all of the supplements listed. If you are unable to take all of them, at least take the first supplement listed in each category. Natural supplements listed in other chapters should be considered secondary; they are important and add benefit, but should not be considered absolutely essential.

Optimal doses of herbal supplements are highly variable from person to person and very dependent on the preparation used. Quite frankly, herbal dosing, as posted on all supplement bottles, is quite arbitrary. It's an estimate of what most herbalists would recommend and what tradition might suggest as an average dose. It's far from absolute; different people will require different dosages to gain benefit. Because most herbs have such low potential for toxicity, the safe dose range is quite broad (as compared to drugs, which have a very narrow dose range because of inherent toxicity).

In general, people who have not been sick very long will not need high doses of herbs; whereas, people who have been very sick for a very long time may need very high doses of herbs for a very long time. That being said, some people who are very sick or are very sensitive to taking anything will need to start with extremely low doses of herbs and gradually increase the doses over time.

The general rule of thumb is start with a low dose and work up to a dose that feels comfortable.

Herbs are traditionally dosed three to four times a day, but this is also arbitrary. Many people have a hard time dosing more than twice a day (me included). Personal experience and experience working with hundreds of people suggest that twice-daily dosing is adequate (though there's nothing wrong with spreading the dose out to three or four times a day).

The doses stated in this chapter are very general recommendations. Doses are quoted for standardized powdered extracts. The amount of herb to take is very dependent on the type of extract used. Less quantity will be needed for a higher-grade extract. If water/alcohol tinctures are chosen instead, dosages range from 15 drops to a full teaspoon several times daily. If you decide to take powdered whole herb, much higher doses will be required. Start slow and work up to a dose that feels comfortable.

Many people with Lyme disease and fibromyalgia have severe gut dysfunction with tender stomachs and sensitive intestinal tracts. In these cases, gut restoration may need to precede taking full doses of herbal supplements (see **Chapters 24** and **25**).

The herbs are separated into categories, but the categories are not absolute. **All herbs have antimicrobial properties. All herbs reduce inflammation and positively affect immune function. All herbs have some adaptogenic properties.** It's the nature of herbs. Some herbs are known for certain properties over others, however. As such, those herbs will be placed in categories to help better organize things.

Herbs have very low potential for toxicity, but allergic reactions and side effects are possible with any herb. Go slow when you first start taking herbs and observe for effects, both positive or negative. Many herbs have antiplatelet properties (blood thinning).

If you are taking blood thinners or have a history of coagulation problems, contact your healthcare provider before taking the herb. Herbs with immunomodulating properties should be avoided by individuals who are taking immunosuppressive drugs or who have had an organ transplant. Discontinue herbal therapy several days to a week before having major surgery.

Use caution with herbal therapy if you are pregnant. Though most herbs pose less risk to pregnancy than most drugs, herbs should be used in pregnancy only if the potential for benefit outweighs potential risks.

HERBAL ANTIMICROBIALS

All herbs express antimicrobial properties, but certain herbs have been defined as being specifically antimicrobial. Herbal antimicrobials are not as potent as prescription antibiotics, but they do offer some distinct advantages in treatment of low-virulence stealth pathogens. Herbs with antimicrobial properties enhance immune function and reduce inflammation. Microbial resistance is less of a problem with herbs than antibiotics.

Herbs provide broad-spectrum antimicrobial properties. Combining different herbs enhances coverage. Specific herbs do not necessarily need to be used for specific microbes. In general, the herbs recommended in this protocol provide benefit for any illness associated with chronic immune dysfunction and stealth microbes.

Because the toxicity of herbs is so low, they can be taken at high concentrations for extended periods of time without concern. In other words, herbs wear the microbes down, instead of killing them aggressively. **For low-virulence stealth microbes, this is the most effective approach.**

Resveratrol from Japanese Knotweed (*Polygonum cuspidatum*). Truly a wonder substance, Japanese knotweed (JKW) offers exceptional antimicrobial activity. JKW is active against a wide range of stealth microbes. It is a primary herbal antimicrobial for both Lyme disease and Mycoplasma treatment. JKW also offers antiviral, anti-Candida (yeast), and antifungal properties. It has been found to disrupt bacterial biofilms.

JKW is a systemic antimicrobial that crosses the blood-brain barrier, and it is protective of the central nervous system. It's also anti-inflammatory and supports immune function.

This is a very important general antimicrobial for Lyme, Mycoplasma, fibromyalgia, and viral infections. JKW provides coverage against Bartonella, Mycoplasma, Candida, and viruses as well.

Suggested dosage: 200-800 mg Japanese knotweed (standardized to 50% trans-resveratrol) two to three times daily.

Side effects: rare with low potential for toxicity. Caution is advised if also taking anticoagulants because resveratrol has blood-thinning properties. Avoid in pregnancy.

Andrographis (*Andrographis paniculata*). Native to India, andrographis offers antiviral, antibacterial, and antiparasitic properties. It is widely used in the treatment of Lyme disease. Beyond Lyme disease, numerous clinical trials have demonstrated the ability of andrographis to reduce the length and severity of common viral illnesses. It has shown activity against viral hepatitis B and C and Chlamydia. Andrographis has been used for dysentery and shows activity against pathogenic strains of *E. coli*. It is active against common roundworms and tapeworms. In a 2011 study, andrographis was found to be beneficial for ulcerative colitis (as compared to drug, mesalazine). Additional benefits include immune enhancement and cardioprotective effects. Andrographis also offers significant liver protection. In vivo and in vitro studies confirm that Andrographis enhances natural killer cells (NK cells) and cell-mediated immunity, while reducing proinflammatory cytokines.

Excellent antiviral and antibacterial properties, important for treating Lyme disease, and important for gastrointestinal restoration. Provides coverage against viral relapse.

Suggested dosage: 200-800 mg, extract standardized to 10-30% andrographolides two to three times daily.

Side effects: About 1% of people who take andrographis develop an allergic reaction with whole-body hives and itching skin (higher percentage than most herbs). The reaction will resolve gradually over several weeks after stopping use of the herb.

Cat's claw (*Uncaria tomentosa*). Native to the Amazon, cat's claw has a long history of traditional use for treatment of a wide range of inflammatory conditions. It also has been adopted by the Lyme community as a primary herb for use in treating Lyme disease. Cat's claw is considered an immunomodulator, meaning it calms an overactive immune system (reducing inflammation), but at the same time, enhances how well the immune system works. Benefits include potent anti-inflammatory properties and historical use for treatment of arthritis. It is known to increase WBCs, including B and T lymphocytes, natural killer (NK) cells, and granulocytes. Cat's claw is also known to enhance a specific type of natural killer cell, called CD 57, which is deficient in Lyme disease. Cat's claw has also demonstrated healing properties for the GI tract (beneficial for healing leaky gut).

Primary herb for Lyme disease and gastrointestinal restoration. Cat's claw is antiprotozoal and may provide coverage against Babesia.

Suggested dosage: 400-800 mg (inner bark standardized to 3% alkaloids or 10:1 concentrate inner bark is preferred) two to three times daily. It is especially important to take this herb with food, as it is activated by stomach acid. If you take acid-blocking drugs, cat's claw will have limited value.

Side effects: occasional stomach upset, but generally very well tolerated.

If you search for cat's claw, sooner or later you will come across information suggesting that "TOA-free" cat's claw is superior to standard cat's claw. **There is no independent research supporting this claim.** All independent experts support use of standard cat's claw as the best option for herbal medicine.

Chinese skullcap (*Scutellaria baicalensis*). Chinese skullcap is a potent synergist (increases benefit of other supplements), a property that is very important when choosing a supplement regimen. In other words, it enhances the value of other herbs, especially those with antimicrobial value. It is, by itself, strongly antiviral (especially against herpes viruses). It also offers antibacterial and antifungal properties. It is one of the primary supplements for use against Mycoplasma and Bartonella. Chinese skullcap is also known for its sedative properties. It contains melatonin, helpful for inducing sleep. It is also strongly protective of nerve tissue and liver function. It is an immunomodulator, which means it calms overactive immune function (reduces cytokine cascades), but improves overall immune function. Some experts consider it useful for autoimmune disease.

Important synergist for Mycoplasma and antiviral protection. Also, provides coverage against Chlamydia.

Suggested dosage: 400-1000 mg two to three times daily. Root extract, preferably 3-year old plant with pronounced yellow color, standardized to >30% baicalin is preferred. (American skullcap does not offer the same antimicrobial properties and should not be substituted.)

Side effects: rare, even at high doses, and are mostly gastrointestinal.

Garlic with stabilized allicin (*Allium sativum*). Garlic has been used as a medicinal since the beginning of recorded time, but the active chemicals in garlic, called allicin, are very volatile. The smell of crushed garlic is allicin; it dissipates as soon as the garlic is crushed, cooked, or consumed. Less than 1% is actually absorbed in active form. Therefore, benefit from standard garlic preparations is highly variable and often minimal.

Through a proprietary process, it is possible to stabilize allicin to increase yield to nearly 100%. Stabilized allicin is now available from several companies. Stabilized garlic has been shown to have potent broad-spectrum activity against gram-positive and gram-negative bacteria and has antiviral, antifungal, and antiparasitic properties. Lyme disease patients have noted significant benefit. Studies have shown allicin to be active against multiple species of Babesia.

It is highly beneficial for chronic fungal infections and Candida (yeast) and has shown activity against MRSA infections. Stabilized garlic also provides remarkable cardiovascular benefits. It lowers cholesterol, inhibits platelet aggregation (stickiness), improves blood flow, reduces blood pressure, and has direct cardiogenic effects.

Excellent general antimicrobial and for gastrointestinal restoration. Provides antiprotozoal (Babesia) and anti-Candida coverage.

Suggested dosage: 180-1200 mg two stabilized allicin product to three times daily (dosage is dependent on garlic preparation used).

Side effects: well tolerated. Raw garlic can cause stomach upset, but stabilized allicin products are associated with few side effects.

Sarsaparilla (*Smilax glabra, medica*). Sarsaparilla is native to South America, but Smilax species with medicinal benefit are common around the world. Sarsaparilla is thought to bind endotoxins. Endotoxins are the debris created when pathogenic bacteria are killed off.

Sarsaparilla also offers antibacterial and antifungal properties. It is commonly used in Lyme disease protocols. Traditionally, it is used for treatment of psoriasis and other skin conditions. Also, sarsaparilla has been used traditionally for treatment of syphilis (another spirochete, like Borrelia). Sarsaparilla increases bioavailability of other herbs and enhances benefit (synergist). Other beneficial properties include potent anti-inflammatory and antioxidant properties. It also enhances immune function.

Synergist for Lyme protocols and important for restoration of gastrointestinal function.

Suggested dosage: 200-1000 mg of standardized root extract two to three times daily.

Side effects: Uncommon. Sarsaparilla is generally well tolerated.

ADAPTOGENS FOR IMMUNE MODULATION

Adaptogens are substances that increase the body's resistance to stress. Adaptogens balance hormonal systems in the body and normalize adrenal function that has been disrupted by stress. They reduce fatigue, restore normal immune function, balance central hormone pathways, and enhance the healing capacity of the body.

Adaptogens are immunomodulators — they calm overactive cytokine cascades and restore effective immune function. Technically, they reduce IL-10 and downregulate Th2, thus shifting from Th2 dominant back to a balanced Th1/Th2 immune response. By normalizing the immune response, they allow the immune system to properly deal with microbes and heal damage done by inflammation. At the same time, these herbs boost natural killer cells (NK cells), which are an important part of immune defense against intracellular microbes. They also provide direct antimicrobial activity. Adaptogens are considered useful for calming an autoimmune response.

Cordyceps (*Cordyceps sinensis*). Native to Tibet, Cordyceps is a fungal species that grows on a specific type of caterpillar during specific times of the year. Historically, its value was equal in weight to gold, and it was specifically reserved for emperors and royalty. Today, fortunately, high-quality Cordyceps can be easily cultivated, and its wonderful benefits are available to anyone.

Cordyceps offers properties of immunomodulation and resistance to any type of stress. It protects mitochondria and is anti-fatigue. It is regularly used by Chinese and Russian athletes. In laboratory studies, Cordyceps was found to reduce heart muscle oxygen consumption and improve aerobic activity. In traditional herbal medicine, it is often used as a kidney tonic. Cordyceps specifically stimulates NK cells and macrophage activity and also enhances cellular immunity. At the same time, it decreases inflammatory cytokine cascades and therefore decreases tissue damage.

Cordyceps also offers antiviral and antibacterial properties. Provides coverage against Bartonella and Mycoplasma.

Suggested dosage: 1-3 grams (1000-3000 mg) whole mushroom Cordyceps powder or 400-800 mg extract (standardized to >7% Cordyceptic acid is preferred) two to three times daily.

Side effects: Mild nausea can occur, but in general, side effects are rare, even with higher doses. Allergic reactions are rare.

Reishi (*Ganoderma lucidum*). Reishi, a mushroom with exceptional immunomodulating and antiviral properties, is a potent adaptogen. Extensively studied in Japan for potential anti-cancer properties, Reishi mushrooms have been found to contain numerous potential cancer-fighting substances. It offers important immune-modulation properties. Reishi reduces inflammatory cytokines and at the same time improves the response against threatening microbes and mutated cancer cells. It is considered useful for calming autoimmune responses. It is calming and improves sleep. Anti-fatigue properties are related to restoration of normal adrenal-cortical function. It offers significant cardiovascular benefit and has been used to alleviate altitude sickness, suggesting that it may also increase oxygenation of tissues (a good thing because many intracellular pathogens thrive in a low-oxygen environment). Reishi is liver and heart protective.

Excellent antiviral and immunomodulator.

Suggested dosage: 1-2 grams (1000-2000 mg) whole mushroom powder or 150-500 mg standardized extract (minimum 20% beta glucans preferred) two to three times daily.

Side effects: Extremely well tolerated with rare side effects and no known toxicity.

Eleuthero (*Eleutherococcus senticosus*). Also known as "Siberian ginseng," eleuthero has been used for thousands of years to fight illnesses associated with microbial infections and increase quality of life. It is immune amphoteric. Offering similar properties to Rhodiola (discussed in Appendix A), the two can be used together or interchangeably; eleuthero, however, may have more potent antiviral and antibacterial properties. Adaptogenic, eleuthero improves stress resistance in all systems of the body. It restores normal adrenal function and normalizes immune function in the face of stress. It is protective against radiation and is liver protective.

Adaptogen with antibacterial and antiviral properties.

Suggested dosage: Herb extract 50-200 mg twice daily (1:1 tincture, Russian extraction, from the root, 15 drops to 1 tsp twice daily can also be used, but it is very stimulating).

Side effects: The primary limiting factor of eleuthero is stimulation. Though it is a wonderful herb, most people with fibromyalgia can only take small amounts of it, if they can take it at all. Otherwise, the herb is well tolerated and has low toxicity.

SUPPORTIVE SUPPLEMENTS

Supportive supplements primarily protect the body from stress factors that contribute to illness. Herbal and other natural supplements can be used to support cellular functions, protect mitochondria, and reduce inflammation (both generally and at specific sites, such as joints, heart and blood vessels, and nerve tissue). This type of support encourages healing and accelerates recovery.

Bioidenticals for Protecting Mitochondria and Cellular Functions
Restoring energy and reducing fatigue is one of the most pressing concerns in chronic Lyme disease and fibromyalgia. Top of the list for restoring energy is protecting mitochondrial function, DNA, and cellular structures against free radicals, toxins, inflammatory processes, and pathogenic microbes. The following list of bioidenticals are supported by scientific evidence showing benefit.

Bioidentical vitamins and minerals. Vitamin supplements are not a substitute for a healthful diet that is rich in vegetables, but supplements can ensure adequate levels of essential nutrients. Vitamins should be presented to the body in natural forms that are readily absorbed and assimilated. The same goes for minerals, which should be present in natural organic forms, not as the inorganic forms found in most multivitamin supplements. B vitamins, including 5-methyltetrahydrofolate, pyridoxal-5-phosphate (B6), and methylcobalamin (B12) are especially important for individuals who have methylation mutations (see Chapter 9, Laboratory Evaluations).

Glutathione. Glutathione is a tripeptide composed of three amino acids, glutamic acid, cysteine, and glycine. It is an essential antioxidant inside cells for protecting mitochondria from free-radical damage during generation of energy. Glutathione is also essential for phase II detoxification in the liver. In vitro and in vivo studies have demonstrated enhancement of detoxification processes, antioxidant properties, and fortification of immune functions. Glutathione increases T-lymphocytes in animal studies. Intestinal absorption occurs by the molecule being broken down into component parts, but also by absorption of the whole molecule. Studies documenting intestinal absorption have been done with the Setria brand of reduced glutathione.

Suggested dosage: 500-1000 mg twice daily of reduced glutathione.

Side effects: Rare.

At one point during my struggle with Lyme disease, I developed a pronounced head and hand tremor. It resolved completely within 2 weeks after starting 1000 mg of the Setria brand of glutathione twice daily. The same effect did not occur with liposomal glutathione.

NAC (n-acetyl cysteine). Another potent antioxidant, NAC is an essential component for formation of glutathione inside cells. It inhibits cytokine cascades (inflammatory messengers stimulated by microbes) It also inhibits the breakdown of collagen. NAC concentrates in lungs and offers antioxidant effects as well as mucolytic properties (breaks down mucus). It also has a reputation for inhibiting biofilms. It is strongly protective of nerve tissue. NAC also protects liver function. Combining therapeutic doses of lipoic acid, vitamin C, and NAC will raise glutathione levels inside cells better than supplementing with glutathione.

Suggested dosage: 500-2000 mg twice daily.

Side effects: Rare.

Alpha lipoic acid. Alpha lipoic acid is a potent antioxidant having the unique property of being both water and fat soluble. This enables it to be easily concentrated in blood, cells, tissues, and extracellular fluids (space and fluid between cells). It is easily absorbed and works with antioxidants already present inside cells to reduce cellular damage from free radicals. It also regenerates glutathione, the cell's most important antioxidant. Alpha lipoic acid enhances antioxidant effects of vitamin C, vitamin E, and NAC. It is protective of liver function and helps remove toxins from the body. It is also protective of nerve tissue and has been shown to reverse diabetic nerve damage. It enhances oxygenation of tissues and immune function. It protects tissues against elevated glucose.

Suggested dosage: 50-300 mg twice daily.

Side effects: Some people experience reflux with alpha lipoic acid and do not feel well when taking high doses.

Vitamin C. Vitamin C aids in too many functions in the body to list, but possibly the most important are function is providing antioxidant properties. When combined with other antioxidants, vitamin C offers a high degree of protection of tissues. Vitamin C is essential for collagen formation and very important for chronic disease recovery. Vitamin C is concentrated in WBCs. It offers antibacterial and antiviral properties. Vitamin C is inexpensive and should be considered a "must take" supplement.

Suggested dosage: 500-1000 mg twice daily during recovery. Lower doses are indicated after wellness is restored. Ascorbate (Ester C) is easier on the stomach.

Side effects: Occasional gastric upset and loose stools at higher doses. If side effects occur, reduce the dose.

Coenzyme Q10 (CoQ10). CoQ10 is an essential component of cellular energy production. CoQ10 is a key component of the machinery responsible for producing energy within mitochondria. Supplemental CoQ10 is another way to keep mitochondria humming, especially in organs requiring high energy, such as the heart. CoQ10 is a potent antioxidant that protects mitochondria; it also inhibits free-radical damage to cell and mitochondrial membrane. The highest normal concentrations of CoQ10 in the body are found in the heart, liver, kidneys and pancreas. CoQ10 is especially protective of heart muscle.

Suggested dosage: 20-100 mg twice daily.

Side effects: Rare.

Vitamin D. The "sunshine vitamin" is important for more than just healthy bones. Vitamin D is essential for too many functions in the body to mention, and **it is essential for normal immune function**. Vitamin D is created in the skin with exposure to UV rays of sunlight. Because most people have low sun exposure (or use sunscreen, which blocks vitamin D production), low vitamin D levels are common.

Full sun exposure, best between 10 am and 2 pm, 30 minutes to an hour every day to the arms, chest, and face without sunscreen is generally adequate to maintain vitamin D levels. Aging and chronic disease also seem to adversely affect the ability of the body to generate vitamin D from sunlight. Though the best source of vitamin D is sunlight, supplementation is often necessary.

During the winter months especially, supplements are the only way to maintain adequate levels. People living in southern locations generally need 1000-2000 IU daily, whereas northern locations often require 4000 IU or greater. Dark-skinned people also often require larger amounts of vitamin D. Vitamin D_3 is the preferred form of supplementation. The best way to know if vitamin D levels are adequate is by having blood levels checked regularly—about every 6 months is ideal. Target a level of > 40 ng/ml.

GENERAL HEALTH AND BLOOD FLOW

Good blood flow is essential for healing to occur. Blood delivers oxygen and vital nutrients. Blood also removes toxic byproducts generated during exercise and debris created by friction-damaged tissues or injury. Blood flow, however, is often constricted by the inflammation that occurs with chronic disease, a toxic and vicious cycle. Chronic pain is the inevitable result. The supplements in this category reduce vascular inflammation and promote optimal blood flow.

Resveratrol from Japanese Knotweed (JKW) (*Polygonum cuspidatum*). JKW is a "double duty" supplement that offers many profound benefits beyond antimicrobial properties. It is a particularly good source of resveratrol, the age-defying substance found in grapes and wine that everybody is talking about. But unlike grapes, **JKW provides *trans*-resveratrol, the form most readily utilized by the body**.

Resveratrol offers a list of benefits including potent antioxidant properties and support of normal heart function. It dilates blood vessels, improves blood flow, inhibits platelet aggregation (thins blood), and mildly lowers LDL cholesterol. Resveratrol is also protective of nerve tissue.

Beyond trans-resveratrol, the whole herb offers a spectrum of chemical substances that have medicinal value. Resveratrol and the whole herb support normal immune function and offer anti-inflammatory and anticancer properties. JKW has been used in traditional forms of Asian medicine for centuries and offers a high level of safety.

Suggested dosage: The commonly recommended dose of resveratrol for vascular benefit is 50-100 mg daily. The traditional dose of JKW and the dose of whole herb to achieve antimicrobial benefit is higher. Dosing is dependent on whether whole herb or standardized extract is used.

Side effects: Rare. Low potential for toxicity.

French Maritime Pine Bark (FMPB). Potent antioxidants and other chemical compounds in FMPB inhibit platelet aggregation (blood thinner), reduce vascular inflammation, and improve the integrity of blood vessels. This improves blood flow to tissues — optimal blood flow is essential for recovering from any chronic illness. Potent anti-inflammatory properties also extend to offer protection for joints and ligaments. FMPB is also beneficial for the immune system. Pycnogenol is the most studied brand of FMPB, but any brand provides the same properties.

Suggested dosage: 50-100 mg daily.

Side effects: Rare. Low potential for toxicity.

Hawthorn (*Crataegus oxyacantha, pinnatifida*). Hawthorn would be best described as a heart tonic. A "tonic" is a substance that has an overall positive effect on a particular organ system. For the heart, hawthorn meets the criteria. Hawthorn increases blood flow to the heart, strengthens contractions of the heart muscle, and improves circulation by dilating blood vessels. This allows increased oxygen delivery to tissues (very important for CF/FMS). It also reduces palpitations and provides a calming effect that reduces adrenaline. It also normalizes blood pressure. Hawthorn lowers LDL cholesterol and has hypoglycemic activity in Type II diabetics.

Suggested dosage: 200-500 mg extract (combined leaf, stem, and flower standardized to 1.8% Vitexin) twice daily.

Side effects: Rare. Hawthorn is very safe for long-term use.

Milk Thistle (*Silybum marianum*). Beyond healthful food, many natural herbal supplements offer liver protection. One of the best is a thistle plant native to southern Europe and North Africa called milk thistle. Milk thistle has been used in its native lands for thousands of years for treatment of jaundice and other liver conditions. Silymarin, the primary active component of milk thistle, offers potent antioxidant protection for liver cells. It also increases natural antioxidants found in liver cells and has been found to induce regeneration of liver cells. It is the most widely researched of all hepatoprotective (liver-protective) herbs and is well known for low toxicity and high safety.

Dosage: 200 mg extract standardized to 80% silymarin twice daily (1200 mg daily if liver enzymes are elevated).

Side effects: Milk thistle is extremely well tolerated. Negative reactions are rare.

Essential Fatty Acids (Omega-3 fatty acids). Omega-3 fatty acids are types of fat that must be obtained from dietary sources. Omega 3s are important for decreasing inflammation in the body and supporting optimum cell membrane function. They also prevent oxidation of cholesterol and platelet aggregation, important factors for maintaining optimal blood flow. Fish, seafood, and vegetables are good sources of omega-3 fatty acids, but taking supplements ensures adequate blood levels of omega 3s. The most beneficial omega-3 fatty acids, EPA (Eicosapentaenoic Acid) and DHA (Docosahexaenoic Acid), come exclusively from marine sources. Both fish oil and krill oil are good sources of DHA and EPA. Krill oil contains astaxanthin, a potent antioxidant. While flax oil does provide health benefits, it takes very large amounts of flax oil to raise omega 3 blood levels.

Dosage: Molecularly distilled fish oil, 1-4 grams (1000-4000 mg) daily, or krill oil, 500-3000 mg daily. Krill oil occurs as a phospholipid (instead of a triglyceride like fish oil), which is easily absorbed through the intestines and more easily utilized by the body. Therefore, lower doses are required.

Side effects: Omega-3 fatty acids thin blood. If you are taking blood thinners or have a bleeding or clotting disorder, discuss taking fish or krill oil supplements with your doctor. Avoid krill or fish oil supplements if you have shellfish or fish allergies.

INTESTINAL PARASITES

If you live in a developed country, the chances of you harboring major infestations of intestinal worms are low, but if you just can't get that worry out of your mind, there are specific herbs to consider. **The best herbs for intestinal parasites are artemisia (wormwood), clove, and black walnut.** These are very potent herbs and should never be used continually for more than 1-2 months. Products that combine these three ingredients are readily available.

CHRONIC YEAST

Most everyone on the planet harbors *Candida*, a common yeast, in his or her intestinal tracts. Chronic illnesses, such as chronic Lyme and fibromyalgia, however, are commonly associated with yeast overgrowth. Typical symptoms include fatigue, bloating, and abdominal discomfort, but separating out symptoms of yeast overgrowth from chronic Lyme disease and intestinal dysfunction symptoms is challenging.

The conventional medical solution to yeast overgrowth is antifungal drugs, most commonly mycostatin (Nystatin) or fluconazole (Diflucan). For chronic yeast, the fluconazole or mycostatin is often prescribed for extended periods of up to 6 months. This has led to a high level of antifungal-resistant strains of yeast. Long-term use of antifungal drugs can cause liver damage.

Most of the time, yeast overgrowth will gradually resolve with improved dietary habits and improved immune function. Avoidance of all sugars and refined starches is essential for overcoming yeast. Avoiding any products made with yeast, including bread and beer, is also important. All of the primary antimicrobial herbs have good activity against *Candida*. Taking a probiotic containing *Saccharomyces boulardii* (a favorable yeast that suppresses *Candida*) can also be beneficial.

15

Establishing a Supplement Routine

CORE PROTOCOL, ABBREVIATED

Here is a summary of all the ingredients for the primary protocol. Each ingredient has been chosen for the value it might offer. Note that herbal therapy induces healing and healing takes time, so you should be patient. Most people, however, will notice significant benefit from taking herbs within a couple of months and many people have gotten their lives back within as little as six months. The more consistent you are with taking the herbs, the better your results will be.

ANTIMICROBIAL

Resveratrol from Japanese Knotweed (*Polygonum cuspidatum*). Suggested dosage: 200-800 mg Japanese knotweed (standardized to 50% trans-resveratrol) two to three times daily.

Andrographis (*Andrographis paniculata*). Suggested dosage: 200-800 mg, standardized extract two to three times daily.

Cat's claw (*Uncaria tomentosa*). Suggested dosage: 400-800 mg of standardized extract two to three times daily with food.

Chinese skullcap (*Scutellaria baicalensis*). Suggested dosage: 400-1000 mg standardized root extract two to three times daily.

Garlic with stabilized allicin (*Allium sativum*). Suggested dosage: 180-1200 mg two to three times daily (dosage is dependent on garlic preparation used).

Sarsaparilla (*Smilax glabra, medica*). Suggested dosage: 200-1000 mg of root extract two to three times daily.

ADAPTOGENS FOR IMMUNE MODULATION

Cordyceps (*Cordyceps sinensis*). Suggested dosage: 400-800 mg standardized mushroom extract two to three times daily.

Reishi (*Ganoderma lucidum*). Suggested dosage: 150-500 mg standardized mushroom extract two to three times daily.

Eleuthero (*Eleutherococcus senticosus*). Standardized herb extract, 50-200 mg twice daily (Optional depending on whether excessive stimulation occurs.)

PROTECTING MITOCHONDRIA AND CELLULAR FUNCTIONS

Bioidentical vitamins and minerals. Vitamins and minerals should be in activated forms that are readily absorbed and utilized by the body.

Glutathione. Suggested dosage: 500-1000 mg twice daily of reduced glutathione.

HAVE **NAC (n-acetyl cysteine).** Suggested dosage: 500-2000 mg twice daily.

Alpha lipoic acid. Suggested dosage: 50-300 mg twice daily.

√ **Vitamin C.** Suggested dosage: 500-1000 mg twice daily during recovery. Ascorbate (Ester C) is easier on the stomach.

√ **Coenzyme Q10 (CoQ10).** Suggested dosage: 20-100 mg twice daily.

√ **Vitamin D.** Suggested dosage: 1000-2000 IU daily (higher doses may be indicated by low vitamin D levels).

GENERAL HEALTH AND BLOOD FLOW

Resveratrol. 50-100 mg (from Japanese knotweed mentioned above).

French Maritime Pine Bark (FMPB). Suggested dosage: 50-100 mg daily.

Hawthorn (*Crataegus oxyacantha, pinnatifida*). Suggested dosage: 100-250 mg extract twice daily.

Milk Thistle (*Silybum marianum*). Suggested dosage: 200 mg extract standardized to 80% silymarin twice daily.

Essential Fatty Acids (Omega-3 fatty acids). Suggested dosage: molecularly distilled fish oil, 1-4 grams (1000-4000 mg) daily, or Krill oil, 500-3000 mg daily.

TIPS FOR TAKING SUPPLEMENTS
START WITH GOOD PRODUCTS

The supplement routine starts with obtaining quality supplements. The steps from fresh grown herb to bottled product include the herb farmer, an ingredient supplier, and a supplement manufacturer. The ingredient supplier buys the raw herb from the farmer and processes it into tincture, whole herb powder, or standardized powdered extract. The manufacturer then buys finished ingredients from the supplier, blends them into unique herbal combinations, encapsulates the mixture, and bottles the final product.

Though it is not necessarily the industry standard, reliable supplement companies will insist on independent third-party testing of ingredients to ensure quality. Independent testing companies test each batch of herbal extract for proper identification, potency, purity, organic toxins, and heavy metals. This information is provided as a "certificate of analysis" (COA) of ingredients. Ingredients that come with a COA are more expensive, but a reliable supplement producer will insist on it for every ingredient.

Having a valid COA is actually more important than having a label of "certified organic". Unlike food plants, herb farming generally does not require heavy use of fertilizer or pesticides. If grown in a clean environment, most herbs are free of chemical pollutants, even if they are not certified as organic. On the other hand, herbs grown "organically" in areas with poor quality air, such as certain areas of China, may still be loaded with toxins. A COA is the best way to confirm that an herbal ingredient is free of significant levels of organic toxins and heavy metals.

Beyond a COA, quality supplement manufacturers have products independently tested several times during the manufacturing process to be sure that the mix of ingredients is consistent (but again, this is not necessarily the industry standard). A reliable supplement company will post this information on the company website. Some companies go the additional step of tracing ingredients all the way back to the farmer to ensure quality and transparency to the consumer.

On the supplement label, the **common name** and **scientific name** of each ingredient should be stated, along with **standardization** and the **quantity** (generally in mg) of each herbal ingredient. If it's not posted on the bottle (sometimes there isn't room), it should be posted on the website. Avoid "proprietary blends" because the quantity of each individual ingredient is not stated (you really don't know what you are getting). There's a lot of hype out there; buy from a reputable source.

Learning about medicinal benefits of specific herbal products is presently being hindered by the FTC (Federal Trade Commission) and the FDA (Food and Drug Administration). In an overzealous attempt to "protect the consumer" (or some would say, protect the drug companies), combined FTC and FDA regulations prevent natural supplements companies from, in any way, implying that the supplements have any effect on treatment of illness or disease. This strictly limits what companies can say about products. In other words, mentioning arthritis on the same page as an herbal ingredient is considered a "drug claim" and is not allowed. Certain words, such as "anti-inflammatory", "recovery", "regeneration", "overcoming" or even "healing" cannot be used in conjunction with discussions about natural products because it implies treatment of disease.

Making matters worse, the FDA and FTC are not enforcing regulations equally. The most visible, reputable, and reliable companies are being hardest hit, whereas fly-by-night companies selling the worst products and making the most outrageous claims are often escaping scrutiny.

When you evaluate a product on a company's website, sometimes you have to read between the lines and understand that they are restricted in what they can say about the therapeutic benefits their products. Learn about the ingredients from other sources and focus on whether the company is offering a quality product for the money.

GETTING INTO A ROUTINE

Be practical. There are multiple ways of taking natural supplements, but for most people, encapsulated herbal extracts are the most practical. Extracts are concentrated and take up less volume than whole herb powder (so fewer capsules to swallow). Capsules eliminate the bitter taste that comes with tinctures.

Stay organized. By default, you end up with multiple different supplement bottles. A shallow box, such as a shoebox, is a convenient place to keep them. Most supplements do not need to be refrigerated, so keep them out on the counter (where you will see them and not forget them). Take a permanent marker and write the number of capsules to be taken on the top of the bottle. A couple of small cups (about jigger size) can be used to separate doses — one for am and one for pm doses.

Only twice a day? If you read much about herbal therapy, you will often come upon recommendations for dosing herbs three to four times daily. Though it is perfectly acceptable to dose three to four times daily, most people find that taking supplements more than twice daily is a real challenge. Working with many patients over the years, I have found twice-daily dosing to be satisfactory (but you do need to be consistent about taking them at least twice daily).

Start slowly. Herbal supplements are generally very well tolerated, and severe adverse reactions are unlikely, but still possible. Therefore, start with only one capsule of each supplement (some people who are very sensitive will have to open a capsule and take only a small amount of the powder). Slowly build up to a full dosage over several days to several weeks (varies from person to person). Avoid taking supplements on an empty stomach. Most supplements can be taken at the same time (unless otherwise specified).

Help them go down. Take your supplements with a viscous (thick) liquid, such as coconut milk. The coconut fat surrounds the powdered particles, which can help absorption. The fat also helps protect the stomach lining (this is why the British drink cream in their tea). Taking the capsules with a smoothie made with coconut milk is even easier! Eat something right after taking the capsules to make sure all the capsules have gone down.

Enhance the protocol with a smoothie. A smoothie is a great way to get down capsules. A great recipe for a nutrient-dense smoothie includes frozen berries (blueberries, blackberries, dark cherries), half of a frozen banana, half of a small peeled cucumber, stalk celery, ice, avocado or avocado oil, stevia, coconut or almond milk, and prune juice (especially if constipation is an issue). Blend in a blender or smoothie maker. You can further enhance your smoothie with herb powders and other natural ingredients. Options might include chaga mushroom powder, ashwagandha powder, turmeric powder, collagen, protein powder, l-arginine, and d-ribose (see **Appendix A** for more information about these ingredients).

If an adverse reaction of any type occurs, stop taking the supplements. Restart each of the supplements independently, so that you will know which ingredient is causing the problem. Start back slowly.

When you travel... If you have to travel, you should take your supplements with you. Place capsules for your daily doses in separate plastic baggies for each of the days you will be away. If you happen to be taking different doses of capsules for the morning and evening, use a marker to label the baggies "am" or "pm".

Hang in there. Often, people start feeling worse before they start feeling better. This is because supplements either kill microbes directly or restore the ability of the immune system to kill microbes. This will temporarily increase symptoms. In Lyme disease treatment, this phenomenon is referred to as a Herxheimer reaction, but it can occur with any microbial infection. If symptoms worsen, reduce the dose of *all* supplements until symptoms ease, and then gradually increase doses over time.

Patience and persistence pay off. Healing takes time. Most people do not start seeing significant benefit for at least a couple of months and sometimes longer. It's an up-and-down ride, but benefits do accrue over time. You will be better in a year than you are now, and even better still, a year after that. It took me a full 5 years to call myself recovered, but things continued to get better every year after that.

Make supplements part of your lifestyle. Recovery from chronic illness is a lifestyle, and natural supplements are an ongoing part of that lifestyle. Even after you are recovered, natural supplements can be continued to support general health and slow the processes of aging. Rotating different types of herbs is a good practice.

Contraindications are rare for any of the supplements listed, but if you are pregnant, on blood thinners, or have any unusual medical concerns, you should consult a healthcare provider with knowledge of natural supplements before using any supplements.

DEALING WITH ADVERSE REACTIONS

Adverse effects associated with taking herbs and other natural therapies are uncommon, but certainly possible. Fortunately, most adverse effects are mild and transient, and you should be able to work around them.

Gut dysfunction. Chronic illness is often associated with gut dysfunction and a sensitive stomach. Restoring stomach health is sometimes a prerequisite for taking supplements at full doses. **Chapter 25, Gut Restoration Protocol**, provides step-by-step advice for restoring gut function.

Upset stomach. The most common adverse effect associated with taking herbal supplements is an upset stomach. The powders dry the stomach lining. If the lining is already irritated, the herbal powders can aggravate the situation further. Symptoms of indigestion include **mild nausea and discomfort mid-chest or on the left side, just under the lower rib cage** (this is where the stomach is located). If upset stomach occurs, **go very slowly** with the supplements until the stomach has started to heal.

- Follow the recommendations in **Chapter 24** and **Chapter 25** for restoring gut function.

- Take **Chlorella**, a freshwater algae, several times a day (1000-3000 mg two to three times daily). It can be found as powder (to add to smoothies), tablets, and capsules. Consistently taking Chlorella does wonders for healing an irritated stomach and re-storing digestive function. Chlorella causes loose stools in some individuals; back off on the dose if loose stools occur. (Avoid products that also contain spirulina; spirulina is a type of blue-green algae that can be stimulating.)

- **Take D-limonene.** D-limonene is the oil found in the peels of lemons or oranges. It is excellent for protecting and healing an inflamed esophagus (damaged by chronic reflux) or an inflamed stomach. It can be purchased as 1000 mg gel capsules. Take a capsule with each meal until healing has occurred. Be sure to eat and drink something immediately after taking a capsule to be sure it goes down all the way. If the capsule opens up while it is still in the esophagus, oil will spurt upward into nasal passages and down into lungs. This can be disastrous.

- Drink **ginger tea** several times a day to start healing the stom-ach. Ginger tea can cause constipation in some individuals. (See **Chapter 24** for a recipe.)

- **Avoid coffee and tea** (green and black) because of the ten-dency to dry out and irritate the stomach lining.

- **Steamed cabbage** is great for soothing an inflamed stomach. Fermented cabbage juice is also wonderful for healing the intes-tinal tract. You can find it in health food stores or make your own.

- **Pepto-Bismol** works great for acute discomfort (but will turn your stools dark).

- **See your healthcare provider if symptoms are severe or per-sistent (do not resolve).**

Herxheimer reactions. Die-offs of bacteria can intensify symptoms of fatigue, muscle pain, and other flu-like feelings. Generally, Herxheimer reactions are more common and more intense with conventional antibiotic therapy, but they can still occur with herbs. If you feel that you are having Herxheimer reactions, back off on the dose of the herbs, and then increase the dose gradually and slowly. (More to come on dealing with Herx reactions in **Chapter 20**.)

Excessive stimulation. The ingredients in the primary supplements have been carefully chosen to not be stimulating. The herb with the highest potential for stimulation is **eleuthero**. Some people are very sensitive to it. If you are, then it is okay to leave this one off the list. If you are only mildly sensitive to it, you may be able to take it early in the day, but not in the evening.

Constipation. If you have tendencies toward constipation, taking herbal supplements may make it worse. Taking chlorella several times a day can help. Prune juice also works wonders; drink an 8-oz. glassful twice daily. If that isn't enough, Miralax (available at any pharmacy) is safe to use regularly, but two to three times the dose recommended on the bottle is often necessary to get results (take it slow at first). Glycerin or Dulcolax suppositories are sometimes necessary to get things going. Saline enemas are also an option. Avoid magnesium products for constipation because regular use of magnesium can make Lyme symptoms worse.

Advanced Support

The core protocol provides a wide spectrum of benefits including suppression of microbes, modulation of immune functions, restoration of homeostasis, antioxidant support, and reduction of inflammation. If runaway inflammation caused by stealth microbes is severe, however, you may want to take additional measures to get it under control acutely. Protecting brain, joints, and eyes is especially important.

CURBING INFLAMMATION

Many symptoms associated with chronic Lyme disease and fibromyalgia result from runaway inflammation — controlling it is essential for advancing your recovery.

Inflammation occurs as part of the healing process. When tissue becomes damaged or infected, white blood cells (WBCs) are called into the area of damage. They congregate and **secrete hypochlorous acid and potent free radicals** to break down damaged tissue and/or kill microbes. The WBCs then engulf and remove all the debris. This must occur before tissues can be mended.

Stealth microbes thrive by taking advantage of the situation. Stealth microbes have the ability to hitch a ride inside WBCs and be transported to sites of damage (such as a strained ankle, knee, or wrist). Upon arrival, the microbes stimulate WBCs to pump out cytokines, which exaggerates the inflammatory response and causes tissues to break down.

Breakdown of tissues allows the microbes to have better access to vital nutrients such as collagen.

Suppressing stealth microbes and restoring normal cytokine balance is, of course, essential for controlling runaway inflammation — the herbs in the core protocol provide more than adequate coverage here.

Antioxidants in the bloodstream also play an important role in reducing the damaging effects of inflammation. Antioxidants, acquired from healthful foods and supplements, counteract free radicals generated by WBCs and reduce damage.

Another way that inflammation can be influenced is by affecting substances called prostaglandins. The entire healing process is orchestrated by a complex network of biochemical messengers; prostaglandins are some of the most important. Certain types of prostaglandins enhance the inflammatory response, while others reduce it. Balance is required for optimal healing.

Diet has a profound effect on which type of prostaglandins predominate in the body. A diet rich in vegetables and omega-3 fatty acids (fish, shellfish, flax, chia seeds) promotes prostaglandins that diminish the inflammatory response. A diet rich in grain products (wheat and corn especially), grain-fed meat, and grain-fed dairy promotes prostaglandins that exaggerate inflammation. (An optimal diet for recovery is discussed in **Chapter 25**.)

A diet rich in vegetables may also reduce inflammation in another way. **Vegetables contain alkalinizing buffers** that may help neutralize acid generated by WBCs as part of the inflammatory process. Though this has not been documented by science, the health benefits associated with an alkalinizing diet are well known.

Inflammation can be directly affected by blocking key enzymes that make prostaglandins. Nonsteroidal Anti-Inflammatory Drugs (NSAIDs), such as ibuprofen and naproxen, artificially control inflammation by blocking a key enzyme, called COX-2. This enzyme is essential for formation of inflammatory prostaglandins. By blocking COX-2, these drugs provide acute relief of swelling, redness, and pain[1].

These drugs, however, are not pure COX-2 blockers. They also block COX-1, which is important for protecting the stomach lining and regulating acid production in the stomach. Not surprisingly, a common side effect with chronic use of these drugs is stomach ulcers.[2] Chronic use of these drugs is also associated with increased risk of cardiovascular events. (All drugs that influence inflammation are discussed at the end of this chapter.)

Interestingly, **many herbs reduce inflammation by inhibiting COX-2**. One of the most studied is turmeric, the spice that defines an Indian curry. **Curcumin, the primary component of turmeric**, has potent anti-inflammatory properties. It has been found to inhibit formation of the COX-2 enzyme (as opposed to blocking it like a drug; therefore it doesn't work as rapidly as NSAID drugs), but does not affect COX-1. Other substances found in turmeric block other inflammatory messengers. Because of this synergistic effect, turmeric not only reduces tissue inflammation, but also heals stomach ulcers and reduces risk of cardiovascular events!

A member of the ginger family, turmeric (*Curcuma longa*) has a long history of use for arthritic conditions. Research has also shown that turmeric has potent anti-cancer and anti-dementia properties. The fact that people in India consume so much turmeric likely explains why

---

1 All cells in the body (with the exception of RBCs) can produce prostaglandins to influence their surrounding environment and the organism as a whole. Production of prostaglandins in undamaged tissues is normally very low, but it increases very rapidly after tissue injury. Therefore, NSAIDs provide the most benefit if taken immediately after an injury or trauma before inflammation becomes established.
2 Pure COX-2-blocking drugs that do not block COX-1 have been developed, but these drugs have the problem of increasing risk of heart attacks. Several have been taken off the market.

they enjoy such low rates of cancer and dementia. Eating food spiced with turmeric is one way to gain the extraordinary benefits of this herb, but you can also add a teaspoon of turmeric powder to smoothies or take it as a supplement. The average dose for a standardized turmeric extract is 200-500 mg twice daily (depending on the type of extract used).

Turmeric, of course, is not the only herb with COX-2 blocking anti-inflammatory properties. Other herbs with similar properties include Boswellia and devil's claw. Known in its native land as Indian frankincense, *Boswellia serrata* has been used for thousands of years for treatment of arthritic conditions (150-300 mg standardized extract twice daily). Native to Southern Africa, devil's claw (*Harpagophytum procumbens*) has long been used for treatment of arthritic conditions and low back pain. The herb gets its name from the hook-like appendages that cover the fruit of the plant, but the root is the part used for medicine (100-200 mg standardized extract twice daily).

Protein-digesting enzymes play a role in the anti-inflammatory process by breaking down inflammatory debris and immune complexes. This can reduce pain and damage associated with inflammation. Enzymes that digest proteins are commonly present in many foods. These enzymes are known to be absorbed through the intestine into the bloodstream where they have anti-inflammatory properties. Some familiar protein-digesting enzymes include **bromelain** from pineapple and **papain** from papaya. Protein-digesting enzymes, such as bromelain, can be also taken as daily supplements (500 mg twice daily).

Turmeric, Boswellia, and devil's claw are often found together with glucosamine and protein-digesting enzymes in anti-inflammatory supplement products.

Protein-digesting enzymes can also be important for breaking down fibrin. It is theorized that severe chronic infection activates coagulation, which increases risk of blood clots. It also causes fibrin to coat blood vessels, which can block absorption of nutrients and passage of hormones such as thyroid hormone. Studies have shown that the natural enzyme, **nattokinase**, taken as a supplement, breaks down fibrin deposition in the body. The blood thinning properties of nattokinase are similar to aspirin, but without the side effects common to aspirin (Jang 2013).

REBUILDING COLLAGEN

The primary tissues affected by inflammation in chronic Lyme disease include joints, ligaments, muscle, brain, eyes, skin, and heart. What these tissues have in common is collagen. Collagen is the most abundant protein in the body. It's what holds you together. **Without collagen, you would be a puddle on the floor.**

Cartilage in joints is made of collagen. Collagen is also present in heart and skeletal muscle. It provides support to bones. The skin is held up by collagen strands. Collagen is a major component of eye tissue. The brain is held together by collagen. Collagen is also a major component of blood vessels.

Collagen is a **prime target of stealth microbes** such as Borrelia and Mycoplasma.

Protecting your collagen is essential for progressing in your recovery.

Adopting a healthful diet is one of the best ways you can protect your collagen. Healthful foods reduce inflammation and provide nutrients to rebuild healthy collagen. **Kale** and other **deep green leafy vegetables, cucumbers, salmon, sardines, eggs, celery,** and **olives** are a few foods that stand out as being especially beneficial for protecting collagen in the body.

Bone broth is the latest health fad for supporting collagen. Bone broth provides all the necessary ingredients for rebuilding cartilage. A basic recipe includes large bones and high-collagen meat parts (marrow, knuckles, feet) from beef, pork, chicken, or lamb; vegetables, such as celery, carrots, and onions; and seasonings, including salt, pepper, herbs, and garlic. Place in a large slow cooker and simmer for 24-48 hours. Add plenty of water. Many restaurants are now making bone broth and pre-made bone broth can be found at many grocery stores. Bone broth is also excellent for healing the gut.

If you don't want to go to all the trouble of bone broth, **eating gelatin** is the easiest way to add an extra supply of collagen to your diet. **Great Lakes Collagen Hydrolysate**, from grass fed cows, is the brand of gelatin to look for. Extra collagen can also be acquired from supplements. **NeoCell Collagen** and **BioCell Collagen** are the most well-known brands. The recommended dose is about 6000 mg daily of the collagen powder mixed in a smoothie.

Silicon is another necessary component of collagen generation. It is also important for repair of myelin nerve sheaths. Natural silicon can be obtained from the herb, **horsetail.** Silicon can also be obtained as stabilized **orthosilicic acid**. This supplement comes in liquid form and is dosed around 20 drops a day. It also can be added to smoothies.

Out of all supplements you can take for supporting collagen and joint function, **glucosamine** has the most scientific evidence to back it up. Glucosamine is a precursor for proteoglycans, the chemicals necessary for smooth and slick joint linings. It also stimulates synthesis of collagen. Glucosamine is formed by a molecule of glucose combined with the amino acid, glutamine. With age, normal glucosamine synthesis decreases. This may be a contributing factor to arthritis. The suggested dose of glucosamine is 500-750 mg twice daily[3].

---

3 Glucosamine HCl is derived from shellfish, but does not contain the proteins that cause reactions in individuals with shellfish allergies. Studies have demonstrated that glucosamine HCl is well tolerated in people with shellfish allergies. Even so, if you have a

RESTORING BRAIN AND NERVE HEALTH

Beyond collagen, microbes commonly scavenge specialized fats in the brain and nervous system. **Myelin**, the fat that surrounds and insulates nerves, is a common target for Borrelia and Mycoplasma. Loss of myelin and other brain fats may cause a range of neurological symptoms, from tingling and burning to brain fog and depression.

Certain foods are especially valuable for supporting optimal brain function. **Eggs** are a good source of lecithin and choline, both essential brain nutrients. **Oysters** supply omega-3 fatty acids and minerals including **zinc**, an essential nutrient for brain function (make sure your oysters are raised in a very clean water source).

Coconut oil provides medium-chain triglycerides (MCTs), which regenerate and heal nerve tissue. Other important anti-inflammatory fats include **olive oil**, **ghee** (clarified butter, limit to 1-2 tsp. per day), and the oil in **avocados**.

Monolaurin, a fatty substance derived from coconut, is known for suppressing microbes, including Borrelia. It penetrates well into fatty tissue (the brain is 60% fat), making it ideal for providing support for neurological Lyme symptoms. Additionally, monolaurin offers anti-inflammatory properties. It comes in a powder that can be mixed with coconut milk or smoothies. The recommended dose is 3000 mg twice daily (work up to the full dose slowly). The most well-known brand is **Lauricidin**.

Certain herbal mushrooms, including **lion's mane** and **chaga** mushrooms, are well known for protecting and restoring brain function. Ground chaga mushroom can be used to make an excellent caffeine-free tea that can be enjoyed instead of coffee or regular tea. **Reishi** and

---

shellfish allergy, use caution when taking glucosamine HCl. Presently, there is no evidence that glucosamine supplements appreciably affect blood glucose levels in diabetics.

Cordyceps mushrooms, from the core protocol, also provide neuroprotective properties.

Other neuroprotective herbs include **ashwagandha** and **bacopa**. These beneficial herbs are further discussed in future chapters and in **Appendix A**.

DHA, one of the omega-3 fatty acids present in marine oils (fish and krill oil), has been associated with improved motor and cognitive function, depression, and insomnia. Higher doses of 3+ grams (3000 mg) of fish oil are often necessary to achieve symptom reduction.

Note that more than 6 grams of fish oil daily has been associated with increased risk of hemorrhagic stroke (blood vessel rupturing in the brain). Do not exceed this dose. If you have a family or personal history of easy bleeding or other bleeding disorders, consult with your healthcare provider before using higher doses of omega-3 fatty acids.

Essential oils are ideal for penetrating into skin, joint, brain, and nerve tissue. Essential oils are primarily administered by aromatherapy. **Lavender, rosemary, and lemon balm** are well known for supporting brain and nerve function. These essential oils also provide anti-inflammatory and antimicrobial properties. (Essential oils are discussed in **Appendix A**.)

START YOUR DAY WITH A **BRAIN HEALTH SMOOTHIE**!

- Cucumber
- Celery stalk
- Frozen blueberries (and/or other berries)
- 2 tbsp. avocado or olive oil

- 1 tsp. ashwagandha (Withania somnifera) powder
- 1 tsp. Lion's mane or chaga mushroom extract powder
- 1 tsp. turmeric powder
- Monolaurin 3000 mg (optional)

Mix all ingredients in a blender or smoothie-making machine and drink daily.

EYE HEALTH

Eye irritation is not uncommon in chronic Lyme disease. Borrelia spirochetes can invade the eye, causing a variety of symptoms, including spots and floaters, eye irritation, blurry vision, and decreased vision. Eye involvement in Lyme disease generally responds to conventional and herbal antibiotic therapy.

Borrelia, Bartonella, and other stealth microbes can cause conjunctivitis, causing redness and irritation of the outer coating of the eye. Conjunctivitis generally responds well to antibiotic and herbal eye drops. Coptis and isatis are herbs commonly used to make eye-wash preparations for alleviating conjunctivitis (see **Appendix A**).

MAST CELL HYPERSENSITIVITY

Many people with chronic Lyme (and similar conditions) experience mast cell hypersensitivity. Borrelia is known to directly stimulate mast cells to produce histamine. Histamine is the substance that mediates allergic-type reactions with skin itching and rash. While many of the herbs offer antihistamine properties, sometimes the potency of a drug is indicated. Antihistamine drugs are some of the most well tolerated and safe drugs. Common, non-drowsy antihistamines include **Claritin (loratadine) and Zyrtec (cetirizine)**. If sedation is desired, **Benadryl (diphenhydramine)** is the best option. **Antihistamines can be taken long term. The biggest drawback is tolerance with decreased benefit over time.**

ENHANCED IMMUNE SUPPORT

For mild to moderate illness, the core herbal protocol alone is generally enough to restore wellness. If illness is severe and symptoms are persistent, however, additional non-herbal measures can be taken to enhance healing.

Low-dose naltrexone. Low doses of the drug, naltrexone, stimulate production of endorphins in the body. This helps normalize the immune response and increases NK cells. Low-dose naltrexone is discussed in **Chapter 18**.

Cannabidiol oil (CBD). Cannabidiol oil is derived from hemp (a variety of *Cannabis sativa*). CBD is an immunomodulatory; it downregulates IL-10 and shifts Th2 to Th1. Cannabidiol oil is also discussed in **Chapter 18**.

Stress reduction. Regular meditation normalizes adrenal function, which supports optimal immune function. Adrenal function and stress management are discussed in **Chapter 28**.

Exercise. Regular moderate exercise stimulates endorphin production and increases NK cells. The benefits of regular exercise are discussed in **Chapter 29**.

Peptides. Peptides are short chains of amino acids that act as messengers in the body. There are many peptide hormones, some of which are known to enhance healing and immune functions in the body. Though functions of various immune-regulating peptides have been well defined by scientific studies, the value of supplementation is less well defined. Even so, the benefit they offer is different than herbs, so if you want added support for healing, peptides may be worth considering. The potential for harm from supplementing with the two following peptides is low.

- *Thymosin Alpha 1 (TA1)*. Secreted naturally by the thymus gland, TA1 stimulates T cell production, increases NK cells, increases antibody production, decreases inflammatory cytokines, and balances Th1/Th2. This reduces inflammation, improves tissue repair, improves stress resistance, increases glutathione, and may increase cancer defense. TA1 is administered as an injection by integrative/functional medical providers. Purified thymic peptide is also available as a sublingual powder (under the tongue) in a product called ProBoost. The dose of ProBoost is 3 packets daily for enhancing immune function and 1 packet daily for maintenance.

- *BPC-157.* This 15-amino acid peptide, isolated from gastric juice, accelerates healing by increasing growth hormone receptors. It has been shown to heal gastric ulcers, improve digestive function, heal nerve tissue, and heal damaged ligaments and joints. BPC-157 is administered as an injection by integrative/functional medical providers. BPC-157 can be injected into joints to stimulate healing.

WHEN TO CONSIDER ANTI-INFLAMMATORY DRUGS

When runaway inflammation is not controlled by diet and supplements, drug therapy is sometimes necessary. Anti-inflammatory drugs are more potent than natural therapies and act more acutely. Chronic use of any anti-inflammatory drugs, however, is limited by significant side effects and disruption of the natural healing process. **Drugs should be considered only if natural therapy options are not satisfactory for controlling symptoms.**

NSAIDs are the primary drugs for reducing inflammation by blocking the COX-2 enzyme. Common over-the-counter NSAIDs include aspirin, ibuprofen, and naproxen. There are also many prescription NSAIDs; meloxicam (Mobic) is the most commonly prescribed. It offers the advantage of high potency and once-daily dosing. Ketorolac (Toradol) is an NSAID administered by injection (IM or IV) for acute management of inflammation.

Acetaminophen (Tylenol) is a distant relative of NSAIDs. Long-term use has been associated with liver damage. Generally, this drug should be avoided.

Steroids strongly suppress inflammation. They do so by strongly suppressing the entire immune system. Broad suppression of immune function not only inhibits inflammation, but also inhibits healing and the ability of the body to fight off infection (especially from stealth microbes). This can result in a wide range of debilitating side effects with prolonged use. Though steroids can be lifesaving if used properly in certain situations, they also have the potential to be severely life disrupting.

Steroids can be administered orally, by injection, by inhalation, or as a topical applied to the skin. Steroids mimic natural cortisol in the body and suppress the immune system. Suppression of immune function is broad, so they are effective for controlling many types of inflammation.

- **Topical steroids** (hydrocortisone, triamcinolone, many others in creams or ointments) are useful for controlling symptoms associated with skin rashes, such as itching and redness. Side effects are mild when they occur. Long-term use is associated mostly with skin thinning and increased risk of skin infections. Persistent rashes may be an indication of a bacterial or fungal infection and should be brought to the attention of a healthcare provider.

- **Steroid injections** can be useful for controlling acute inflammation reactions, such as whole-body allergic reactions, severe bronchitis, or poison ivy. Single injections are associated with few side effects and minimal risk of long-term problems.

- **Local injections of steroids into joints** can also help with localized inflammation. Chronic use of steroid injections, however, can be destructive to joints.

- **Inhaled steroids** are used for control of asthma and acute sinusitis. Long-term use is associated with thinning of bones and increased risk of infection.

- **Prednisone** is the most commonly used oral steroid (but there are many others). Long-term use of oral steroids (for weeks or months) is sometimes beneficial for calming out-of-control, whole-body inflammation (autoimmune disease). Oral steroid therapy, however, deeply suppresses the entire immune system, resulting in an increased risk of infection and poor healing. Oral steroids can definitely inhibit recovery from Lyme disease. Other common side effects include disruption of normal sleep, bone loss, mood changes, and irritability, to name a few.

  Oral steroids should be used only when absolutely necessary, in the lowest dose possible to achieve positive benefit, and for the shortest duration possible. Once steroids are started, they should be weaned very slowly.

Humira and similar drugs block targeted pathways of the immune system and therefore are more specific in action than steroids. These drugs, however, block key healing pathways, potentially resulting in catastrophic side effects, such as life-threatening infections and cancer.

Use of immune-suppressing drug therapy (steroids, other immune-suppressing agents) should be reserved for situations where immune dysfunction is overwhelming. Suppression of immune function to control symptoms carries risk of compromising the ability of the immune system to suppress microbes and also inhibits healing systems in the body. Overzealous use of these types of drugs can lead to worsening of illness.

Talk to your doctor about potential side effects and complications before using any medication.

17

Sleep, Anxiety, and Depression

Starting and ending every day, day after day, feeling like you have the flu, is depressing. Seeing no hope for it ever getting better generates fear, which is the root of anxiety. Chronic anxiety disrupts normal sleep. Sleep is further disrupted by inflammation irritating the brain, which also contributes to stress intolerance and depression. Lack of sleep lowers the threshold for anxiety and depression to occur.

Lack of sleep disrupts immune function. Chronic immune dysfunction is the root cause of chronic illness.

A vicious cycle if there ever was one.

You cannot get well without normal sleep. For your body to recover, you need at least 7-9 hours of good sleep every night (including at least 4 hours of deep sleep).

Often, this is easier said than done. Even though your body wants to sleep, all the factors that cause chronic Lyme disease or fibromyalgia prevent sleep from happening. The long-term solution is reducing inflammation and balancing hormones, but natural restorative therapies take time to work — you need a sleep solution right now. Sometimes heroic measures are indicated.

Factors causing sleep disturbances associated with chronic Lyme disease:

- **Elevated adrenaline** and over-activity of the sympathetic nervous system from chronic stress

- Disruption of adrenal function from chronic stress causing **imbalances in cortisol secretion**

- **Inflammation of the brain** resulting from your body's response to low-grade infection by stealth microbes

QUICK TIPS FOR BETTER SLEEP

Be very particular about your sleep habits. A dark, quiet room is essential. A fan by your bedside for generating white noise can help you stay asleep at night. White noise generators also work well. A favorite of mine is the LectroFan generator.

Allow enough time for sleep. You may need to allow 10 hours to get 8 hours of sleep. By 9 o'clock, you should be winding down and starting a bedtime ritual. TV and computers should be off.

Avoid alarm clocks. Try to schedule your days such that you are able to wake up naturally with daylight instead of an alarm clock.

Avoid caffeine and alcohol. Caffeine builds up in your system. It should be avoided completely during your recovery. The metabolites of alcohol are stimulants that will not only keep you awake, but also inhibit your recovery.

Are drugs keeping you awake? Selective serotonin reuptake inhibitors (SSRIs) used for anxiety and depression are notorious for causing insomnia in people with brain inflammation. If you are taking one of these drugs (Prozac, Paxil, Lexapro, Zoloft, Effexor, Wellbutrin, others), it may be the reason for your insomnia. Wean off slowly.

Turn off your brain. This is a skill that can be mastered through regular practice of breathing exercises and relaxation techniques. If you don't have these skills just yet, don't worry about it. Just focus on the things that you can do easily.

If you need more, consider natural options first. Natural supplements are not as potent as drugs for sleep, but also are not habituating and do not cause dependence.

- **Herbal supplements**. A tried-and-true combination of **baco-pa**, **passionflower**, and **motherwort** is a very safe alternative for improving sleep (see **Appendix A** for an in-depth discussion of these herbs). These herbs are also effective for acute relief of anxiety episodes. All three herbs can be taken together. Combination supplements are available; follow the recommended dosages for the product. The dose can be repeated upon wakening in the middle of the night.

  Valerian and kava are also popular herbal options, but both have higher potential to cause side effects and have been associated with liver damage. Kava is as habituating as drug therapy. A combination of bacopa, passionflower, and motherwort generally works just as well and is safer.

- **Melatonin.** Often used as a sleep aid, melatonin is primarily beneficial for *inducing* sleep, but less beneficial for *maintaining* sleep. It can be used in combination with drugs or supplements. Start with 1 mg sublingual (under the tongue) dosing. It is preferred because it more closely mimics natural melatonin secretion. The dose can be repeated with wakening in the middle of the night to re-initiate sleep. Limit to a maximum dose of 5 mg over a 24-hour period.

- Inadequate serotonin is sometimes associated with poor sleep. The most natural way to raise serotonin levels in the brain is by taking **5-HTP** as a supplement. The normal dose is 100-300 mg before bedtime.

- **Methylation problems**. Many toxic substances irritate the brain and prevent good sleep. The body gets rid of toxins by "methylating" them. For this, you need an adequate supply of methyl donors. **SAMe**, 400-800 mg in the evening, is a great methyl donor known to improve sleep.

- Irritation caused by inflammation of brain tissues is a primary cause of sleep disturbances. **Omega-3 fatty acid** supplements help reduce inflammation. **Fish oil and krill oil** are the most popular options for omega-3 supplementation. (Individuals on blood thinners or who are having a history of easy bleeding should discuss taking of omega-3 supplements with a health-care provider prior to use).

MEDICATIONS FOR SLEEP AND ANXIETY

Sleep is essential for your recovery, and on occasion, you may need something potent to get you there. Generally, this means drug therapy. While drug therapy is never the ideal solution, sometimes it's the only solution. When drugs do become part of the solution, however, they need to be used carefully and respectfully to avoid long-term consequences. All drugs used for sleep and anxiety carry the potential for habituation. Drug habituation will slow your recovery!

The **classic sleeping pills (Ambien, Lunesta, Sonata) are generally best avoided.** They are very effective for inducing sleep, but use of them one night causes rebound insomnia on the next night. This provides an ever-present incentive to use them on the following night and every night thereafter. Habituation occurs rapidly and, once you are habituated, sleeping pills are extremely hard to stop. Eventually, they quit working completely, and insomnia becomes a nightmare of the worst kind.

When your nervous system so agitated that sleep just won't come, the long-acting benzodiazepine, **Valium (diazepam),** is a better choice for breaking the cycle. Because it stays in your system for over 30 hours, next night rebound insomnia is less apt to occur. Valium also provides muscle relaxing properties that are not provided by classic sleeping pills. Like all drugs in this class, however, Valium is extremely habituating. Save it for when you really need it and avoid regular use. Ask your doctor for the 5-mg tablet. A half-tablet will often work, but you can safely take up to 10 mg (two 5-mg tablets) in a 24-hour period. Klonopin is a similar long-acting benzodiazepine.

Xanax (alprazolam) or **Ativan (lorazepam)** are short-acting benzodiazepines that are ideal for acute anxiety or panic attacks. These drugs stay in your system for 6-12 hours. Because they are short acting, they are less useful for sleep; rebound insomnia becomes a problem. The average dose for these drugs is 0.25 to 1 mg up to every 6 hours. Use the lowest dose possible to achieve benefit.

> **As much as benzodiazepines can be your best friend when used acutely and occasionally,** *they become your worst nightmare if used every day (or every night).* **Benzodiazepines are possibly the most habituating substances on earth (even more than heroin). The habituating tendency of these drugs must be respected!** *Reserve use of these drugs for crisis situations only.*

Lioresal (baclofen) is a muscle relaxant that also can be used for sleep and anxiety. It does have habituating tendencies, but less so than sleeping pills or benzodiazepines. Ask for 10-mg tablets, but start with only half a tablet. The top dose for muscle spasm is 20 mg three times daily, but you should try to avoid using that much. Avoid regular use.

Neurontin (gabapentin) is typically used for treating nerve pain in extremities, but it also has sedative properties; some people find it valuable for sleep and anxiety. It is less habituating and does not cause addiction problems like classic sleeping pills and benzodiazepines. It can be taken continually, but it loses sedative properties with chronic use. Most often, it is prescribed as a 300-mg capsule, three times daily. There is a 100-mg capsule available; ask for the 100-mg capsules, and start with the lowest dose that provides benefit. You may be able to get by with one to two 100-mg capsules at bedtime.

Remeron (mirtazapine) is classified as an antidepressant, but has strong sedative properties. It is one of the few drugs that can be used on a regular basis for insomnia. It doesn't cause perfect sleep, and most people do have significant next-day sedation, but it is less habituating and easier to discontinue than classic sleeping pills. Some people tolerate it; others do not. Ask your doctor for the 15-mg tablet, but you will typically only have to use ⅛ to ½ of the tablet. Use as little as possible.

Many doctors have become fond of writing prescriptions for a drug called **Trazodone** as an alternative to sleeping pills. Trazodone has many undesirable side effects and suppresses immune function. It is also very habituating and very hard to discontinue. **Stay clear of this one if you can.** Also, stay clear of anti-seizure drugs, which are commonly written for insomnia. They also carry a lot of side effects and suppress immune function.

Belsomra (suvorexant) is a newly released drug for treating insomnia (as of January 2015). This drug blocks orexins, chemical substances produced by the brain to keep us awake. It is not related to benzodiazepines or other sleep medications, and it is not associated with habituation. Early on, the drug looked promising, but reports from users have not been positive. In one Internet survey, 50% of users gave it one star out of five. The most commonly reported side effect was horrible nightmares. You are better off passing this one by.

GUIDELINES FOR SAFE MEDICATION USE

- Before considering drugs, do everything you can to promote a calm brain (you will get better at it as time goes by).

- Have a standard bedtime ritual that starts about 8-9 pm. Take advantage of natural supplements and melatonin, as needed, to promote calm. Have a medication on hand, however. Sometimes just knowing that you have it, is enough to prevent you from needing to take it.

- If it looks like it's going to be one of those nights when sleep isn't going to come easily or you have a big event the next day that requires you to be rested, go ahead and take a half of a 5 mg diazepam tablet (you can also substitute baclofen or gabapentin).

- If your brain is still agitated, and you do not fall asleep by 11 pm, take the other half of the dose. You can safely take up to 10 mg of diazepam within a 24-hour period.

- If you awake with an agitated brain at 3 am, you can repeat the half dose (but be prepared to be groggy the next morning).

- Do everything you can be avoid repeating this same process night after night. It's better just to suffer through and do the best you can.

- If chronic insomnia is so severe that you have no choice but to take a medication every night, try Remeron. Start with ⅛ - ¼ tablet of Remeron 15 mg. Take it around 8 pm; it takes about 2 hours to start working. As soon as your sleep situation is better, start weaning off it.

- There is no single drug choice that works for everyone. You may have to try different drugs.

- Talk to your doctor about potential side effects and complications before using any medication.

DRUG HABITUATION

If you can get through your recovery without becoming habituated to a drug, you will be better off, but many people with chronic Lyme or fibromyalgia end up habituated to medications. If you are already habituated to a habit-forming drug, note that many symptoms caused by drug dependence can mimic Lyme disease symptoms. As the spiral of dependency tightens, severe withdrawal symptoms can occur if the dose of the drug is not continually increased, until a point is reached when increasing the dose does not get rid of the symptoms.

The best strategy for dealing with habituation to sleep medications or benzodiazepines is stabilizing on a regular dose of a long-acting drug (such as Valium), and save weaning off of the drug until you have mastered all other aspects of your recovery. Once you are very stable and your recovery is progressing in a positive direction, you can carefully and gradually start the weaning process. If you try to do it too soon or too fast, it will throw you into a tailspin.

When you come around to considering weaning off the drug (or drugs), please take the time to review *The Ashton Manual,* found at www.benzo.org.uk. It is the ultimate guide for understanding habituation and defining a safe protocol for weaning off these types of drugs. Many people print the manual and give it to their doctor for reference.

Weaning off sleeping pills or benzodiazepines is a rocky road. Two therapies, however, that can ease the process include **Cranial Electrotherapy Stimulation** (discussed later in this chapter) and **cannabidiol oil** (THC-free, CBD-rich hemp oil), which will be discussed in the next chapter.

MEDICATIONS FOR DEPRESSION

Some people have more of a tendency toward depression than others, but dealing with any chronic disease process, especially chronic Lyme disease or fibromyalgia, can be depressing. Usually depression lifts as health improves, but during the thick of things, drug therapy for depression can sometimes be beneficial.

Selective serotonin reuptake inhibitors (SSRIs) are the most commonly prescribed non-habituating drugs for anxiety and depression. Common SSRIs include **Prozac (fluoxetine), Lexapro (escitalopram),**

Zoloft (sertraline), Paxil (paroxetine), and **Celexa (citalopram)**. These drugs cause buildup of serotonin (the mood hormone) in the brain. This can have the positive effect of relieving anxiety as well as depression. SSRIs also provide pain-relieving qualities.

Wellbutrin (bupropion) and **Buspar (buspirone)** are similar to SSRIs, but also affect dopamine in the brain. Often, they provide better relief for anxiety than SSRIs.

Closely related to SSRIs, **Serotonin-Norepinephrine Reuptake Inhibitors (SNRIs),** cause both serotonin and norepinephrine to build up in the brain, promoting a mood-elevating effect. **Cymbalta (duloxetine)** is the most useful of these drugs because it has strong pain-inhibiting qualities. **Effexor (venlafaxine)** and **Pristiq (desvenlafaxine),** two closely related drugs also in this class, should be avoided because of tendency for excessive stimulation (insomnia) and the potential for dependence.

The **most concerning side effect of all of these drugs is insomnia,** which occurs in 20-40% of chronic Lyme sufferers who use these drugs. If it occurs with one of these drugs, it will occur with any and all of these drugs (even St. John's wort, which works similarly to the drugs). Other common side effects include weight gain, decreased libido, lethargy, and constipation.

An older class of drugs, **tricyclic antidepressants,** have limited use because of significant side effects including daytime sedation, lethargy, dry mouth, and constipation. Of this group, **Elavil (amitriptyline)** is sometimes useful to control nerve pain.

NATURAL OPTIONS FOR ANXIETY AND DEPRESSION
St. John's wort is the classic substitute for antidepressants, but it actually works very much like the SSRIs. St. John's wort enhances liver enzymes, which can affect metabolism of other drugs and supplements

(See **Appendix A** for more information). Like SSRIs, the biggest limitation of St. John's wort is inhibition of normal sleep.

Rhodiola is an adaptogenic herb with antidepressive properties. It also is anti-fatigue and immune modulating, another great herbal choice for chronic Lyme disease or fibromyalgia (See **Appendix A** for more information).

Cannabidiol oil (CBD) can be useful for controlling anxiety and depression. For some people, it also helps with sleep. In addition, it has also shown benefit for reducing drug-withdrawal symptoms. The pros and cons of cannabis will be discussed in **Chapter 18**, Dealing with Pain.

AN ELECTRICAL ALTERNATIVE

Cranial Electrotherapy Stimulation (CES) is a simple device that utilizes low-intensity, pulsed electrical current across the head to induce a relaxed state or sleep. It is a gentle, safe, and non-invasive method of normalizing the neurotransmitters in the brain. It can provide relief from anxiety, insomnia, depression, and habituation to medications.

Processes in the body are usually explained in terms of chemical reactions, but they are also electrical. All chemical reactions involve the transfer of electrons from one molecule to another. Electricity is the movement of electrons.

Disease (and inflammation), in electrical terms, is a deficiency of electrons in the system (a loss of energy). Therefore, it shouldn't be a surprise to find that placing a low-intensity electrical current across the head has a positive benefit when brain functions are out of balance.

That's what CES does. A current of 100 pulses/sec (Hz) in a modified square wave of less than 1 mAmp of current is generated by a portable battery-powered device and delivered across the head with electrodes attached to the scalp or ear lobes. Treatments are painless and last 30-60 minutes, once or twice daily (depending on the device used). Benefit is cumulative and lasting.

The technology has been available since 1953. There are scores of studies documenting the benefit of CES for treatment of insomnia, anxiety, and depression. It is FDA-approved for treatment of those disorders. It has also shown benefit for relieving pain, improving cognitive function, reducing spasticity associated with MS and Parkinson's, relieving migraine and tension headaches, and helping patients with narcotic addiction.

It is very safe and is free of side effects. Over 150 clinical studies and many thousands of patient encounters have not revealed significant side effects or long-term ill effects from regular use of CES. Most common side effect: 2% of users report tingling sensation or mild headache during use.

The FDA requires the written order (but not necessarily a prescription) from a healthcare provider for use of a CES device. In Europe, CES does not require the approval of a healthcare provider.

SOURCES OF DEVICES
Reliable CES devices are available from three primary companies: CES Ultra, Alpha-Stim, and Fisher-Wallace. The devices differ in amplitude of current delivered and pulse rate.

The Alpha-Stim (www.alpha-stim.com) and Fisher-Wallace (www.fisher-wallace.com) devices offer digital readouts and are the most commonly used devices in current clinical research, but they are also the most expensive, running about $750. Alpha-Stim also makes a more expensive device that includes treatment of localized muscle pain. Fisher-Wallace is focusing on reducing spasm associated with MS and Parkinson's disease (but all devices offer similar benefits).

Neuro-Fitness, LLC, the company making CES Ultra (www.cesultra.com), has stuck to the basics. Their simple device conforms to specifications used in the original research on CES. The device has been available for over 15 years and is supported by scores of positive testimonials. By keeping things simple, they are able to offer the device for less than half the price of the other devices ($350). Customer support and the company's return policies are excellent. For most people, the lower cost of the CES Ultra allows access to this valuable technology.

18

Dealing with Pain

Pain is possibly the most disabling symptom of chronic Lyme disease. The only upside of pain is knowing you are still alive. And if you are alive, then there is hope you can recover a normal state of pain-free health. Otherwise, pain is just something to deal with.

MEDICATIONS FOR PAIN

No one likes to be in pain, especially when the pain never goes away. To escape pain, people often turn to narcotics. Chronic use of any type of narcotic, however, leads to habituation and dependence. Most studies show that narcotics are poorly effective for controlling chronic pain. Regular use of narcotics suppresses natural endorphins, which are essential to your recovery. Use of narcotics to control chronic pain is a dead-end cycle that will leave you going nowhere forever.

Narcotics should be reserved for treatment of acute pain caused by trauma only. Many narcotic products **(Percocet, Vicodin)** contain acetaminophen and should be avoided completely.

The safest option for narcotic-like relief is a drug called Ultram (tramadol). Tramadol carries slightly less habituating tendencies than standard narcotics, but it still should be reserved for intermittent use. Disrupted sleep is a common side effect of tramadol.

Ketamine, a potent anesthetic agent, can be used topically with lidocaine and anti-inflammatory agents to relieve pain in joints and muscles. This combination must be prescribed by a healthcare provider and dispensed by a compounding pharmacy. Some integrative providers also administer it by injection.

Muscle relaxers can be effective for riding out episodes of muscle pain. Sedating muscle relaxers include **Flexeril (cyclobenzaprine)** and **Lioresal (baclofen)**. These drugs can also be used as sleep aids, especially when muscle pain is an issue. Use them intermittently, and try to get by with a half dose (half of a 10-mg tablet). Less sedating muscle relaxers include **Skelaxin (metaxalone)** and **Zanaflex (tizanidine)**. Again, try to get by with the lowest dose possible. For Skelaxin, use half of a 200-mg tablet, and for Zanaflex, use one quarter (1 mg) of a 4-mg tablet. **Note that all of these drugs are habituating and should be used only on a limited basis.**

Two closely related drugs, **Neurontin (gabapentin)** and **Lyrica (pregabalin)**, can provide effective relief for nerve pain and bothersome neurological symptoms include burning and tingling in extremities. The standard dose of gabapentin is 300-mg capsules three times daily, but 100-mg capsules are also available. Ask for the smaller capsules, and try to get by with a lower dose. The initial dose of pregabalin is 75 mg twice daily, but larger doses are often required. The biggest problem with these drugs is tolerance and reduced benefit over time.

Talk to your doctor about potential side effects and complications before using any medication.

NATURAL THERAPIES FOR PAIN

Natural herbal alternatives that work specifically for pain include **corydalis** and **Indian pipe**. **Corydalis** (many species worldwide), from

Traditional Chinese Medicine, offers only about 1% of the pain-relieving ability of morphine, but it can still be valuable for pain control. It is non-narcotic and is not reported to have habituating tendencies. **Indian pipe (Rauwolfia serpentina)** has been used on the Asian subcontinent for relief of pain and as a sleep aid for thousands of years. **Passionflower** is excellent for relieving muscle spasm. (See **Appendix A** for in-depth discussions on these herbs.)

Turmeric and **boswellia** offer potent anti-inflammatory properties and can also relieve pain. (See **Chapter 16** for more information).

Essential oils rubbed into joints can be very beneficial for soothing joint pain. Non-irritating oils that can be used for topical application include **frankincense, ginger, white birch, lavender, peppermint, helichrysum, and German chamomile**. Oils can be mixed together or used individually. Before topical use, dilute the oil mixture 4:1 with a carrier oil, such as jojoba or coconut oil. (Essential oils are further discussed in **Appendix A**).

Raising endorphin levels is important for controlling pain. Having normal endorphin levels is intimately tied to good health and well-being. Baseline secretion of endorphins can be increased with regular exercise, vigorous massage, and acupuncture. The ancient Chinese movement exercises (Qigong and tai chi) and yoga are a great way to get started. Chronic stress decreases endorphins and, not surprisingly, regular practice of meditation or relaxation techniques stimulates endorphins. Just having a warm and friendly attitude will also increase endorphins.

CANNABIS

Cannabis sativa has been cultivated by people throughout recorded history. A very versatile plant, cannabis has been used for food, medicine, religious and spiritual purposes, industrial fiber, and, of course, recreational use. Medicinal use of cannabis includes management of pain, anxiety, and depression.

Different varieties of cannabis provide different uses. What is known as marijuana is only one variety of *Cannabis sativa*. Hemp, another variety of *Cannabis sativa* lacking properties of intoxication and euphoria, is known for high-tensile-strength fibers that are ideal for making rope and other textiles. Hemp seeds and sprouts are a nutritionally complete food offering high-quality protein and beneficial omega-3 fatty acids.

Only recently have the potential medicinal benefits of each of these varieties of cannabis (and many new varieties in between) been fully recognized.

The remarkable difference between marijuana and hemp has to do with the presence or absence of one of two enzymes. In marijuana, an enzyme is present that converts a precursor substance called cannabigerolic acid (CBGA) into tetrahydrocannabinol, better known as THC. The enzyme in hemp converts the same substance into cannabidiol (CBD). Marijuana contains both THC and CBD, but hemp contains almost exclusively CBD. There are many strains in between, however, with varying concentrations of THC and CBD.

THC is the infamous substance found in marijuana that is associated with euphoric and intoxicating properties. THC mimics a natural mood-altering substance in the body called anandamide. Having normal levels of anandamide in the brain is associated with a rosy disposition. Because THC binds to anandamide receptors in the brain more intensely than anandamide, an exaggerated or euphoric response occurs (you get high).

There are different receptors for cannabinoids (CB receptors) found throughout the body. Scientists are still sorting out how it all works. CB1 receptors are found in high concentrations in the brain and nervous system. CB2 receptors are found predominantly within the lower body and immune system. Endocannabinoids (natural cannabinoid-like compounds including anandamide) appear to work by modulating or modifying the activity of other neurotransmitters in the body (but not by acting directly).

Cannabidiol (CBD) has very different properties than THC. It binds very weakly to both CB1 and CB2 receptors (both mildly stimulating and blocking the receptors at the same time). The end result of taking CBD is positive mood and improved pain tolerance without euphoria (you don't get high).

CBD also modulates other receptors in the body. Modulation of the 5-HT1A receptor (involved with serotonin) provides anti-anxiety, anti-depressant, and neuroprotective properties. Modulation of opioid receptors provides pain relief and anti-inflammatory properties. **CBD is neither stimulating nor sedating (neutral), but some people find that CBD improves sleep.**

Beyond THC and CBD, *Cannabis sativa* contains other chemical substances with medicinal properties. Other cannabinoids (THC is the only one with intoxicating properties) and a host of antioxidant and anti-inflammatory substances are found in the plant. In this respect, cannabis is like other herbs used for recovery.

How to take medicinal cannabis

Cannabis for recreational use is generally inhaled as a vapor or smoke. Inhalation provides a rapid peak in blood levels that are ideal for recreational purposes, but less useful for medicinal purposes because blood levels are only sustained for a short period of time.

Cannabinoids (THC and CBD) are fat-soluble compounds (they dissolve in oil). For medicinal purposes, cannabis extracts are dissolved in oil (coconut oil and ghee are commonly used) and administered by dropper orally. Cannabis compounds are absorbed into the tissues of the mouth (under the tongue is ideal) and the intestinal tract. This provides for a slower peak and prolonged dose response. Euphoria is not a targeted medicinal response; therefore, CBD-rich cannabis with minimal or trace THC is preferred.

Cannabis side effects and concerns

With the recent legalization of marijuana in several states and the legalization of CBD-rich, THC-free cannabidiol in all states, the industry has exploded. Production methods and quality control in the industry vary a great deal. Chemical solvents (including hexane, which can cause severe liver damage) are often used in the extraction process. Quality control and concentrations of CBD and THC vary widely between producers and even within the same products. If cannabis is considered for a medicinal use, it is very important to find a pure product.

It should be noted that recreational use of marijuana (high-THC, low-CBD cannabis) does result in dependence, but not as debilitating as narcotics or alcohol. Because there are no endocannabinoid receptors in the brainstem, overdose of cannabis does not cause respiratory depression (stop breathing) like narcotics and alcohol. Chronic use of THC may be associated with atrophy in certain areas of the brain and reduction of certain cognitive functions (at this point, studies are inconclusive).

Some people experience agitation and insomnia instead of euphoria with THC; it's not for everyone. A few people have this effect with CBD also.

Cannabis and Lyme disease

The fact that CBD has the potential to relieve pain without causing euphoria or intoxication makes it interesting from a medicinal point of view. In fact, CBD-rich cannabis may be the ideal option for acute management of pain and sleep dysfunction associated with Lyme disease and fibromyalgia. Though cannabis should be considered primarily valuable for controlling symptoms (and not as primary therapy for treatment of

Lyme disease), CBD and other phytochemicals in cannabis also support immune function and provide other health benefits.

THC-free cannabidiol (CBD) products are legal in all 50 states, but the cost of quality products can be high. A month of product with high enough concentrations of CBD to be therapeutically beneficial can run $150-$500. Avoid products containing only synthetic CBD; whole plant extractions standardized to CBD also contain all the other beneficial phytochemicals found in cannabis. Concentrations of CBD range from 250 mg to 1500 mg per fluid oz. (See **Resources** for Cannabis sources.)

LOW-DOSE NALTREXONE (LDN)

Naltrexone is a drug designed to block opioid receptors in the body. Opioid receptors block pain and are activated by endorphins. Opioid receptors are also activated by opioid drugs, such as morphine and heroin (that's why they're called opioid receptors).

Naltrexone was created back in the 70s to help addicts get off heroin. At a standard dose of 50 mg, the drug blocks all opioid receptors in the body. In other words, it blocks all the effects of heroin. In theory, the addict would find heroin useless and would stop using it, but it never took off as a popular drug.

Interestingly, someone noticed that a very low dose of naltrexone (1.5-4.5 mg) had a very different effect. At a very low dose, opioid receptors in the body are only blocked for only a short period of time, and the body responds with surges in endorphin production. Endorphins enhance immune function and increase tolerance to pain. If naltrexone is taken daily, elevated endorphin secretion is sustained.

Use of naltrexone at this dose is very safe and is associated with minimal side effects. It has no narcotic effects and carries zero potential for dependence and habituation. Novel application of naltrexone use has shown benefit for a wide range of conditions including chronic Lyme disease and fibromyalgia. Use of low-dose naltrexone is well supported by research documented at lowdosenaltrexone.org.

Naltrexone requires a prescription from a healthcare provider. **To use low-dose naltrexone, you must be off all narcotics for at least a week.** The lowdosenaltrexone.org website regularly posts compounding pharmacies that compound it. They may be able to help you find a local provider who can see you and write a prescription.

NON-PHARMACEUTICAL DEVICES

Devices using low-intensity electrical current to modulate pain pathways have been available for almost a hundred years. The focus on drug therapy during that period, however, suppressed research on anything but drugs. Fortunately, the tide has turned, and attention is now being paid to this potentially valuable and non-invasive modality.

Transcutaneous Electrical Nerve Stimulation (TENS). A TENS unit is a battery-powered device that delivers an electrical current between two electrodes attached with sticky pads to the skin. Pulse width, frequency, and intensity of current are variable and depend on the application. In theory, the electrical impulses disrupt pain signals transmitted to the brain. Studies have shown TENS to be effective for controlling certain types of pain, including muscle pain and pain associated with migraines.

There are a wide range of TENS units available, ranging from simple, inexpensive devices available without prescription at a pharmacy or on the Internet, to more sophisticated devices available exclusively at a doctor's office.

These devices are safe and relatively inexpensive (less than $100). You should not expect total pain relief, but you may gain enough benefit to warrant the expense.

ACUPUNCTURE

This form of Traditional Chinese Medicine involves the application of very fine needles at key acupuncture points on the body. Scientific studies have documented pain relief, but results are somewhat dependent on the skills of the practitioner. Acupuncture has been associated with increased endorphin production. Best results require multiple applications regularly. Placement of the needles is not painful, and side effects are rare.

Acupuncture points on the body can also be affected by holding pressure on that spot. While acupressure is not as potent as acupuncture, learning acupressure points and performing self-acupressure regularly each day (or night) can be effective for conditions like insomnia or pain. Numerous books and Internet resources are available for learning self-administered acupressure.

19

Heroic Therapies and Other Alternatives

People have thrown everything but the kitchen sink at Lyme disease, all with the purpose of killing whatever microbe or microbes might be present. But if any one of these options worked consistently or absolutely, there wouldn't be so many possibilities, and there wouldn't be so many people searching the Internet for workable solutions.

To get well, you must do more than just kill microbes — normal immune function must be restored.

Therefore, restorative herbal therapy is your best initial approach to recovery. If steady progress is not being made, the careful addition of a heroic therapy may be reasonable. Heroic therapies are potent. And sometimes, for brief periods of time, the potency of heroic therapies can be valuable.

The biggest limitation of heroic therapies is collateral damage. Heroic therapies may kill microbes, but they may also damage tissues, suppress immune function, and disrupt the balance of the microbiome. The toxicity of heroic therapies must be respected.

For therapies focused primarily on killing microbes, the potential for killing microbes is generally proportional to the toxicity of the therapy — that is, the more potent a therapy is, the more toxic it is.

The purpose of this chapter is to explore heroic therapies that are currently being used for treatment of chronic Lyme disease or fibromyalgia. It is not meant to be an exhaustive list of all heroic therapies, but simply an introduction to the wide spectrum of different possibilities. Similarly, it is not an endorsement of any one single heroic therapy option.

CHEMICAL WARFARE

- **Synthetic antibiotics.** A lot has been said about antibiotics already. **The primary indications for synthetic antibiotics include early-phase infections, manifestations of Lyme with cardiac or neurologic symptoms, and during relapses that do not respond to natural therapy.** Long-term use of antibiotic therapy has not been documented. Synthetic antibiotics are best used intermittently along with herbal therapy continuously to keep putting pressure on microbes, but minimize toxicity of the antibiotics.

- **Synthetic antivirals.** These drugs can sometimes be beneficial for suppressing reactivation of herpes-type viruses (EBV, CMV, HHV). The class of antiviral drugs specific for herpes-type viruses includes ganciclovir/valganciclovir (primarily CMV), acyclovir (resistance is now very common), valacyclovir, and famciclovir. Limitations include difficulty in identifying symptoms associated with viral reactivation and other symptoms associated with chronic Lyme disease and fibromyalgia. Viruses reproduce much faster than bacteria, and resistance to antiviral drugs is common.

- **Vaccines.** Several attempts have been made to create a vaccine against Borrelia, but none have been successful. This isn't surprising because **Borrelia is continually changing its antigenic presentation**. Also, vaccines are species specific, and we now know there a many species of Borrelia that can cause Lyme disease.

In general, vaccines are most valuable for highly virulent microbes, such as the microbes that cause smallpox, polio, and other dreaded infectious diseases. Vaccines are much less reliable for low-virulence microbes.

- **Colloidal silver.** Historically, silver was widely used both externally and internally prior to the discovery of synthetic antibiotics in the 1940s. It does have antimicrobial properties, but not as much as synthetic antibiotics. For suppressing hidden stealth microbes, it is certainly no better than herbal therapy and offers none of the other benefits inherent to herbs. The body does not use silver for any metabolic processes and has a hard time getting rid of it. Silver builds up in tissues with regular use, resulting in blue-gray discoloration of the skin known as *argyria*. Colloidal silver is classified by the FDA as being unsafe for internal use.

- **Turpentine.** Yes, some people are actually drinking turpentine to get rid of Lyme disease, but it's not the stuff from the hardware store. The type of turpentine being used is 100% pure distilled gum spirits from pine resin. Any other type of turpentine is extremely unsafe for consumption. Though people are reporting benefit from the 100% pure product, turpentine in any form is a strong skin and mucous membrane irritant and can cause allergic reactions. Turpentine use has been associated with severe kidney and liver damage. There are better natural alternatives for overcoming Lyme disease (see Essential Oils in **Appendix A**).

OXIDATIVE THERAPY

Life requires energy, and biological life forms derive energy from breaking down hydrocarbon molecules. The energy provided by hydrocarbons alone was enough to get life started on earth, but it took the addition of oxygen for life to truly flourish on the planet. Oxygen added to the hydrocarbon reaction allows 10 times as much energy to be produced. It was the catalyst that allowed higher life forms to exist.

For oxygen to work as a catalyst, it must break down into highly reactive components. These reactive components are electron greedy and pluck electrons off hydrocarbon molecules, such as glucose. When exposed to these reactive components, the glucose molecule becomes unstable, and the chemical bonds are easily broken, thus releasing energy.

The tradeoff is that electron-greedy reactive oxygen species (the most potent type of free radical) also pluck electrons off any other molecules in the vicinity, potentially damaging all cellular structures, including cell membranes and DNA. Unconstrained free radicals can quickly destroy the cell. Therefore, all cells contain potent antioxidants (glutathione, vitamins, and other antioxidants) to gain protection and prevent destruction of the cell.

Many bacteria do not use oxygen to produce energy. Bacteria in general are more susceptible to damage by oxygen-generated free radicals. This is the basis of using different forms of oxygen free radicals to kill microbes. As such, it may be the most beneficial form of heroic therapy for Lyme disease. Even so, oxidative therapies alone are unlikely to eradicate all Borrelia microbes and/or other stealth microbes that are present. The benefits of therapy should be weighed against the risk of toxicity to tissues.

In general, heroic oxidative therapies should be reserved for occasions when restorative herbal therapy alone does not result in wellness. You may get benefit from oxidative therapies, but the benefits are unlikely to be sustained when the therapy is terminated. Long-term risks are unknown. Because these therapies are expensive and toxic to tissues, long-term use is not recommended. Restorative herbal therapy is much more likely to result in sustained long-term improvement. Therefore, if you choose to use oxidative therapies, it is best to continue restorative herbal therapies during and beyond oxidative treatments.

- **Hyperbaric oxygen.** The air we breathe is only 20% oxygen and 80% inert nitrogen gas. Pure oxygen is highly toxic to bacteria, but also tissues of the body, especially the lungs. Hyperbaric oxygen is administered by delivering 100% oxygen into a pressurized chamber.

  In a study published informally in 1998 (Fife 1998), the benefits of hyperbaric oxygen were documented in Lyme disease patients. Ninety-one participants in the study received 1 hour of hyperbaric oxygen treatments on 5 days out of 7 for an average of 145 total treatments. Eighty-five percent of the participants reported significantly decreased symptoms while undergoing therapy. There was no follow-up noted to document any long-term positive or negative effects.

  A study published in 2015 showed significant reduction of symptoms using hyperbaric oxygen therapy in a female population of fibromyalgia sufferers. This important study supports the link between fibromyalgia and stealth microbes (Efrati 2015).

- **Ozone/hydrogen peroxide.** Ozone is a molecule composed of three oxygen atoms fused together. It is an extremely reactive free radical. There is no doubt that ozone kills microbes, but it can also destroy any living tissue. Ozone gas is very effective for eradicating mold from a building, but concentrated ozone gas is very toxic to the lungs. Most mainstream medical applications include dental procedures and skin ulcer treatment.

  For Lyme disease, ozone is primarily administered dissolved in liquid solution or delivered intravenously. It is theorized that ozone presents an oxidant challenge to the body, and the body responds by increasing production of antioxidant enzymes (glutathione peroxidase, reductase, superoxide dismutase, and catalase) for an overall beneficial effect. Also in theory, bacteria, viruses, and unhealthy cells are killed, while healthy cells remain less affected. It is unknown how ozone might affect the total microbiome. Ozone can also be administered by insufflation of (blowing) ozone gas into the rectum.

Many people report significant benefit from ozone therapy, but benefits decline several weeks to months after treatment. There are no formal studies evaluating ozone therapy (either rectally or intravenously) for Lyme disease, and the short-term and long-term harmful effects are unknown at this time. Ozone therapy is not approved by the FDA and is not allowed in many states. Ozone can damage rectal and colon tissue when administered rectally and can damage veins when administered intravenously. Even so, ozone is probably a better heroic choice than long term antibiotic therapy.

Ozone naturally reacts with water vapor to form hydrogen peroxide (H_2O_2). Hydrogen peroxide is also a potent oxidant that can be used externally to clean and disinfect wounds (3% solution). Some medical clinics administer hydrogen peroxide orally and intravenously, but it should not be self-administered in this fashion. Hydrogen peroxide has similar toxicity and risks as ozone.

- **MMS.** Of all the oxidative therapies, this one is the least credible (but possibly the most reasonable from a cost standpoint). Miracle Mineral Solution (MMS) has long been championed by Jim Humble. As the story goes, while on a trip to the Amazon, he used a solution of chlorine dioxide (derived from sodium chlorite mixed with citric acid) to purify his water. He saw that others in his party who did not use the water purifier came down with malaria, and he did not. From there, he launched a campaign to promote the wonders of chlorine dioxide, which he named the Miracle Mineral Solution.

  Humble has published several books and has quite a few loyal followers. Most of his writing, however, has the ring of a snake-oil salesman. In one of his books, he actually claims that Lyme disease was hatched in a lab as a biological weapon. Humble is not a trained scientist; scientific scrutiny of the many claims made about MMS have been marginal at best. There are no published studies supporting chlorine dioxide for treating Lyme disease or anything else. Because of his often-outrageous claims, he has alienated both the scientific community and the FDA.

Critics of MMS often refer to it as "drinking bleach." It is true that drinking either straight bleach (sodium hypochlorite) or chlorine dioxide (MMS) would be extremely hazardous. But adding 1/8 teaspoon of household bleach to a gallon of water is a perfectly safe way to purify water for drinking (according to the CDC). About the same dilution of chlorine dioxide is used for purifying drinking water (and for therapy).

Unfortunately, all of the snake oil-style hype surrounding chlorine dioxide may halt ever finding out if it has any true therapeutic value. The FDA is doing everything it can to ban sale of the substance for any purpose (though it is making no effort to ban household bleach, which is no less hazardous).

In the meantime, if you decide to use MMS, know that there are no studies defining risks or benefits. It does kill microbes in water when used as a water purifier, but no one knows whether it does so in the human body. There are potentially serious harmful effects that can occur if chlorine dioxide is used in anything but minute quantities. The dose must be carefully controlled. As compared to ozone, however, it is not as strong an oxidizing agent (and may be safer).

- **Herbal therapy.** Many herbs, including Cordyceps and Rhodiola are known to improve oxygenation of tissues. Chlorella also increases delivery of oxygen to tissues. While this would not be considered heroic therapy to kill microbes, use of these herbs likely does provide a beneficial effect.

ELECTRICAL/ENERGY THERAPIES

- **Rife machine.** Royal Raymond Rife was an American inventor who, in the early 1930s, invented a "beam ray" machine that supposedly killed hidden microbes he felt were the underlying cause of certain cancers. The machine, which utilizes a DC electrical current to produce an electromagnetic wave of energy (radio frequency EMF), is tuned to the frequency of viruses and bacteria that were suspected as the underlying cause of cancer, resulting in destruction of the microbes. The device was dismissed by the medical community of the time.

  Use of the device was revived in the 1980s by the Lyme community and is sold by many companies for use in treatment of Lyme disease.

  Though Royal Rife was ahead of his time in suggesting that many chronic illnesses (including many cancers) are linked to hidden microbes, there are no clinical studies evaluating use of Rife machines for Lyme disease. There are limited scientific evaluations, however, showing benefit of radio frequency EMF in cancer treatment (Zimmerman 2013), thus validating some of Dr. Rife's work. As research in this area strengthens, more will be known about uses, capabilities, and limitations of radio frequency EMF technology.

  Whether Rife technology kills microbes is unknown. Benefits may be primarily related to reducing inflammation. Inflammation, in electrical terms, is an electron-deficient state (see Earthling later in this chapter). The "beam ray" may contribute electrons and therefore reduce inflammation in the body.

  One question today is whether Rife machines currently on the market are satisfactory for treating Lyme disease. Many Rife machines apparently are low frequency and low output compared to Dr. Rife's original machine (and as compared to

RF EMF machines used in cancer therapy). Rife machines are not approved by the FDA or any similar agency worldwide. Finding a reliable machine is not a straightforward process.

Even so, the risk of using Rife technology is low, and users of Rife technology do report benefit with regular use (though most people report only transient relief of symptoms and not being cured). The biggest risk of buying Rife technology is ending up with an expensive machine that doesn't do anything. Rife machines can run anywhere from a $1000 for a low powered machine to $4000 for a higher power machine.

- **Pulsed Electromagnetic Field (PEMF).** Similar to a Rife machine, the PEMF uses a pulsed electromagnetic AC current to generate a magnetic field of energy. While claims are made by companies selling the device that the technology kills microbes, there is no proof to support such claims. PEMF may reduce inflammation by donating electrons, possibly more so than Rife because the current is stronger. People report benefit, but benefit is transient and only related directly to treatment. Risks of use are unknown.

- **Whole-Body Hyperthermia Treatment (WHBT; raising body temperature).** Fever is the body's response to infection, and it is theorized that high temperature kills microbes (what type of microbes and whether it destroys normal flora is not defined) and unhealthy or abnormal cells. Theoretically, it also stimulates healing systems in the body. Whole-body hyperthermia treatment (WBHT) has been applied to a variety of conditions, including Lyme disease and cancer (in conjunction with chemotherapy).

The procedure is performed under general anesthesia. Body temperature is raised to between 105° and 107°F and maintained for 60-90 minutes. Typically, more than one treatment is administered, spread apart by a week or more.

Clinical studies about WBHT are available for cancer treatment and depression, but not for Lyme disease. The procedure is not FDA-approved for treating Lyme disease. People who undergo WBHT generally go to Germany to have the procedure done.

Extreme heat is a severe stress on the body. There are also risks associated with general anesthesia. It's another case of "can I kill the microbes before the treatment kills me." Though many people report feeling better after the procedure (once they recover from the procedure), that improvement is generally short lived. It is unlikely that the procedure eradicates all Borrelia microbes (or other stealth microbes). If a decision is made to undergo WBHT, it should be accompanied by comprehensive measures to boost the natural healing capacity of the body.

- **Earthing.** From a chemical point of view, inflammation is excessive free radicals produced by WBCs. Free radicals steal electrons from other molecules, thus creating damage to cellular structures. From an electrical point of view, all this stealing of electrons creates an electron-deficient state — therefore, inflammation is an electron-deficient state.

The earth is a great source of electrons. Proponents of earthing suggest that being grounded to the earth will relieve an electron-deficient state (inflammation). Grounding is done during sleep with a pad or special sheet that has been connected to the grounding wire in an electrical socket (not the electrical plug), which is connected to the ground.

There are many reports of benefit posted on the Internet, but also complaints that the sheets lose effectiveness after they are washed. The biggest risk is electrical shock during a lightning storm (though there are no reports of this yet).

You can get the same effect by walking barefoot in the grass (plastic soled shoes insulate and block transfer of electrons from the earth). You can also get electrons by breathing negative ions in air present in pine forests and by open water (most enclosed buildings, including gyms, are loaded with positive ions from toxic air, which steal electrons).

NATURAL HEROIC THERAPIES

- **Bee sting therapy.** Bee venom has been used for relief of joint pain for thousands of years. Benefits derived from bee venom are attributed to an anti-inflammatory substance called melli-tinin, which is 100x more potent than cortisone.

  Bee venom is administered as direct bee sting or injection of bee venom at the site of pain. Treatment is typically adminis-tered twice weekly. Patients with Lyme disease, fibromyalgia, or other similar chronic illnesses associated with pain have report-ed significant benefit.

  Unfortunately, **bee sting therapy has been associated with se-vere allergic reactions, severe liver toxicity, kidney damage, and myocardial infarction**. Side effects may be evident imme-diately or appear weeks after exposure.

- **Immunoglobulin.** This therapy involves transfusing immuno-globulins from another person to enhance another person's immunity. It can also be done with a specific immunoglobulin against a specific microbe. Immunoglobulin therapy has shown benefit for certain types of viral infections. There are no studies evaluating this practice for treating Lyme disease, and there is little on the Internet about patient experiences.

- **Heparin therapy.** Chronic infection with stealth microbes, es-pecially Babesia, can stimulate low grade coagulation in the body (clotting). This causes fibrin (what scars are made of) to coat the inside of blood vessels, limiting diffusion of oxygen, nutrients, and hormones such as thyroid hormone into tissues. Some integrative providers advocate use of protein-digesting enzymes such as nattokinase with heparin therapy to correct the problem. Heparin is a natural anti-coagulant that is commonly used in conventional medicine for treatment of blood clots. It is administered as a subcutaneous injection (injection just under the skin) in doses of 1000-5000 IU twice daily. The presence of low grade coagulation can be evaluated by lab studies (see **Chapter 9**, under "Coagulation Factors").

- **Stem cell therapy.** Injections of stem cells are theorized to stimulate the immune system and stimulate repair of tissues. At present, stem cell therapy is not recognized in the United States and therefore, some people travel to China, Mexico, or India for treatments. There is no evidence that stem cell therapy eradicates Borrelia or other stealth microbes. Treatments can cost as much as $40K.

  While this may prove to be a very promising therapy for Lyme disease, it's too early to tell. No formal studies have been done to evaluate the benefit of stem cell therapy in Lyme disease. The potential for adverse reactions is unknown. A study of a single patient with Crohn's disease did show benefit (Shroff 2016).

- **Fecal transplant.** *Clostridium difficile* (also known as *C. diff*) overgrowth is becoming a widespread problem in North America and Europe as a result of antibiotic overuse. Fecal implantation has proven to be effective therapy for *C. diff* overgrowth and other gut microbiome disturbances associated with intestinal disease.

  Donor stool from a healthy person is infused into the gut of the sufferer either by nasogastric tube or colonoscopy. Fecal transplant displaces the imbalanced gut flora in a symptomatic patient with the entire gut flora of another person by way of a fecal load.

The biggest concern associated with fecal transplant is the many diseases that are transmitted by fecal contamination. Though donors are screened extensively for microbial diseases and are healthy, who knows what they might be carrying without having symptoms. The FDA classifies fecal implant as an experimental procedure.

This heroic procedure may be worth considering if you end up with a terrible case of *C. diff* overgrowth that nothing else will get rid of, but otherwise, how much are you willing to trust that some other person's feces isn't carrying something you don't want?

20

Setbacks are an inevitable part of recovery. **Recovery from any chronic illness is an up-and-down process.**

Just when you think everything is turning around, you have a setback for seemingly no reason. One top of that comes the fear of slipping back into a cycle of never-ending misery. *How long will this last? Will it ever get better, or will I have to live this way for the rest of my life?*

Know this: It's just a bump in the road. Sometimes a big bump, but still just a bump, and not a mountain. You'll get back on track.

Fortunately, with time, setbacks gradually become less common and less intense. As you become better at self-analysis and self-correcting, your recovery will quicken each time. When a setback occurs, do not become mired in depression and fear; that will hold you back. Pull up your bootstraps and become proactive.

Look for causes. Everything that happens results from a cause. There are always factors that precipitate a setback. Self-reflection and a little detective work are necessary to trace out why the setback occurred. Get in the habit of going through the **list of system disruptors** looking for causes. You will generally find your answers there:

1. **Poor Nourishment.** Have you been taking excessive dietary liberties? Have you been eating on the run? Are leaky gut or food sensitivities a problem?

2. **Toxins.** Have you had higher than usual toxin exposure, such as painting a room in your house or removing mold from a bathroom with toxic chemicals? Sometimes the effects do not show up for several days. Look for any sources of added toxin exposure.

3. **Emotional Stress.** Stress is frequently the cause of a setback. Has your stress load been unusual? Are you getting enough sleep? Have you had to travel recently? Is someone else's stress causing you stress? Do you have deadlines (self-imposed or real) that are keeping your adrenaline and cortisol elevated?

4. **Physical Stress.** Often people use intense exercise as stress relief. While this can be beneficial, if the exercise is too intense, it can cause a setback. Know your limits, and do not go beyond them. Follow the 70% rule: do not exercise beyond 70% of your total capacity. This is different for every person.

5. **Oxidative Stress.** Generally, this one is harder to self-evaluate, but do you feel inflamed? The solution to this one is taking all the supplements vigilantly and following an extra-healthy diet.

6. **Destructive Energy (Radiation).** Have you been sitting by a computer or on your cell phone more than average? Have you been cooped up indoors more than usual? Have you been getting enough sun to make vitamin D, or are you taking in adequate levels of vitamin D?

7. **Microbiome Imbalance.** Have you been exposed to a new microbe? Have you had a new tick bite? Are you coming down with a cold or the flu? Are you having a Herxheimer reaction?

HERXHEIMER REACTIONS

One of the most common reasons for a setback is a Herxheimer reaction (often referred to as Herx or Herxing). The classic explanation of a Herxheimer reaction is that when bacteria are killed by antibiotic therapy, parts of dead bacteria are shed (called endotoxins), causing an intense, whole-body inflammatory reaction...but it may not be quite that simple.

Symptoms associated with chronic Lyme disease are mostly caused by the reaction of the immune system to the presence of the microbes. It amounts to a small war going on inside the body. The addition of therapy to suppress or kill microbes intensifies that war. Intensification of the immune reaction may be as much a part of it as bacterial die-off. Also, herbal or antibiotic therapy may flush microbes out of hidden niches and into the bloodstream.

The result is intensification of all symptoms, especially pain and fatigue. Though disconcerting, it is often a sign that the therapy is working.

Distinguishing a Herxheimer reaction from something else can sometimes be challenging. In general, a **Herxheimer reaction will come on within a day of starting a new therapy and will intensify as the dose is increased**.

Herxheimer reactions are classically associated with Borrelia, but they can also occur with some (but not all) types of bacteria (Mycoplasma and Bartonella are less associated with Herxing). Herxheimer reactions are generally more common with conventional antibiotic use than with the use of herbs, where the bacterial die-off is more gradual and the immune response is less intense. Herxheimer reactions are highly variable from person to person.

If Herxing is intense, back down on the dose of therapy until symptoms are tolerable. As symptoms abate, gradually increase the dose again. Follow the guidelines at the end of this chapter to reduce the intensity of the reaction.

BACTERIAL AND VIRAL FLARE-UPS

Stealth microbes are opportunists. Every time you let your guard down, they are going to take advantage of the situation. Any kind of extra stress can precipitate a flare-up. For Borrelia and Mycoplasma, common flare-up symptoms are intensification of arthritis and fatigue. Reactivation of viruses, such as Epstein-Barr virus, CMV, or other herpes-type viruses from immune suppression, can cause intense flu-like symptoms and muscle pain.

Any type of stress to your system (emotional stress, poor diet, toxins, physical stress, or chronic excessive exposure to electromagnetic (EM) devices) can disrupt immune function and cause a flare-up.

A new tick bite can also cause a bacterial flare-up. If you have tick-borne microbes, such as Borrelia, in your system, when you get bitten by a tick, the saliva from the tick rapidly circulates throughout the body and causes mobilization of bacteria to the tick site. This can cause intense symptoms.

Sometimes it's actually hard to differentiate a Herx reaction from a bacterial flare-up, but in general, a Herx reaction will start after supplements are initiated or the dose is increased; whereas, a bacterial flare-up will occur while taking a stable dose of supplements. Generally, a bacterial reaction is a reaction to some type of stress.

The solution to a bacterial flare-up is consistently taking the herbal supplements at the same dose or higher dose. Anti-inflammatory supplements can also be beneficial.

TOLERANCE TO THERAPY

When a plateau or backslide occurs while consistently taking supplements in the absence of other stress factors that could precipitate a flare-up, it may be a sign that the microbes have developed resistance to the herbs. This doesn't happen very often, but it can happen after long-term use of the same herbs (usually for years). One solution is increasing the dose of the herbs. Another (and better) solution is rotating the different herbs altogether. Fortunately, there are almost unlimited choices for other antimicrobial herbs. Essential oils are also a reasonable choice. See **Appendix A** for other herb choices and a discussion about essential oils.

ACUTE VIRAL INFECTIONS
Exposure to cold or flu-type viruses is a common affair. Most of them are mild enough that no obvious symptoms occur; a few can cause typical cold or flu symptoms. Any of them have the potential to cause a dip in your recovery.

Something else to be aware of: if herbal therapy is your primary therapy, cold and flu viruses often do not cause typical cold and flu symptoms, but instead cause a setback in recovery. It will pass with time.

FOOD REACTIONS
If the intestinal tract is inflamed, and the gut microbiome is imbalanced, reactions to foods are common. Often, they are related to foods that are consumed most commonly. Food reactions are typically delayed hours or even days and are associated with overall intensification of symptoms.

Food sensitivities will be covered in **Chapter 24,** Digestive Dysfunction.

FLU VACCINE
A flu vaccine can disrupt immune function and allow a severe flare-up, but a severe flu can certainly cause a significant setback. Whether to get a flu vaccine is an individual decision. In general, it may not be worth the risk in mild flu years, but it may be worth consideration if a severe flu season is predicted.

DRUG REACTIONS

Most drugs come with a long list of potential side effects, and many of those side effects resemble fibromyalgia symptoms. Withdrawal symptoms associated with habituation to drugs, such as benzodiazepines and sleeping pills, can be very similar to chronic Lyme disease symptoms. Symptoms are intensified if the dose of the drug (or drugs) is reduced. Symptoms are relieved if the dose of the drug is increased.

ALLERGIC REACTIONS TO HERBS OR DRUGS

True allergic reactions to supplements, foods, or drugs will generally be associated with itching skin reactions, along with intensification of other symptoms. Many people with Lyme disease have mast cell hypersensitivity, which causes enhanced allergic reactions. Often, an antihistamine, such as Claritin or Zyrtec, will provide relief. Antihistamines are one of the safer classes of medications and will not disrupt immune function.

INADEQUATE SLEEP

Most people with chronic Lyme find that sleep is very fragile. Not getting sleep will definitely set you back. Be very particular about your sleep habits, and guard your sleep time carefully. Often, it takes 9-10 hours to get 7 hours of sleep. Make sure you allow yourself plenty of time.

Note than many drugs can disrupt sleep. Many people find that tramadol, a common pain medication, causes poor sleep. Drugs such as Prozac and Zoloft also disrupt sleep in many people. **Do not use alcohol to induce sleep.** Alcohol is sedating for a couple of hours, but the metabolites of alcohol are very stimulating and will keep you awake.

TRAVEL AND/OR STRESSFUL EVENTS

Travel is especially difficult for people with Lyme disease and fibromyalgia. It can certainly cause setbacks, so avoid travel if you can.

If you must travel, try to control situations as much as you can in your favor. Rest often, and avoid unhealthy food. Be sure to take all your supplements with you. Try to make the environment around you as much like home as possible.

COMPLACENCY

It happens to the best of us: You start feeling better, and then you take more liberties with unhealthy foods and allow stress to creep back into your life. You stay up a little later at night and protect your sleep a little less. You skip supplement doses more often and forget to order refills before the supplements run out. The next thing you know, you get walloped with a huge setback. And you know why. Time to start paying attention again.

GENERAL GUIDELINES FOR SETBACKS AND RELAPSES

- If the flare-up seems like a Herx reaction, back down on the therapy dose until symptoms are tolerable. As symptoms abate, gradually increase the dose again.

- **Lots of liquids** in general are a good idea. Fresh ginger tea is a good choice because it has potent, systemic anti-inflammatory properties for reducing Herxheimer symptoms. Ginger tea is easy to make. Simply peel a large piece of ginger, thinly slice the peeled pieces, place them in large pot filled with a half-gallon of spring water, heat the water to a boil, turn off the heat, cool, strain the liquid, and sweeten with honey or stevia. It can be consumed warm or iced.

- **Vitamin C**, 500-1000 mg twice daily can help support immune function during times of excessive stress (Ester C is better tolerated than standard vitamin C).

- **Turmeric and boswellia** are excellent for reducing systemic inflammation associated with Herxheimer reactions. These two important anti-inflammatory substances can be found in combination supplements for joint health. It's hard to take too much. Consider adding a teaspoon of turmeric (found in any grocery store in the spice aisle) to smoothies.

- **Enzymes that digest proteins** help break down immune complexes and reduce inflammation. There are a variety of different enzymes that will work, including enzyme supplements used for digestion. Bromelain (from pineapple) is a good choice. The dose is 500-1000 mg, one to two times daily. Bromelain is sometimes found in combination supplements for joint health including turmeric and boswellia.

- **Marine-source omega-3 fatty acids** offer anti-inflammatory support, especially for high-fat tissues, such as the brain. Both fish oil and krill oil reduce inflammation, but krill is better absorbed and also contains the antioxidant astaxanthin, which provides extra anti-inflammatory support.

- **Red root** is an herb that is very good for stimulating the clearing of dead cellular debris from the lymphatic system. It also helps reduce inflammation in the liver and spleen. Support of the spleen is very important for infections with Babesia. Red root also supports optimal immune function. Red root is especially indicated for swollen lymph nodes. It can help alleviate Herxheimer reactions.

  Generally, red root is obtained as a 1:5 tincture dosed at 30 drops three to four times daily. Use only during acute events, and discontinue when symptoms subside. Red root increases blood coagulation and should be avoided by anyone with a history of a clotting disorder. (See **Appendix A** for additional information.)

- **Heat can be very soothing** during Herxheimer reactions. A far infrared (FIR) sauna is a practical way to apply whole-body heat, but a hot bath will also do nicely. A FIR sauna is also excellent for removing toxins from the body and boosting immune function. (See **Chapter 21**, Turn up the Heat on Your Recovery!)

- **Standard anti-inflammatory medications**, such as ibuprofen and naproxen, can be beneficial, but these medications should not be used long term.

- **Cannabidiol oil (CBD)** can be beneficial for controlling pain and also boosts immune function (see **Chapter 18**).

- Go down the list and try to **minimize any potential system disruptors** than could be contributing to the setback.

- If your diet has not been optimal, review the guidelines in **Chapter 24**, Digestive Dysfunction. This should help identify and eliminate food sensitivities as a cause. If food sensitivities are a problem, be especially careful with those foods during a setback.

- **Take herbal supplements regularly**. Adaptogenic herbs especially will help reduce Herx reactions and moderate the effects of stress. Herbs also contain potent anti-inflammatory substances that can help resolve a setback. (Reduce herbs that are primarily antimicrobial during a suspected Herx reaction.)

- **Get outside and breathe fresh air**. Forests and beaches/shores along open water are especially beneficial. Take your shoes off, and walk barefoot. "Grounding" is a good practice for reducing inflammation in your body.

- **Meditation and relaxation** are important for normalizing the adrenaline/cortisol response.

- Make sure that you **allow for plenty of sleep**.

- **Make your world small.** Take care of absolute necessities, and let everything else go until you are back on your feet.

- **Generate endorphins.** Endorphins suppress pain and enhance immune function, which will help break you out of a setback. Any type of exercise generates endorphins, but **regular practice of Qigong or yoga** is one of the best ways to work through a setback and keep endorphins flowing. If exercise on any level is not practical, FIR sauna is another way to generate endorphins.

- **Massage, acupuncture, and energy healing** can be very beneficial for working through a setback.

- **Having a plan and being proactive reduces fear**, which, in itself can help overcome a setback. Sometimes you have to do multiple things intensely to break free and get back on track.

- For a **persistent bacterial flare-up, when nothing else seems to work**, some form of oxidative therapy (hyperbaric oxygen, ozone), in combination with continued herbal therapy, may be your best bet. MMS would be considered "poor man's oxidative therapy;" if you cannot afford other options (note that risks are unknown). A short course of synthetic antibiotics is another option that can sometimes help you break free and get you back on course.

21

Turn up the Heat on Your Recovery!

Brief episodes of elevated body temperature may inhibit microbe reproduction and enhance the effectiveness of therapy. Elevated body temperature is one natural way your body fights infection (fever).

For some people, increased body temperature helps alleviate Herxheimer reactions. Raising your body temperature results in increased blood flow and sweating, which both help to **remove toxins from your body and stimulate endorphin secretion.** The best part? It feels good.

The simplest way to measure body temperature is a thermometer in your mouth or under your arm (raising your body temperature to above 100° F, but never above 102° F for 10-20 minutes daily is often the recommended target). For techies, a few products designed for monitoring body functions include skin temperature and heart rate. Expect to pay around $100-200 for these types of devices.

Far-infrared sauna (FIR) is possibly the most precise way to raise your body temperature. Temperature of the sauna can be very specifically regulated, such that it can be gradually increased as tolerance to heat improves. FIR sauna is dry, which tends to be better tolerated by Lyme disease and fibromyalgia patients than a steam sauna. FIR sauna is backed by scientific studies demonstrating **removal of toxins, including**

heavy metals, from the body. In fact, it may be the safest and most efficient way of removing heavy metals from the body.

On the positive side, **raising body temperature with FIR sauna may suppress microbes, enhance immune function, stimulate endorphin production, and remove toxins via sweat.** On the other hand, intense heat is a significant stress factor. You must balance benefit with the potential for harm. This can differ from person to person; it really depends on your state of health and stamina.

Start with short episodes of less intense heat, and gradually build up as your stamina improves. The time period for this to happen varies widely. Don't overdo it! Whether you do it daily or less frequently is up to you. Most people find that they progress faster if the sauna is done less intensely, but consistently on a daily basis when possible. A starting goal is 30 minutes per session.

If you do not have access to a sauna, **a hot bath can provide a similar effect.** The addition of **Epsom salts** (magnesium sulfate salts) may enhance detoxification. For a hot bath, it is best to get into the tub before turning on the water. Start with warm water and gradually increase the heat as your body acclimates.

The ultimate heat treatment (and also the most expensive) is the **Migun thermal bed**. This sophisticated device combines heat, massage, and acupressure to treat the entire body. The device is FDA-approved, and the company claims it provides relief for chronic pain and muscle tension. For a less pricey option, the company also makes several versions of thermal mats that provide localized heat and acupressure.

If your health is significantly compromised, you should discuss using sauna or hot baths with your healthcare provider. Excessive heat is a stress factor, and you should **work up to an elevated body temperature very**

slowly. If you feel stressed or dizzy, you should exit the sauna or hot bath immediately.

Once your health rebounds, **moderate exercise** is another way to favorably raise body temperature, improve blood flow, and induce sweating. It is the best natural way to stimulate endorphins. Regular exercise can gradually replace the need for sauna or regular hot baths.

Hot yoga is an excellent way to step back into exercise. This variation of yoga is performed in a hot environment. Temperatures vary from 85° to 110° F. Heat induces sweating, which removes toxins from the body. Heat also relaxes and soothes sore muscles. Many patients with chronic Lyme disease or fibromyalgia report decreased fatigue and pain with regular practice of hot yoga. Care, of course, must be taken not to get overheated. Start with a brief exposure at lower temperatures. Stop the session if you start to feel bad. Some days are going to be better than others. Never exceed more than an hour of exposure.

In every case, make sure you drink plenty of clean filtered water!

22

Understanding Biofilm

Though there's been a lot of talk about it in Lyme communities, you may not understand exactly what it is and how it fits into the picture of chronic Lyme disease. And some of what you have heard may be counterproductive to your recovery. This chapter covers everything you need to know about biofilm for your recovery.

WHAT EXACTLY IS A BIOFILM?

Biofilms are colonies of microbes. They chiefly contain bacteria, but biofilms can also include viruses, protozoa, and fungi. Biofilms can form anywhere there is moisture and a surface. In other words, everywhere, including many surfaces inside the human body.

The ring inside your toilet bowl and plaque on your teeth are examples of biofilm.

Biofilms are initiated by certain types of bacteria that are able to attach to a moist surface with special adhesion structures called **pili**. Once adhered to the surface, bacteria stick together and begin producing a matrix of a substance called an extracellular polymeric substance (EPS), otherwise known as slime. Once the matrix is established, other kinds of microbes can join in.

Imagine a crowded dance floor with bodies squeezed together forming a uniform mass swaying to the rhythm of the music. That's the feel of a biofilm.

A polysaccharide shell on the surface of the biofilm protects the organisms inside from starvation, drying out, the immune system, and antibiotics. The surface can include minerals, such as calcium, and blood products, including fibrin.

Safe inside the biofilm, microbes are free to mingle and exchange information. Communication between microbes, called quorum sensing, is accomplished by signaling molecules. Once a community is formed, certain groups of microbes take on specialized roles of performing metabolic functions for the entire unit. Water channels develop within the biofilm for moving nutrients and signaling molecules. The biofilm grows by cell division and recruitment of new individuals.

In essence, the biofilm becomes an organism in itself.

Biofilms are as ancient as any lifeform. They were likely the bridge between single-cell organisms and complex multicellular organisms.

The immune system of the human body is well adapted to dealing with biofilms. Someone with a healthy immune system will not need to be concerned about biofilm (except for needing teeth cleaning a couple of times a year).

Biofilms that occur in the intestinal tract are actually important for normal health. Intestinal biofilms protect the lining of the gut. Biofilms in the colon and appendix are supported by the immune system and play a role in re-inoculating the gut with favorable bacteria. Prolonged antibiotic use and heroic therapies, such as rectal ozone, break down protective biofilms in the gut.

COMMON BIOFILM DISEASES
Chronic immune dysfunction is a prerequisite for forming threatening biofilms in the body. If immune function is compromised, biofilm can form on surfaces in the body.

Typical biofilm diseases occur where there are surfaces for biofilm to form. Surfaces that can harbor biofilm in the body include teeth, heart valves, intestinal lining, sinuses and bronchial airways, bladder, vagina, brain ventricles, and synovial lining of joints. Biofilm damages the surface and causes localized symptoms where the biofilm forms (sinusitis is a good example).

Common biofilm illnesses include bacterial vaginosis (bacterial vaginal infection), chronic urinary tract infections, chronic sinusitis and chronic bronchitis, and middle ear infections in children. Chronic vertigo caused by calcium deposits in the inner ear may be a form of biofilm. Dental plaque and gingivitis are classic examples of biofilm. Arterial plaques causing heart attacks and stroke have many characteristics of biofilm and are often found to harbor bacteria. Heart valve infections are biofilms. Hospital infections involving indwelling devices, such as catheters, are associated with biofilms.

If a biofilm becomes massive enough, it can cause obstruction (a plaque inside an artery). Once a biofilm reaches a certain size, it disperses, allowing inhabitants to spread and colonize other surfaces. Spreading biofilms accelerate damage. Bacteria in the body are constantly trying to form new biofilms, and the immune system is constantly breaking them down.

BIOFILM AND LYME DISEASE

Contrary to a popular dialogue going on in the Lyme community, **Lyme disease is *not* primarily a biofilm disease**. The thought that it is comes from a study showing that Borrelia *could* form a biofilm in a test tube. This isn't very remarkable, however. Biofilm formation is Bacteria Survival 101. **Many bacteria, including Borrelia, can form biofilm under just the right circumstances.**

What happens in a test tube, however, is very different from what happens inside a living body. Symptoms of Lyme disease are caused by the bacteria manipulating the immune system to generate inflammation. It invades tissues directly and lives inside cells. Inflammation breaks down tissues and allows the bacteria to access vital nutrients. This causes typical Lyme symptoms (fatigue, brain fog, pain, etc.).

When it comes to biofilms in the body, it wouldn't be surprising to find that Borrelia often joins the party, but **once inside the biofilm, it would be less active in manipulating immune functions and causing symptoms.**

Immune dysfunction caused by Borrelia, however, *could* allow biofilms generated by other bacteria to flourish. This may be a factor in intestinal disease that commonly accompanies Lyme disease and skin diseases sometimes associated with Lyme disease. Dizziness that is common with Lyme disease may be related to biofilm formation with calcium deposits in the inner ear (but probably caused by other bacteria).

As to whether biofilms prevent antibiotics from eliminating Borrelia, other factors previously mentioned (slow growth, isolated locations, intracellular) possibly play a greater role in allowing antibiotic resistance. Biofilm may also be a factor, but determining how much is very hard to define.

The primary places where biofilms may be a concern in Lyme disease are joints, skin, and the brain. Damage to joint linings may be aggravated by formation of biofilm (involving Borrelia and other microbes). Biofilm is also a factor in chronic skin conditions associated with Lyme disease. Borrelia has also been found in amyloid plaque (basically a biofilm in the brain) associated with Alzheimer's (Allen 2016). When biofilms form in Lyme disease, it suggests a high level of chronic immune dysfunction.

HOW TO OVERCOME BIOFILMS
Though Lyme disease is not primarily a biofilm disease, it is a good idea to support the body's ability to deal with biofilms during any illness.

A healthy immune system is the best way to slow formation of biofilm in the body. The immune system is constantly breaking down new biofilms that start to form. It's part of the everyday struggle of life.

Any **herbal therapies** with antimicrobial and immune-enhancing properties are beneficial for controlling biofilm. This may be the most important thing you can do for preventing biofilms from being a problem.

Essential oils can be beneficial for breaking down biofilms in nasal and sinus cavities. Eucalyptus and thyme oils are good choices administered by aromatherapy (See **Appendix A**).

Protein-digesting enzymes can help break down biofilm in the gut. They may also help break down other biofilms in the body. There are many protein-digesting enzymes. The ones most widely available in supplement form include bromelain, serrapeptidase, and nattokinase.

Monolaurin is thought to help break up biofilm (mentioned in **Chapter 16**). Because monolaurin is fat soluble, it penetrates into brain tissue.

N-acetyl cysteine (NAC) is known to break up mucous and may also play a role in dissolving biofilm.

EDTA, a chelating agent, is commonly recommended for breaking down biofilms. It removes minerals from the biofilm surface and can help break up a biofilm, but it can also remove essential minerals from the body at large. EDTA enemas may break down beneficial biofilms in the gut. Therefore, it may not be the best choice for use in chronic Lyme disease.

Oxygen and nitric oxide penetrating into the biofilm can help degrade the biofilm. Oxygen therapies, especially rectal ozone, however, also break down beneficial biofilms in the colon.

Blasting biofilms with strong chemicals and potent antibiotics doesn't work because it suppresses immune function. Supporting healthy immune function and etching away until the biofilms are gone is the best approach.

PART FOUR
Essential Support

Mindset for Getting Well

It's not uncommon for people to go from one therapeutic option to another, always getting better for a while, only to inevitably slide backward again into a life of misery. This is especially true with heroic options, but it can also happen with natural therapy.

Stealth microbes win by persistence; they have an uncanny ability to hang on. As long as immune function is depressed, they can keep coming back. Every time the pressure lets up, they gradually gain ground again until you're back where you started.

The only way to win is by restoring robust immune function. Herbs do a much better job of restoring immune function than any other therapy, but sometimes taking herbs alone is not enough.

Everything you've done up until this point has been mostly passive — you take something or have something done to you. To truly get well, you must play an active role in your recovery.

It's a matter of reining in those system disruptors to take the pressure off the immune system and allowing it to rebound. Natural killer cells must be boosted, and other immune functions must be normalized.

There are four primary areas to focus on: 1) Poor diet and gut problems can definitely hold you back. 2) Toxins and radiation, both natural and unnatural, can inhibit immune function enough to prevent full recovery. 3) Excessive stress is the worst type of immune depressant. 4) The wrong approach to exercise or not moving enough can strongly inhibit your recovery.

Being proactive is something you have to put your mind to. It's not going to happen unless you make it happen. No one else can do it for you.

You have to take ownership of your situation. Taking ownership means taking on responsibility and risk. It's natural, however, to put this kind of responsibility off on someone else's shoulders; that way, if failure occurs, it's their fault and not yours.

But to get well, you must get beyond the fear of failure. No one knows your situation better than you do. And no one is more capable than you are. You don't have to go it alone, but you must take responsibility for your own well-being.

You must do everything in your power to boost your immune function and stimulate healing within your body.

The next section of the book is devoted to helping you take a proactive approach to your recovery. Intestinal dysfunction, food sensitivities, and intestinal bacterial imbalances are common factors that can hold back progress. **Chapter 24** defines why gut dysfunction occurs, and **Chapter 25** provides a detailed protocol for overcoming gut dysfunction.

Chapter 26 provides guidelines for cleaning up your living environment and purging toxins from your body. This is more about optimizing detoxification for the long haul than doing a week-long detox. The negative effects of unnatural electromagnetic radiation are also addressed.

For some people, mold and mycotoxins are the two main factors preventing wellness from occurring. **Chapter 27** will help you determine if mold is an issue in your recovery.

You can't get rid of all stress in your life, but you must learn to work around it. **Chapter 28** addresses the role that stress plays in recovery. Adrenals, thyroid, and menopause/andropause are discussed.

You have to move to get well. Move too much and you increase inflammation and cause damage that can hold you back. The key is moving just enough every day to generate endorphins and boost natural killer cells. **Chapter 29** will tell you how to do it just right.

MAKING IT HAPPEN

Creating an optimal environment for healing within your body is not an overnight transformation. It's something that you grow into gradually. Your situation is different from everyone else's, and therefore it may require different solutions. The sooner you get started, however, the sooner you can get back to living a normal life.

Get organized. After reading the chapters in this section, make a list of factors in your life that may be roadblocks to getting well. Define them in terms of degree of difficulty in solving the problem. You may want to tackle the easy things first. Chip away at the big ones to solve them over time.

Gather your resources. You don't have to go at this alone. Rely on people who you can trust. Friends and family can help. Help them understand how to best help you. Give them direction. The healthcare community and online support groups are always there for you. Just be careful about using other people and other outlets as a place to chronically complain. A negative attitude and complaining will get you nowhere.

Think positively. A positive attitude generates endorphins and enhances immune function. You can't afford to be negative. Start every day with the attitude that you are going to get well and get your life back!

Be patient, but persistent. The entire transformation can take years, but every year can be better than the last. You don't have to stop improving. Generally, most people who embrace a healthful approach to life find that their lives are enriched by it in unexpected ways. People who overcome chronic illnesses like chronic Lyme are more centered and less tied to the superficial trappings of life.

Don't get discouraged. Every day isn't going to be great, and some days are going to be awful. There will be setbacks and relapses. Every time it happens, you must gather your resources and start moving forward again. Strive to make every day better than the last.

Keep pressure on the microbes. Natural therapies, such as herbs and essential oils, are the best way to keep constant pressure on the microbes. Constantly pushing them down while your immune system is recovering is essential for winning in the long run. Occasionally, short courses of antibiotics may be necessary to break free from a setback.

Make your world small. Try to condense your world down to your immediate needs. All that should matter are things that directly affect your recovery.

Live in the present. What happened yesterday or what might happen tomorrow has little significance on your recovery. Try to unplan your life and unplug yourself from schedules and obligations as much as possible. It's hard to do, but it may be more important for your recovery than anything else.

Reduce the stress of everyday life. To overcome invisible threats that are the root of chronic illness, you must reduce perceived threats and learn not to be driven or consumed by conflict. Let things roll off your shoulders as much as possible.

Limit stress associated with work as much as possible. Applying for complete disability is generally not necessary, but limiting the demands of work as much as possible should help your recovery. This may mean cutting back on certain luxuries and expenses, but it will pay off in the long run. The more time you can call your own, the better. A long-term goal may be changing the way you work.

Put your bills on automatic. Have monthly bills placed on direct withdrawal. Pay your daily expenses with a credit card. Stick to a budget. Absolutely do not spend more than what you can pay off at the end of the month. Having to pay the bank interest on an overextended credit card is the worst type of financial stress. If you are already financially overextended, work with a financial planner, and do whatever it takes to overcome the situation — and don't ever get into that situation again.

Keep moving forward...you can be well again!

24

Digestive Dysfunction

For many people, one of the biggest roadblocks to becoming well is digestive dysfunction. It seems to go hand in hand with many chronic disease processes. Without normal digestion, absorption of critical nutrients and removal of toxins is compromised. The digestive system is intricately connected with every other system in the body. When digestion suffers, nothing works well.

Your recovery cannot move forward until you restore normal digestive function.

This chapter is devoted to helping you understand the factors that cause digestive dysfunction, how these factors come together to disrupt digestive function, and what to do about it.

IS LECTIN-LOADED FOOD MAKING YOU SICK?

Lectins are not something you hear much about. Maybe that is because they affect so many foods people enjoy. Most nutrition books and books on intestinal health don't even mention lectins. Even so, lectins are a topic that anyone with any sort of digestive issue should be paying attention to.

What are Lectins?

Lectins are specialized proteins present in *all* plants and plant seeds. They work as a deterrent against creatures consuming the plant or the seeds. They cause harm by binding to carbohydrate molecules present in cell membranes in the gut. This disrupts the cell membranes and irritates the gut lining.

Of course, humans have been eating plants for a long time (but less so with seeds). And, not surprisingly, humans have a natural protection built in. The lining of the gut is coated with a protective barrier of specialized carbohydrate molecules, better known as mucus. The carbohydrate molecules act as decoys that neutralize the plant lectins.

High concentrations of lectins disrupt the mucous barrier and damage the intestinal lining. The barrier contains friendly microbes and can be considered a form of biofilm, so chronic use of antibiotics also break down the barrier and allow the intestinal lining to be damaged.

The primary sources of problematic lectins include:

- Grains, especially wheat and corn
- Beans/legumes, especially soybeans, kidney beans, black beans, and peanuts
- Tree nuts, such as almonds, pecans, walnuts, cashews, and pistachios
- Nightshade vegetables, including tomatoes, potatoes, eggplant, and peppers
- Dairy from cows raised on corn and soybeans

Lectins: The Same Thing as Gluten?
Though both lectin proteins and gluten proteins have potential to damage the gut lining, they are not the same. Lectin proteins are found in the outer protective covering of the seed, called bran (whole grain products are actually higher in lectins).

Gluten is a plant storage protein found in the endosperm of a seed. The purpose of gluten is storing amino acids necessary for the sprouting of a seed. Because plant storage proteins are of different structure than animal proteins, they are typically hard to digest and very irritating to the intestinal tract of animals. All seeds contain storage proteins, but gluten proteins are the most irritating.

Gluten is actually not one protein but, instead, a family of proteins. Exclusive to wheat and grains related to wheat (rye, barley, kamut/ancient forms of wheat), gluten provides the stickiness that allows bread to rise. Gliadin, a component of gluten found only in wheat (not barley or rye), is the most reactive protein of all.

Because fluffy bread is so desirable, modern wheat has been specifically cultivated for high gluten concentrations. Modern gluten proteins are highly allergenic (allergy-causing). Not surprisingly, wheat gluten is notoriously hard on the digestive tract (think eating glue). **Most people do not tolerate wheat in any significant amount**.

Other Seed Hazards

Beyond glutens and lectins, grains, beans, and nuts contain phytate (phytic acid). Phytic acid is present in the seed to store phosphorus for the growing plant. This molecule also binds to minerals, such as calcium, iron, and zinc, and prevents absorption by the body when consumed. While this is not an extreme food hazard, it is something to take note of.

Excessive Carbohydrates

You would think that with all the associated problems, seeds would never have become a primary food source for humans. But seeds are a ready and reliable source of the one necessity of life that stands out over all others: energy. No other natural foods supply raw energy like seeds.

Seeds can also be easily cultivated and store well for long periods of time. Cultivation of seeds was the primary factor that propelled expansion of human civilization. Grains and beans were especially attractive because of high concentrations of starch.

Nothing on earth tempts our taste buds like starch and sugar. As a result, the modern food supply is loaded with sugar from sugar cane and starches from grain, beans, and potatoes. Excessive carbohydrate consumption **causes insulin resistance, disrupts hormone systems** in the body, and **suppresses immune function**. If it goes on long enough, diabetes is inevitable.

Beyond contributing to an epidemic of diabetes, the types of carbohydrates present in grains and beans feed abnormal bacteria in the gut. **This not only causes overgrowth of bacteria, but also stimulates growth of disease-causing bacteria (pathogens) in the gut.** Overgrowth of pathogens damages the intestinal lining and contributes to the vicious cycle of digestive dysfunction. Excessive carbohydrates may also provide a fuel source of opportunistic microbes that cause many chronic illnesses.

Fortunately, Nature Provides Exceptions
Rice is an exceptional grain. The storage proteins in rice are much less allergenic than glutens and other storage proteins. Rice lectins are much less irritating to the intestinal tract, and white rice is very low in lectins (lectins are present in the outer bran, which is removed in white rice, but present in brown rice). The starches in white rice are rapidly broken down and absorbed into the bloodstream. Therefore, white rice (in reasonable quantities) does not contribute to overgrowth of bacteria in the gut. When a caloric source of energy is required beyond vegetables and lean meat, white rice is possibly the best choice.

MORE FOOD HAZARDS TO AVOID
Goitrogens
These substances block thyroid function by interfering with iodine uptake. There are many foods that are mild goitrogens, but the primary ones to know about are **cruciferous vegetables, soy and soy products**

(including fermented soy), peanuts, and strawberries**. Generally, the effect is mild and mostly a concern only to people with poorly controlled thyroid disease. Goitrogens are reduced in food by steaming and boiling. Wheat gluten is not labeled as a goitrogen, but it is also closely linked to autoimmune thyroid disease.

Mycotoxins (Mold)

Mycotoxins are toxins produced by fungi (molds) growing on food. There are many varieties of mold that can grow on food. **Any vegetables or fruit beyond the fresh stage can grow mold, even in the refrigerator**. **Peanuts and mushrooms** are notorious for harboring toxin-producing fungi. **All dairy products, with the exception of cultured dairy** (yogurt, kefir), grow fungi rapidly. Cottage cheese contains the highest concentration of mold toxins.

Produced by **black mold, the most notorious mold toxin is trichothecene**. Black mold is a common problem in moist areas of homes and workplaces, but trichothecene toxins are also produced by a fungus that **commonly contaminates wheat, corn, and oats**.

People who have become sensitive to black mold from exposure at home or at work will be especially sensitive to mold growing in foods.

Toxic Fat

Fat (oil) is not only something you ingest as an energy source; it literally becomes part of you. The membranes surrounding each of the trillions of cells in your body are made of fat. **Any fats or oils that you consume end up in your cell membranes**.

Polyunsaturated oils from vegetable sources (corn, soybean) are particularly susceptible to damage by high heat (frying or high temperatures used in processing). Heating polyunsaturated oil to high temperature also creates *trans* fats, a type of fat that disrupts cell membranes. When consumed, damaged oil particles are laced into the membranes of all cells in the body. Damaged oil particles are **potent free radicals that set off destructive chain reactions in cell membranes** — certainly not how you want to treat your cell membranes!

Monounsaturated oils, such as olive, sesame, and avocado, are less susceptible (but not immune) to this process. Therefore, these oils are preferred in cooking and preparing food. Even monounsaturated oils, however, can be damaged by high heat. High temperatures on the stove should never be used when cooking with vegetable oil. **When purchasing oils, make sure they have been minimally refined (no chemicals used in processing) and cold-pressed (it will say so on the bottle).**

Saturated oil is the least susceptible to damage by high heat causing free-radical formation. The most well-known vegetable source of saturated fat is **coconut oil**. Unlike saturated fat from animal sources, which consists of long chains of fat, coconut oil contains saturated fat of only medium length. Called **medium-chain triglycerides (MCTs)**, these fats are burned immediately for energy and have lower potential to cause arterial plaques. Coconut oil also contains fats that suppress viruses (monolaurin).

The saturated fat found in red meat (beef, pork) occurs in long chains. The potential for harm associated with saturated fat is dose-related. **In low concentrations, saturated fat is anti-inflammatory and stabilizes cell membranes in the body.** When consumed in excessive amounts, however, saturated fats make cell membranes stiff and inflexible. They also thicken blood (think lard mixed in water), which can contribute to arterial plaque formation. Grain-fed beef and (especially) pork are excessively fatty. Undigested animal fat stimulates growth of certain types of unfavorable bacteria in the colon (called putrefaction dysbiosis), causing odorous flatulence and increasing risk of colon cancer.

Grain-fed beef and pork are also very high in inflammatory omega-6 fatty acids. Omega-6 fatty acids are cousins to omega-3 fatty acids. Omega-3 fatty acids reduce inflammation, and omega-6 fatty acids promote inflammation. You need a balance of both to be healthy. **Corn and corn-fed meat are particularly high in omega-6 fatty acids**. Regular consumption tips the balance toward inflammation in the body. Grass-fed meat has higher concentrations of omega-3 fatty acids.

Before you decide to become a vegetarian, however, know that **animal-source protein is the least allergenic and best tolerated of all protein sources**. The trick to gaining the most benefit with the least amount of harm depends on the source of meat chosen.

Fish and seafood are top choices (especially wild caught) because of the high levels of omega-3 fatty acids. These special fats reduce inflammation in the body and protect cell membranes.

Poultry (chicken, turkey, eggs) is next on the list with a blend of polyunsaturated and saturated fats. Pasture-raised is preferred, however, in both poultry and eggs. Corn-fed, hormone-injected chickens are plump and inexpensive sources of protein, but are unhealthy. Antibiotic use in the industry is heavy, and most poultry meat is now contaminated with antibiotic-resistant bacteria (all poultry and eggs should be thoroughly cooked before consumption).

A small amount of animal-source dietary saturated fat may actually be a good thing. Low concentrations of saturated fat (accompanied by a mostly vegetarian diet) are favorable for cell membrane health, reduce inflammation, and provide a favorable balance of omega fatty acids. Occasionally (two to four times per month), putting pasture-fed (beef, bison) or wild sources (elk, venison) of lean red meat on the table is a reasonable protein choice. Portions matter, however; 6 ounces (the size of a deck of cards) is enough to meet daily protein requirements.

Meat from animals raised on small farms with open pastures or wild-caught fish and seafood are the best choices.

Problems with Dairy

Dairy carries multiple concerns. Many people do not have adequate enzymes to break down the primary sugar in milk called lactose. **Lactose intolerance** contributes to intestinal discomfort, gas and bloating, and loose stools when dairy is consumed.

Casein proteins in milk are as difficult to digest as gluten; they irritate the gut and are highly allergenic. Whey proteins, which make up 20% of milk proteins, are generally well tolerated (protein powders made from fractionated whey protein are tolerated well by most people).

Grain-fed dairy also contains lectins from the grains. Toxins, hormones, and antibiotics are also commonly used in industrial milk production. In addition, dairy products (other than fermented dairy) are **more apt to grow toxin-producing fungus than any other food source** (cottage cheese, again, is the worst).

The best tolerated dairy products include fermented dairy (yogurt, kefir) and ghee (clarified butter used for cooking). Hard cheese, such as parmesan, is generally well tolerated in small amounts.

Alpha-gal Allergy

Alpha-gal allergy is an allergic reaction to a carbohydrate called Galactose-alpha-1,3-galactose. The carbohydrate is present in tick saliva of the Lone star ticks (and other ticks) that have been feeding on mammals. Alpha-gal is found in all mammals, with the exception of old world monkeys, apes, and humans. Tick bites transferring this carbohydrate in saliva can sensitize the individual to alpha-gal. Once sensitized, the individual will have an allergic reaction anytime red meat is consumed. Poultry and fish do not cause allergic reactions.

Artificial Toxins in Food

Pesticides and herbicides are heavily used in agriculture. These substances are concentrated in thin-skinned vegetables and fruits, such as berries and tomatoes, but are less of the problem in thick-skinned vegetables, such as watermelon. Beyond agricultural toxins, processed food products are loaded with artificial preservatives and coloring agents.

Grain-fed livestock not only contains agricultural toxins from the grain, but also **hormones and drugs** used during the life of the animal. These toxins are concentrated in the fatty tissues of the animal. Excessively fatty meat contains higher concentrations of toxins. Heavy use of antibiotics in the livestock industry creates antibiotic-resistant pathogens that commonly contaminate meat (especially chicken).

Food toxins place extra pressure on the liver and have a negative effect on digestion overall.

Beyond toxins found in food, many drugs inhibit digestive function:

- **Acid-inhibiting drugs**, commonly used for reflux and stomach complaints, inhibit digestion of proteins and slow gastric emptying.

- **Sedative drugs and narcotic pain medications** inhibit the movement of food material through the intestinal tract.

- **Non-steroidal anti-inflammatory drugs (NSAIDs)**, such as ibuprofen and naproxen compromise the protective barrier in the stomach and promote inflammation and ulceration of the lining of the stomach.

- **Antibiotic therapy** destroys normal flora in the gut, allowing overgrowth of disease-causing bacteria and yeast. This suppresses immune function and allows low-virulence microbes to flourish.

- **Antifungal drugs** are notorious for compromising normal liver function.

DETAILS OF DIGESTIVE DYSFUNCTION

A Recipe for Digestive Dysfunction

Spoon in lectin-loaded food laced with other food hazards, three times a day. Snack on gluten products loaded with plenty of sugar for good measure. Top it off with a generous dose of chronic tension that comes with everyday life. And be sure to eat on the run.

Chronic stress and eating on the run make a bad situation worse. Stress slows movement of food through the intestinal tract. **Food materials stagnate and sour**. This compounds the erosive properties of lectins, gluten, and other food hazards.

Digestive Problems Start in the Stomach

When stomach emptying is compromised, the erosive properties of lectin-loaded processed foods strip away the protective barrier of the stomach lining. Irritated and inflamed, the stomach lining becomes susceptible to infection from microbes, such as Mycoplasma and *H. pylori*.[1] **This is how ulcers form**.

The normal flow of digestive enzymes and acid is also inhibited. Everything gets backed up. **Reflux, heartburn, and chronic stomach discomfort are the inevitable result**.

Without acid and enzymes, proteins are not properly digested. Most proteins in foods are foreign to the body. If not properly broken down by the digestive process, food proteins can stimulate an allergic response.

Processed food and chronic stress also inhibit bile flow in the liver and gallbladder. Bile is necessary for digestion of fat. It is also the vehicle for

---

1 Many doctors consider H. pylori to be the primary cause of stomach ulcers. H. pylori microbes, however, are normal flora in 40% of the population. Infection with H. pylori associated with ulcers occurs only if the protective lining of the stomach has been disrupted by other factors. If those factors are not addressed, ulcers will recur, despite antibiotic therapy.

carrying neutralized toxins out of the body. **Inhibited bile flow leads to liver congestion, retention of toxins, gallbladder dysfunction, formation of gallstones, and poor digestion of fat**.

Small Intestinal Bacterial Overgrowth (SIBO)

Processed food products are loaded with starch and sugar — much more than the body can use or absorb. Additionally, wheat and corn are loaded with starches that are not broken down and absorbed by the body. Excess sugar and starches are fodder for intestinal bacteria.

Undigested starches and sugars **stimulate overgrowth of bacteria in the small intestine** (concentrations of bacteria in the small intestine are normally very low). Fermentation of starches and sugar by bacteria causes symptoms of bloating and trapped gas. Bacterial overgrowth compromises the protective barrier of the intestine. This process is referred to as Small Intestinal Bacterial Overgrowth.

Starches and sugars also **stimulate growth of yeast**. Yeast is always present in the intestines, but growth is normally inhibited by friendly bacteria. The presence of undigested carbohydrates allows yeast to flourish. Yeast overgrowth is also toxic to the intestinal lining and intensifies immune dysfunction.

Once the outer barrier is stripped away, **intestinal cells are left unprotected**. Lectins and other proteins, such as gluten, are then able to attach to and disrupt cell membranes of intestinal cells. Microvilli, the microscopic finger-like protrusions covering the surface of intestinal cells, are destroyed, and the **ability of the cells to absorb vital nutrients is compromised**.

This **damage can be intensified by stealth pathogens** — Mycoplasma is notorious for destroying intestinal villi. Even normal friendly flora are opportunists. Once the barrier is down, intestinal microbes can infect intestinal cells and cause damage.

Leaky Gut
Once the intestinal lining (mucosa) has been totally compromised, undigested foreign proteins (including lectins and other plant proteins not broken down by normal digestion) **leak into the bloodstream in high concentrations**. This is commonly referred to as leaky gut.

Foreign proteins, especially lectins, **stimulate the immune system into overdrive.** Lectins stimulate antibody production (IgA antibodies), activate cytokine cascades (chemical messengers of the immune system), **initiate histamine response and contribute to mast-cell hypersensitivity** (causing nonspecific allergic-type responses, including skin rashes). Lectins may play a significant role in rheumatoid arthritis and other autoimmune diseases.

Beyond lectins, all foods contain proteins that can potentially cause sensitivity. **Sensitivity to food proteins occurs only in the presence of leaky gut.** Sensitivity to a particular food can be mild to severe. Multiple sensitivities are common. The most common food sensitivities include **wheat, dairy, corn, nuts, yeast, tomatoes, citrus, eggs, soy, bananas, beans, potatoes, pork,** and **beef.** As long as leaky gut is present, food sensitivities will typically shift to whatever foods are commonly consumed.

Food sensitivities are the result of antibodies (IgA and IgG) binding to foreign proteins (lectins and other food proteins) that have leaked into the bloodstream in excessive amounts (small amounts are normal). The immune complexes that form circulate throughout the body, **clogging up the lymph system and causing inflammation in all organs and tissues.** Lectins that have leaked into the bloodstream can also attach to cell membranes of RBCs, causing clumping (called hemagglutination).

System-wide symptoms can occur, including fatigue, brain fog, flu-like symptoms, muscle pain, joint pain, anemia, and a wide range of other nonspecific symptoms (which, of course, makes fibromyalgia or Lyme disease symptoms even worse). Symptoms can occur 1-2 hours after eating, but often do not show up until 1 or 2 days later. Considering the nonspecific nature and delayed onset of symptoms, defining the specific offending food is quite a challenge.

Leaky Gut and Oxalates
If that were not enough, increased intestinal permeability (leaky gut) allows a plant substance called **oxalate** to "leak" across the intestinal barrier. Oxalate is an **end-product of metabolism** in both plants and animals.

Many foods are high in oxalate, but if the gut barrier is intact, oxalate is not absorbed to any significant degree. In other words, people with a normal healthy gut can eat foods that are high in oxalate and not have a problem. **With leaky gut, however, large amounts of oxalate can be absorbed**.

Excess **oxalate binds with calcium in the body, forming sharp crystals** that build up in tissues. **Muscle pain and joint pain** associated with movement and fatigue are possible associated symptoms.

Oxalate is excreted by the kidneys. Excessive oxalate is associated with increased risk of **kidney stones** (70% of kidney stones are calcium oxalate). Interestingly, people with Crohn's disease, known for increased intestinal permeability (leaky gut), have a threefold increased risk for kidney stones. Crohn's disease is also commonly associated with muscle pain and fatigue.

Oxalate crystals can also concentrate in the bladder and vulvar/vaginal area in women, causing **chronic bladder irritability** and **chronic vulvar**

pain (called vulvodynia). At least a third of women with this condition respond well to a low-oxalate diet.

The **primary high-oxalate foods** include nuts (especially almonds), most grains, most legumes (especially soybeans and peanuts), beets and beet greens, potatoes, tomatoes, sweet potatoes, chard, spinach, parsley, rhubarb, starfruit, strawberries, raspberries, black tea, and dark chocolate. Visit www.lowoxalate.info for more information on the low-oxalate diet.

Once the gut heals and leaky gut resolves, moderate to high oxalate foods become less of a problem.

Toxin Build-Up in the Colon (Dysbiosis)
Everything eventually works its way downstream to the colon. Excess dietary starch stimulates overgrowth of bad bacteria in the colon (called **dysbiosis**). Toxins shed by bad bacteria irritate the colon, causing loose stools. Alternately, toxins can inhibit motility, causing constipation. Many people alternate between the two.

Damage in the walls of the colon allows pouches called diverticula to form. When multiple diverticula are present, it is called **diverticulosis**. If diverticula become infected, the condition is called **diverticulitis**. Some people do have a genetic tendency toward forming diverticula.

Buildup of toxins and undigested animal fat can contribute to formation of colon cancer.

Simple Steps to Enjoy Normal Digestion!
You can't eradicate all threats to normal digestive function, but you can minimize them — it's the price of becoming well. How much is your health worth?

Plant lectins are not nearly as much of a problem as seed lectins. For this and a long list of other reasons, at least half of your food should come from vegetables. Vegetables provide essential nutrients without excess carbohydrates. The type of fiber present in plants does not stimulate overgrowth of bacteria; it's the ideal type of fiber necessary for normal digestion. Fish, eggs, and poultry (red meat is a bit harder to digest) do not contain lectins or other damaging substances and therefore are your best sources of protein.

Cooking most of your food is a good idea. Cooking helps break down lectins, toxins, threatening microbes, and mold. Steaming is the most effective method of cooking vegetables. Steaming provides enough intense heat to destroy toxins and break down fiber, but seals in nutrients.

Lectins can be reduced in grains by sprouting and boiling, but not eliminated completely. Baking does not significantly reduce the high concentration of lectins or gluten in wheat products. For this reason, **grains and beans are best eliminated while regaining health or overcoming digestive dysfunction**. Some grain and bean products can be resumed after recovery is complete.

Fortunately, there is an exception to every rule. The lectins and storage proteins in white rice have a low potential for harm, and the carbohydrates in rice are broken down completely and do not contribute to overgrowth of bacteria in the gut. For individuals suffering from severe digestive dysfunction who are underweight and having difficulty gaining weight, white rice can be a good source of calories.

Gut Restoration Protocol

Digestive dysfunction is common with chronic illness, but the degree of dysfunction is highly variable. The effort necessary to restore normal function depends on the overall health of the gut. For some people, gut restoration will be a major part of the overall recovery process.

A diet for optimal health and a diet for overcoming digestive dysfunction are not necessarily one and the same. Many otherwise healthful foods can irritate an inflamed gut. Also, the foods that contribute to digestive dysfunction can vary from person to person.

To get well, foods that irritate the gut must be avoided long enough for healing to occur.

During the Gut Restoration Protocol, **only foods that have a low potential for harm** to the digestive tract are allowed. Once grains, beans, nuts, nightshade vegetables, high-oxalate foods, red meat, and dairy are excluded, the menu does seem fairly limited. Fortunately, there are enough exceptions to allow for a healthful and nutritious diet. Once healing progresses, a wider variety of foods can be added back in. If digestive dysfunction is significant, you may also have to hold back on herbal supplements until digestive function improves.

All food (with only a few exceptions) should be cooked, preferably boiled, steamed, or sautéed using low heat. Cooking breaks down the cell wall in plants and releases nutrients. Cooking also **reduces lectin concentrations, kills mold and other microbes, neutralizes many toxins**, and **makes food easier to digest**. Baking and grilling should be avoided during this phase.

Your general approach to eating also matters. **Eating quality food, eating less at one time, eating more slowly, and chewing food adequately** all support not only a healthy stomach, but also a healthy GI tract overall. A 12-hour fast each day from 6 pm to 6 am allows for optimal digestive function.

Eating organic whenever possible is also a commendable practice, but fresh sometimes trumps organic. A fresh conventional vegetable or fruit is superior to an organic vegetable or fruit past its prime and growing mold. **Organic is most important for thin-skinned fruit or vegetables, such as berries or celery.** Thick-skinned vegetables or fruit that can be peeled, such as avocado or melons, generally do not need to be organic. The Environmental Working Group (ewg.org) posts current recommendations on which fruits and vegetables you should buy organic.

Note that the food lists provided in this chapter are not all inclusive or absolute. The lists simply reflect the most commonly available foods at an average grocery store. It is up to you to expand the list as you desire. Researching the potential for harm that a particular food may carry is generally easy with an Internet search.

This introductory gut-healing protocol typically lasts 2 weeks to 2 months, or until symptoms have improved. After the healing process is established, other foods can gradually be reintroduced.

For a more comprehensive gut restoration protocol, visit RawlsMD.com.

Monitoring Progress
Progress is defined by a reduction in symptoms.

Intestinal symptoms include **abdominal/stomach discomfort**, **nausea**, **bloating**, **trapped gas**, **loose stools with undigested food**, **constipation**, **flatulence**, and **chronic pain at the lower right side of the abdomen**.

Systemic symptoms include **fatigue**, **muscle pain**, **joint pain**, **headache**, **itching rash (allergic-type skin reaction) and exacerbation of Lyme/fibromyalgia symptoms**.

Symptoms occurring 1-2 hours after eating are definitely food-related, but food sensitivities can be delayed to the next day (or even later if you have a chronic condition).

Sometimes it is difficult to differentiate from Lyme/fibromyalgia symptoms, but as healing progresses, it will be easier to distinguish where the symptoms are coming from.

Stool characteristics can be helpful for monitoring. Normal stools come spontaneously with little abdominal straining, are formed, are soft, are brown in color, and sink. Floating stools indicate poor fat digestion. Grey stools indicate inhibited bile flow. Loose stools with undigested food indicate poor digestive function overall. Extremely odorous stools indicate bacterial imbalance. Constipation with hard stools indicates poor intestinal motility.

Of course, any severe or unusual symptoms, such as vomiting, vomiting blood, passing blood from the rectum, severe cramping, severe abdominal pain, or any other symptom that seems serious should be immediately reported to your healthcare provider.

Things You Can Have

The following is a list of foods low in lectins, oxalate, toxins, and other factors contributing to food reactions. It is possible, however, for certain individuals to react to even these foods. Rotate foods around, and look for subtle reactions that may alert you to a food that does not agree with you (or if food-sensitivity testing is positive for that food). Primary foods that can be staples are listed in **bold** type. Other foods can be eaten as tolerated.

Vegetables

- Low-oxalate cooked vegetables, including **asparagus** (promotes gut-friendly bacteria)**, turnips, acorn/butternut squash, pumpkin, and zucchini**
- Seed pods and seeds from pods, including **peas, green beans, and snow pea pods** are low in lectins and generally well tolerated
- Well-cooked **cabbage** is generally well tolerated (avoid if Hashimoto's thyroiditis is an issue)
- Fermented cabbage, found in **Kimchi** (a Korean dish) and **sauerkraut**, promote favorable bacteria in the gut
- Vegetables from the allium family **(onions, garlic, leeks)** promote growth of favorable bacteria in the intestines and offer antimicrobial properties
- **Mushrooms** (brown button, shiitake, Portobello) are good sources of nutrition and contain immune-enhancing substances called beta-glucans
- **Sea vegetables** help protect the intestinal lining and are a good natural source of iodine (admittedly an acquired taste, but great for your GI tract!)
- **Raw cucumber** is the only raw vegetable allowed
- **Pickles** are also just fine; brine curing promotes friendly bacteria in the gut

Seeds (Grains)

- **Cooked white rice** (white rice is the well-tolerated exception)
- **Cooked wild rice**
- Puffed rice cereal

Fruits

- Temperate fruits, including **cooked apples, pears, plums, and apricots** (peeled or cooked)
- Fresh berries, including **dark cherries and blueberries** (raw or cooked)
- **Avocados**

Meat

- Poultry, including **chicken and turkey** (organic, pasture-raised preferred)
- Fish, including wild-caught **salmon, cod, halibut, flounder, grouper**, and other white fish

Dairy-like

- **Oat milk** or rice milk
- Almond milk and coconut milk if nut sensitivities are not a problem
- Goat's milk is tolerated well by some people

Oils

- **Olive oil**
- **Grapeseed oil**
- Coconut oil

- Ghee (clarified butter) is generally well tolerated in small amounts (1-2 teaspoons per day)

Condiments

- **Egg-free mayonnaise made from grapeseed oil** (Vegenaise, usually found in the fresh produce section of upscale grocery stores)
- **Vinegar**, any type
- Mustard

Herbs and spices

- **Fresh herbs**, such as basil, oregano, thyme, dill, sage, cilantro, and lemon grass
- **Dry spices**, such as cinnamon, cumin, coriander, turmeric, ginger, and nutmeg

Sweeteners

- **Erythritol**/xylitol
- **Stevia**
- **Honey**

Beverages

- **Ginger tea** — excellent for reducing inflammation in the entire intestinal tract
- **Water** with a squeeze of lime, lemon, or orange
- **Herbal teas**
- **Roasted dandelion root tea** is a tasteful substitute for coffee that promotes favorable bacteria
- **Chaga mushroom tea** is excellent

Things You Should Avoid

Primary foods to be avoided are listed in **bold** type. Other foods listed can be added back once gut recovery has progressed.

Vegetables

- Nightshade vegetables, including **potatoes, tomatoes, peppers, and eggplant**
- High-oxalate foods, including **beets, carrots, celery, collards, kale, leeks, okra, spinach, yellow squash, Swiss chard, sweet potatoes, parsley, rhubarb, and figs**

Seeds

- **All gluten grain products** (white wheat, whole-grain wheat, rye, and barley) should be strictly eliminated during your recovery and beyond
- **Bread, pastry, cakes, and pasta** made from gluten grains
- Products made from **any type of flour**, including gluten-free flour
- **Breakfast cereals** (except puffed rice)
- Legumes (**beans** of any variety, dried or canned)
- Soy products
- Products made from **GMO soy and corn**
- Tree nuts and nut butters
- **Peanuts** (which are actually legumes)
- Chocolate (sorry about this one...but it's only temporary)

Fruits

- **Tropical fruits**, such as bananas, pineapple, and mango
- **Grapes** (very high in sugar)
- **Figs** (high in oxalate)

- **Canned pineapple** (high oxalate and sugar)
- **Dates** (high oxalate)
- **Prunes** (high oxalate)
- **Raspberries** (high oxalate)
- **Strawberries** (high oxalate)

Meat

- **Grain-fed beef**
- **Pork**
- All **processed meats**, such as sausage, hot dogs, and bologna
- **Salted meat** of any variety (country ham, beef jerky, salted fish)
- Eggs (common food allergen, but most people can add them back later)

Dairy

- All **non-cultured dairy products**
- Hard cheese, such as Parmesan cheese
- **Soy milk**

Oils

- **Refined vegetable oils**, such as corn oil or soybean oil
- Canola, sunflower, and sesame oil should also be avoided at this time

Condiments

- Ketchup
- Mustard
- **Salad dressing with soybean oil**

Herbs and spices

- Hot spices, such as hot pepper sauce, with greater gut-irritating potential should initially be avoided

Sweeteners

- **Table sugar**
- **Organic cane sugar**
- **All artificial sweeteners**

Beverages

- **Soft drinks** (saturated with sugar or artificial sweeteners)
- **Fruit drinks** (excessive sugar)
- Coffee (gastric irritant)
- Black and green tea (strip away the mucous barrier [astringent])
- Beer, wine, other alcohol-containing drinks

Alcohol is a toxin that in any amount will hold back your recovery. If caffeine is a habit, wean down slowly using green tea mixed with ginger tea.

It is nearly impossible to absolutely avoid all offending foods, especially all at one time. The objective is to minimize reactive foods until healing can occur and identify the foods that cause the most problems.

Once healing occurs, many foods can gradually be reintroduced. The reintroduction process can take weeks to months. Attention must be paid to the occurrence of food reactions as foods are added back.

Ultimately, a high vegetable, low grain or no grain diet, such as the Paleo diet, is the best choice for long-term maintenance. Another option is going ketogenic (consuming <50 grams of carbohydrate a day) once your recovery is well progressed. Many endurance athletes are citing the benefits of ketogenic diets and scientists are finding links to lowered cancer risk. Ketogenic diets, however, are challenging to follow consistently, especially during the early stages of recovery.

ADDITIONAL SUPPORT FOR GUT HEALING

Manage Stress

Stress management. Uncontrolled stress is often a primary driving force behind digestive dysfunction. Putting stress back in the box is essential for allowing the gastrointestinal tract to perform its job. Stress management is addressed in **Chapter 28**.

Protect and Repair Intestinal Mucosa

Gut healing. The freshwater algae, **chlorella**, is excellent for healing the stomach and intestinal lining. It is possibly more important than any other supplement for gut restoration. It also binds organic toxins for removal from the body. Chlorella can cause loose stools in some individuals. Dosage: 1000-3000 mg two to three times daily. It can be found as powder (to add to smoothies), tablets, and capsules. **Look for chlorella that has had the cell wall disrupted by mechanical methods and not by using heat or chemicals.** This information should be provided on the label of the product.

Ginger has excellent anti-inflammatory properties and is great for healing an inflamed stomach. It is well known for settling the stomach and reducing nausea. It also offers antiviral and other antimicrobial properties. To top it off, ginger is a synergist that helps other herbs work better. Ginger tea should be your regular beverage during recovery. (Some people experience burning with drinking ginger tea if the stomach is very inflamed; if this happens, stop the ginger tea, and wait until the gut has healed a bit.)

Making ginger tea by the gallon is easy. Take a large piece of ginger, and peel it by scraping it with the edge of a spoon. Slice/chop it into small pieces, enough for a double handful. Pour a gallon of spring water into a large pot, and toss in the ginger pieces. Bring to a boil, and then reduce to simmer for about 10 minutes. Sweeten with honey or stevia. Allow to cool. Strain/filter the tea back into the jug. Store in the refrigerator, and enjoy several times a day. If caffeine is a necessity, add a couple of bags of green tea.

Demulcents. Demulcents are natural substances that reestablish the mucous barrier protecting the gut. Specialized carbohydrates in these substances act like decoys (very similar to the natural barrier that has been stripped away) and bind lectins before they can do damage. Either of the two following options provide benefit.

- *Deglycyrrhizinated licorice (DGL).* DGL is a special form of licorice with the substance that affects adrenal function (and can raise blood pressure) removed. Usually found as a lozenge, DGL can be chewed several times a day. (Note that some people experience stimulation and sleeplessness with DGL.)

- *Slippery elm.* Contains a substance called mucilage that provides protection for the lining of the entire gastrointestinal tract.

Protectants. If ulcerations are suspected in the stomach or intestines, additional protection may be required.

- *D-limonene.* The oil from orange or lemon peel, called d-limonene, is excellent for protecting the esophagus and stomach lining and inducing healing. D-limonene can be found in 1000 mg gel-capsules. Take one with each meal until healing has occurred. Always follow the capsule with food and drink to make sure it goes down all the way.

- *Pepto-Bismol.* Over-the-counter medication for protecting the stomach lining.

- *Sangre de Gardo (Dragon's Blood).* Dragon's blood is the sap of a South American tree. In liquid form, it is deep red, but when the natural latex in the sap dries, it forms a protective beige-colored layer. It is excellent for application to cuts and scrapes on the skin, but also is commonly used internally for protecting the lining of the stomach. **Every natural medicine kit should contain a bottle of dragon's blood. (It tastes terrible, but works great!)**

- Avoid use of anti-inflammatory drugs (ibuprofen, naproxen, numerous prescription drugs) and alcohol, which contribute to ulcer formation in the stomach.

Carminatives. Substances that soothe the intestinal wall, ease intestinal cramping, and reduce intestinal gas production.

- *Ginger* is one of the best carminatives.

- *Cardamom and fennel* are excellent for reducing intestinal spasm and decreasing cramping.

- *Peppermint oil capsules* are very effective for decreasing spasm and cramping in the small intestine. Take a capsule form whenever spasm occurs. The oil can irritate the intestinal lining if overused, however.

- Other carminatives include *celery seed, chamomile tea, cinnamon, garlic, lemon balm,* and *motherwort.*

Restore Normal Digestive Function
Digestive enzymes. A complement of enzymes for enhancing digestion of fats, carbohydrates, and enzymes can improve the digestive process.

Improve stomach acidity. *Apple cider vinegar (ACV)* improves digestion in the stomach by increasing acidity. Acetic acid in vinegar is then neutralized in the small intestine to acetate, which is absorbed into the bloodstream. Acetate can help dissolve calcium oxalate crystals in tissues. ACV is also known to help control abnormal blood sugar. Take 2 tbsp in 6 oz of water with a drizzle of honey with each meal. (If burning or discomfort occurs, use of ACV should be discontinued until healing is more advanced.)

Limit absorption of oxalate. *Calcium citrate* taken with meals can reduce absorption of oxalate. The calcium binds with oxalate in the gut and prevents absorption through the intestines. The citrate is absorbed and helps dissolve calcium oxalate crystals already present in tissues. 500-mg calcium citrate tablets are inexpensive and available at any pharmacy. Take one with each meal. Good bacteria in the gut degrade oxalate.

Restore normal liver and gallbladder function. The herb, *milk thistle* (400-1200 mg daily) is well known for improving biliary flow, protecting liver cells, and actually promoting regeneration of liver cells. Andrographis and artichoke extract provide similar properties.

Nourishment for the gut. To heal properly, the gut needs a ready supply of vital nutrients.

- The amino acid, *l-glutamine*, is a primary energy source for intestinal mucosa. Supplementation can enhance healing. The average daily dose of glutamine in powder form is 1000-6000 mg, depending upon severity of disease.

- *A, C, and B vitamins and minerals* are also essential for normal bowel function.

- *Omega-3 essential fatty acids* (krill oil, fish oil, flax oil, or borage oil) reduce inflammation in the gut and encourage normal bowel movements.

Restore Normal Intestinal Microbiome (Intestinal Flora)

Dietary modifications alone are not always enough to restore bacterial balance in the stomach and intestinal tract. Even when extra measures are necessary, select herbs and probiotics can accelerate the restoration process. Once well established, balance can generally be maintained with diet alone.

Eliminate abnormal microbial overgrowth. For significant intestinal dysfunction, antimicrobial supplements may be necessary to reduce the burden of abnormal bacterial overgrowth. Herbs are especially useful for controlling symptoms of small intestinal bacterial overgrowth (SIBO). Herbs with antimicrobial properties offer the advantage of inhibiting growth of pathogenic organisms, without adversely affecting normal bacterial flora. Natural herbs also normalize the immune system.

- **Gut-friendly herbs include berberine, andrographis, cat's claw, sarsaparilla, and garlic.** This synergistic combination of herbal ingredients supports growth of friendly normal flora and suppresses growth of pathogenic bacteria. Coverage includes common pathogenic bacteria, yeast, and protozoa. These same ingredients enhance healing of the gut.

- *Artemisia annua (wormwood)* is a useful addition when protozoa and ameba are a concern (500-700 mg twice daily for no more than 1 week).

- *Ginger* offers activity against many common gut pathogens.

Note that herbal therapies have the potential to irritate the gut if significant damage is present. If intestinal symptoms increase after taking herbal therapy, stop or reduce the dose until healing occurs, and then resume cautiously.

Prebiotics. Foods that promote growth of favorable microbes in the gut are called prebiotics. These foods contain *inulin and fructo-oligosaccharides* that provide nourishment for favorable bacteria. These substances are found in onions, garlic, chicory, and Jerusalem artichoke.

Fermented foods. Daily consumption of yogurt and/or other fermented foods is important for seeding the intestinal tract with favorable bacteria, but concentrations of bacteria in yogurt are often not adequate if significant dysbiosis is present. Fermented vegetable juices, such as fermented cabbage juice, are excellent for promoting gut healing. These products can be purchased at health food stores or you can make them yourself. Probiotic supplements can provide additional support.

Probiotics. Probiotic supplements provide concentrated doses of live bacteria. Special capsules ensure the bacteria are not destroyed by stomach acid. Best quality supplements provide several strains and species of favorable bacteria, including **Lactobacilli** and **Bifidobacteria**. If yeast overgrowth is a problem or you have a history of C. diff, ***Saccharomyces boulardii***, a favorable probiotic yeast (5-10 billion cfu daily), is a good choice.

Optimal dosing ranges from 10 to 50 cfu (colony-forming units) daily for standard probiotics. Probiotic supplements should be taken with food. Freeze-dried powdered supplements in capsules are just as effective as live preparations and have a much longer shelf life. Probiotics are especially important with and after use of synthetic antibiotics (but not necessarily herbs with antimicrobial properties).

Note that use of probiotics can sometimes be a tricky business. Because every person's microbiome (bacteria makeup) is unique, what works for one person may not work for the next. It should also be noted that probiotics containing lactobacilli can cause worsening of trapped gas, bloating, and intestinal spasm associated with SIBO. If this occurs, switch to a lower dose of a single species probiotic containing only Bifidobacterium, but not Lactobacillus.

Manage Constipation
Magnesium is the usual go-to solution for constipation, but many people with Lyme disease experience flare-ups with regular use of magnesium. There are better choices for managing constipation.

For chronic constipation, it is important to restore normal function to the colon. Avoiding processed food products is especially important. Wheat fiber (raisin bran and whole-wheat products) actually makes constipation worse instead of better. Vegetable fiber is what you need. Also, tea and coffee are really hard on the lining of the intestinal tract and should be avoided while you are healing. Ginger tea is great stuff, but sometimes it can make constipation worse.

As mentioned previously, **chlorella** is great for healing the gut, and it can help ease constipation. You need 2-3 grams (2000-3000 mg) two to three times daily. **Prune juice twice daily** also works wonders. *Swiss Kriss* is a natural laxative product that can be used while things are getting back to normal. Initially, however, none of this may be enough. For stubborn constipation, Miralax powder is the best solution (available at any pharmacy), but you have to take two to four times as much as is recommended on the bottle for it to work.

You can work from the other end at the same time. Glycerin or Dulcolax suppositories or enemas soften stool and stimulate the colon. They only work on the very lower portion of the colon, however, and are not a total solution. Enemas should not be used chronically.

Once you get things going, start taking **triphala 500-1500 mg twice daily** (larger doses are generally well tolerated and not harmful). Triphala is an Ayurvedic (traditional medicine in India) herbal remedy that gradually restores tone and function to the colon. It has a mild laxative effect, but does not damage the colon.

26

Curbing Toxic Threats

Detoxification is not a one-day or even a one-week event. Detoxification is an ongoing process that occurs continually every minute of every day. It's a simple matter of limiting toxins entering the body and enhancing the ability of the body to remove toxins. When *out* is greater than *in*, the body will gradually be purged of toxins.

Toxins can only enter the body three ways: from what you drink and eat, with air you breathe, and by absorption through the skin. If the amount of toxins being taken in exceeds the capacity of the body's ability to remove toxins, then toxins build up in tissues.

The first step in purging the body of excess toxins is reducing the inflow — not for just a one-week detox, but continually. It's a matter of cleaning up your diet, breathing clean air, and being mindful of any toxic substances coming in contact with your skin. This will allow the detoxification systems of the body to get ahead, but it's not enough alone to get the job done.

Toxins built up in your tissues are like sediment on the bottom of a polluted pond. Just cleaning the surface water only superficially addresses the problem. You have to agitate the sediment and then clean the water, over and over, until all the sediment is gone.

In the human body, toxic sediment is held mostly in fatty tissue. Increased blood flow, on a regular daily basis is necessary to mobilize toxins from tissues and gradually purge toxins from the body. Regular exercise is the best way to increase blood flow, but in the beginning when exercise (**Chapter 29**) is less practical, far-infrared sauna is an adequate substitute (**Chapter 21**, Turn up the Heat on Your Recovery).

CLEANING UP THE INFLOW

Toxic threats are subtly attached to things we do in life. Reducing the inflow of toxins is a matter of making minor adjustments to how you go about life. **If smoking and excessive alcohol consumption are not issues, then you are already two steps ahead.** All you really have to do is become more aware of where toxic threats come from and make a conscious effort to avoid them.

Giving up processed food and embracing a clean diet is a good place to start. Fiber from vegetables binds toxins for removal. Strive to make fresh vegetables more than half of your diet. Fruit, meat, beans, and healthful grains should make up a much smaller portion of your diet.

Healthful meat comes from animals raised humanely and fed natural food. Wild caught is preferred for fish and seafood. The cost is worth it, as most grocery store meat is a source of hidden toxins. EatWild (www. eatwild.com) provides lists of local farms producing better quality meat products.

Chlorella, a type of freshwater algae, is a great purifying agent that can be taken as a supplement to expedite the process. Chlorella contains many health-enhancing substances, but chlorophyll may be the most important for removing toxins. Detoxification of the body is also supported by herbs and natural substances, such as glutathione, vitamin C, NAC, and alpha lipoic acid.

Buying organic is a good practice whenever it's affordable. The most important foods to buy organic are thin-skinned vegetables and fruit; berries, apples, peaches, celery, peppers, spinach, lettuce, tomatoes, and potatoes are some examples. Thick-skinned vegetables and fruit, such as citrus, melons, and avocados, generally do not have to be organic. Vegetables and fruit, organic or otherwise, should be either cooked thoroughly, peeled, or thoroughly washed before consumption. The Environmental Working Group (www.ewg.org) provides reasonable guidelines for food choices.

Use filtered water. Reverse osmosis (RO) water filter systems are the most effective for removing toxins from tap water. RO filter systems can be purchased from any home improvement store and easily installed within a couple of hours. The small investment is worth the peace of mind. If RO is not possible or available, use filtered bottled water.

Clean outdoor air is a matter of selecting a location known for clean air and supporting clean air legislation. If you live in an area where clean air is not guaranteed, be mindful of smog alerts and times of day when it is not a good idea to spend time outdoors. Also, get out of the city as frequently as possible, and enjoy clean air.

Read labels on skin care products. Seek out products derived from natural sources. Deodorant products not containing aluminum are preferred. Creams, lotions, and other topically applied substances are often overlooked as sources of toxins and allergens. The Environmental Working Group (www.ewg.org) regularly posts lists of safe skin care products.

Go natural for hair and nails. Most hairdressers use toxic chemicals for hair treatments. Manicure and pedicure treatments are also very toxic and best avoided during your recovery.

Quit smoking. Use of tobacco products should be discontinued permanently; your recovery absolutely depends on it. It is impossible to smoke tobacco products and recover from chronic illness. Electronic cigarettes may be better, but they still contain toxins. Get help if you need it (acupuncture, hypnosis), but you must stop!

Curb alcohol. Alcohol is a toxin and should be avoided while recovering from any sort of chronic disease. Your body just can't handle any toxins right now. If you drink regularly, wean off slowly.

Use prescription drugs carefully. Most prescription drugs are therapeutically dosed toxins. They can be useful and important, but at the same time, drug toxicity must be respected. Most synthetic pharmaceuticals have direct toxic effects on tissues and contribute to a decline in liver function. If prescription drug therapy is indicated, use the lowest dose possible to achieve the desired result. As your health improves, drug therapy can often be reduced or discontinued. Always talk to your healthcare provider about changing doses or stopping a drug.

HEAVY METAL CONCERNS

Historically, heavy metals have not been present on the surface of the planet to any significant degree, but manufacturing and burning coal for energy have ensured exposure of heavy metals (lead, mercury, cadmium) to virtually every living organism on earth. Mercury in large fish actually comes from mercury released into the atmosphere from burning coal and then concentrated up the food chain. Tobacco is a notorious source of heavy metals, especially cadmium.

What to do about heavy metals is hotly debated. While studies in healthy individuals show that mercury intake from environmental sources does not exceed the natural ability of the body to rid itself of heavy metals, this may be less true in individuals with chronic illness where detoxification is impaired. While this often inspires people to go through elaborate detoxification protocols to rid themselves of heavy metals, these types of practices may pose more harm than benefit.

The most logical solution is reducing intake and supporting the natural ability of the body to get rid of heavy metals. Even when detoxification is impaired, the body will still slowly and gradually purge heavy metals, as long as less metal is coming in than going out. Eating organic, avoiding tobacco, breathing clean air, being mindful of occupational exposure, and avoiding large deep sea fish will reduce the heavy metal burden. Glutathione is excellent for pulling heavy metals out of tissues. A FIR sauna and regular exercise expedite the process. Because heavy metal toxins accumulate in fatty tissue, staying thin is not a bad idea.

Many people are concerned about **amalgam fillings**. Amalgam consists of an alloy of silver, copper, tin, and zinc combined with mercury. The FDA has concluded that mercury present in amalgam fillings does not pose any harm. Studies have shown that mercury absorbed from amalgam fillings is under the tolerable limits of 30 micrograms per day established by the World Health Organization.

Autopsy specimens, however, show mercury levels 2-12 times higher in individuals with amalgam fillings. The mercury is found concentrated in brains and kidneys. High levels were also found in pituitary and thyroid glands.

Whether to replace amalgam fillings is a challenging question to answer. The process is difficult and potentially hazardous. Most dentists will tell you that polymers used to replace amalgam just aren't very good. They don't hold up very well. There is also building evidence that the polymers are toxic to cells and cause a higher incidence of allergic reactions than amalgam.

A conservative approach is reasonable. If you have amalgam fillings, reduce other potential sources of mercury, and take supplements to enhance detoxification. If your health is not rebounding completely, you may have to make the very difficult decision to have amalgams replaced, but do everything else possible to restore your health first. Many people have amalgam fillings without having any health problems.

DETOX YOUR HOME AND WORKPLACE

Most people spend more time indoors than outdoors, and indoor air quality is easy to maintain. **Change AC filters regularly.** Write a date on the filter, so you know when it was placed. **Self-contained, free-standing HEPA air filters** for individual rooms, especially the bedroom, are very effective for cleaning indoor air.

Replace indoor cleaning products with natural cleaners, such as white vinegar and ammonia. Avoid using sprayed pesticides for crawling pests; use traps and solid baits instead.

If you have carpet, invest in a first-class vacuum cleaner. Also have carpets professionally cleaned regularly. Even better, have carpets replaced with wood or cork floors.

Have upholstered furniture cleaned regularly.

Declutter your home. Clutter collects dust and mold.

Get houseplants. Plants clean the air and add a pleasant feel to a home. Do not overwater plants, and make sure pots are not a source of mold.

Wash your bedsheets regularly. Unclean sheets harbor dust and mites.

Musty indoor odor signals a mold problem. (See **Chapter 27**, Mold and Mycotoxins, for advice.)

Be wary of exposing skin to toxic chemicals. If you must chemicals, wear gloves and a mask with a chemical filter. Replace toxic cleaners with safer natural alternatives.

For years, the government required **flame retardants to be applied on all upholstered furniture**. It turns out that the chemicals were extremely toxic and did not prevent fires. They are no longer required, but many upholstering cloth manufacturers still use them. You probably have furniture in your home that contains toxic fire retardants. If you buy new furniture or have furniture reupholstered, make sure the cloth does not contain fire retardants.

PROTECTION FROM ARTIFICIAL RADIATION

In the modern world, we are constantly exposed to artificial electromagnetic radiation in the form of radio waves, microwaves, and radiation from electrical devices, such as computers and cell phones. Eliminating exposure is impractical, but reducing exposure and gaining protection from this type of radiation is not only possible, but smart.

Create distance. If you can, avoid living near cell phone towers, radio towers, or large electric power grids. Distance is the only way to limit this type of exposure.

Protect your vitals. Laptops put out copious radiation. If you have ever experienced the "toasted legs" feeling that occurs while using a laptop, you know what I mean. Fortunately, there are shields available, that when placed under the laptop, block some of the radiation. There are various different shields on the market.

Desktops are a little easier. The processor can be located far enough away from your body so as not to be a problem. This is advisable, both at home and work. A shield can also be placed between you and the processor.

Take breaks. If your livelihood has you strapped to a computer, try to break up the time you spend staring at a screen. Beyond the radiation, you get from the computer, staring at a screen for long hours disrupts hormone balance and suppresses immune function. For every 1-2 hours you spend on the computer, try to spend 15-30 minutes doing something else that does not involve staring at a screen, preferably something active.

Be smart about your phone. Cell phones are smaller, but are used often and are kept near or on the body continually. Shields can now also be purchased for cell phones. Other ways to limit radiation exposure include the following:

- Use remote wireless headsets and car speaker/microphone kits whenever possible.

- Text instead of talk (except while driving, of course).

- Do not charge the cell phone directly beside the bed.

- Avoid carrying a cell phone in a pocket with close contact to skin.

- Radiation shields are also available for cell phones, but their effectiveness is not well documented.

Supplement for safety. Radiation causes damage that is very similar to that of free radicals. Antioxidant supplements can offer protection. Certain natural supplements have been defined by studies to offer protection from different types of radiation. Not surprisingly, many of the recommended herbs offer protection against damage from radiation.

Review your radon risk. If you live in a high-risk area for radon gas, have the crawlspace of the home checked. Testing kits can be ordered over the Internet. A simple Internet search for "radon gas high-risk areas" will tell you if there is need for concern.

Sun protection. The sun is a potent force; spending a day in bright sunshine, even with sunscreen and protective clothing, can be quite debilitating. Clothing offers the best protection. Protection can also be gained from eating certain vegetables. Chemical compounds called carotenoids, found in yellow-orange vegetables, build up in the skin and retina of the eyes and counteract the damaging effects of sun exposure. Two carrots a day is a good practice. Lutein/zeaxanthin supplements offer additional protection.

Though using sunscreen is a good idea, many sunscreens contain chemical compounds that can become carcinogenic when exposed to UV light. The Environmental Working Group (www.ewg.org) regularly posts lists of sunscreens that are free of potentially harmful chemical compounds.

Sunscreens also block vitamin D synthesis. Limited exposure (20-30 minutes several days a week) without protection is not harmful and is enough to generate daily requirements of Vitamin D. Even with sun exposure, having your vitamin D levels checked and supplementing as indicated make sense.

All the little things add up. Living in a clean environment is not only better for you, it is a gift to the rest of the world.

27

Mold and Mycotoxins

Mold...it's everywhere.

And if you are not yet improving, chronic exposure to mycotoxins (mold toxins) may be an issue.

For someone struggling with chronic Lyme disease, chronic exposure to mycotoxins can worsen immune dysfunction, inhibit the healing process, and stall recovery. Mycotoxins also disturb hormone balance in the body and reduce tolerance to any type of stress. Sometimes **exposure to mycotoxins is the factor that initiates chronic immune dysfunction** in the first place.

Mycotoxins alone can cause symptoms very similar to chronic Lyme disease and fibromyalgia. Common symptoms include chronic burning in the throat and nasal passages, coughing, wheezing, shortness of breath, vision changes, headache, eye irritation, dizziness, hearing loss, fatigue, muscle weakness, heightened sensitivity to chemicals and foods, joint pain, muscle pain, irregular heartbeat, depression, anxiety, skin rashes, and sleep problems.

Symptoms can occur directly from exposure to mycotoxins or from an allergy to mold spores in the environment. Some people have both. Mold allergy symptoms tend to be associated with chronic sinus and respiratory problems. Symptoms associated with sensitivity to mycotoxins are systemic and nonspecific.

If mold is present in your living environment (or food), and you are sick with symptoms common to immune dysfunction disorders (Lyme, fibromyalgia, chronic fatigue, or autoimmune), then you are probably mold sensitive. Eradicating mold from your environment should be part of your recovery strategy. Your recovery will not progress until the mold problem is eradicated.

Hundreds of different mycotoxins are produced by a variety of different molds. Molds can grow in many environments, but especially in warm, moist environments and inside buildings.

If mold is present, mycotoxins saturate the air. **The best sign of mycotoxins being present is the stale smell of mold and mildew.** Mold-sensitive individuals are often alerted to the presence of mold by developing irritation of the throat and nasal passages (often immediately with exposure). Sometimes, however, the presence of mold is hidden.

FINDING MOLD WHERE YOU LIVE AND WORK
Seeing mold and smelling it are good initial search options. Start your search with ceilings above showers and in bathrooms. Moisture is necessary for mold to grow.

Mold, however, can remain hidden in walls, crawl spaces, and attics. Often bathroom fans that draw moisture from the bathroom are vented into the attic instead of outside the house. Accumulation of moisture can turn an attic black with mold. Moist crawl spaces can also be sources of mold. Drywall in old houses is notorious for harboring mold. Air-conditioning systems and ductwork commonly accumulate mold.

Black mold (stachybotrys) produces a potent mycotoxin called trichot-hecene that can make you very sick. There are other forms of toxic mold, however, that are less easy to identify.

There are two main ways of testing for mold in a dwelling. **Mold plates** contain a growing medium specifically for mold. The plates are placed at different locations around the dwelling, and mold spores in the air fall on the plate and start to grow. It can work, but it is not very sensitive.

A more sensitive method of testing uses species-specific PCR analysis. Dust from key areas in the dwelling is placed on a test strip. The results are immediate. The Healthful Home 5-Minute Mold Test tests for 32 species of mold, including stachybotrys, aspergillus, cladosporium, alternaria, and penicillium, the most common forms of household mold (Amazon, $50). Testing can also be done by professionals.

Automobiles are an often-overlooked source of mold. Modern humans spend a lot of time in cars, and the ventilation systems in cars can harbor mold. When you go in for regular service for your car, have them check and clean the ventilation system. Some newer cars have ventilation air filters that need to be changed regularly (otherwise, they will harbor mold).

It is possible to test for mycotoxins in your body (by testing urine), but, if you have mold exposure and you feel bad, you are probably mold sensitive and have mycotoxins in your system (though even healthy people have a certain number of mycotoxins). The solution is still the same — eradicate mold from your environment.

MOLD IN FOOD

Mold is actually present in all foods, and all foods contain small amounts of mycotoxins. The longer food sits out, especially after cooking, the more apt it is to grow mold. Refrigeration can slow, but not eliminate growth of mold.

Nuts (peanuts especially), all grains, dried beans, and all dairy products (except yogurt, kefir) are the most notorious for harboring mold. These products are associated with molds that produce aflatoxin, a mycotoxin that can cause cancer. Grains, especially wheat and corn, can harbor several species of mold, including black mold. Dried fruits can also harbor mold.

Processed meats are also notorious for harboring mold.

There has been a lot of Internet discussion about mold in coffee. **Like most foods, coffee does harbor some mold, but not more than any other foods.** In other words, the levels are not exceptionally high as compared to foods known for harboring mold. Hot water used to make coffee actually gets rid of some of the mycotoxins present. Decaffeinated coffee has higher levels of mycotoxins than regular coffee. If you are extremely mold sensitive, however, it is best to look for higher grades of coffee (which have lower levels of mold) or avoid coffee altogether.

The solution to mold in food is buying fresh and avoiding foods that are apt to harbor mold. Thorough cooking helps reduce the concentration of mycotoxins in food.

ELIMINATING MOLD FROM YOUR ENVIRONMENT
In most cases, it's best to hire a professional to help with locating and dealing with mold. Areas to concentrate on include the following:

- Inspect crawl spaces, and use a dehumidifier if necessary. Have any visual evidence of mold removed by a professional.
- Make sure attics are dry and moisture is not being vented into the attic.

- Have heating and air-conditioning systems checked for mold and cleaned.

- Make sure carpets are not damp and growing mold. Replace carpet with wood or cork if you can afford it.

- If you have removed all visible mold, and mold smell is still present or testing is still positive, the mold may be embedded in drywall, inside walls, in crawl spaces, or in attics. In this case, the only recourse is removing the drywall and insulation completely and replacing it with mold-resistant drywall and insulation. This should be done by professionals. DIY projects can cause severe exacerbation of symptoms in a sensitive individual.

- Temporary measures for reducing mold spores and mycotoxins in the air include placing HEPA filters in rooms where mold is present, ozone treatment, or diffusion of essential oils into the air (done when the building is unoccupied), but these measures will not eradicate mold.

ELIMINATING MOLD FROM YOUR BODY

Mold cannot grow inside your body unless you are extremely ill. Mold can, however, grow inside body cavities. Nasal passages and sinuses offer a perfect warm, moist environment for growing mold. If immune function has been compromised by exposure to mycotoxins and stealth microbes, mold can take hold. Once mold becomes established, burning and irritation of throat and nasal passages become chronic. Mycotoxins produced by the mold add to the misery.

The primary solution is minimizing exposure to mycotoxins and mold spores. You will never get rid of the problem unless you rid your environment of mold. You will still probably have to treat the mold directly, however. The best approach is nasal washes with antifungal medications. Sometimes nasal steroids are necessary to reduce inflammation, but will not cure the problem. It is sometimes valuable to do cultures to distinguish between a bacterial and a fungal problem. Antibiotics alone can make the situation worse.

Natural solutions include **xylitol nasal wash** and **Allimax (Allisure garlic) liquid solution**. **Grapefruit seed extract** used as a liquid nasal wash is also excellent for treating sinusitis and reducing mold.

Everyone has Candida, a yeast (a fungus, but not a mold) that is ubiquitously present in the human intestinal tract. Generally, low levels of yeast are not a problem unless immune dysfunction and imbalance in gut flora are present. In this case, overgrowth of yeast can occur. Yeast overgrowth causes problems directly and also produces a mycotoxin, which can cause systemic symptoms. In addition, fermentation of carbohydrates in the gut by yeast produces aldehyde, a potent toxin that can make you feel terrible.

The primary solution for yeast overgrowth in the gut is restricting the processed carbohydrates and sugar that feed them. In addition, yeast is suppressed by probiotics and herbal products. Antifungal drugs (Diflucan) are sometimes necessary if yeast overgrowth is severe.

Mycotoxins are present in every person on the planet, but some people retain mycotoxins more than others. Having symptoms is mostly associated with having higher concentrations of mycotoxins, but certain mold-sensitive individuals can be symptomatic from low levels of mycotoxins. The solution in either case is reducing concentrations of mycotoxins in the body.

The primary way to reduce mycotoxin concentrations in the body is reducing exposure, but mycotoxins can be recirculated for some time (years). Food substances that bind mycotoxins for removal from the body are important. Dietary fiber is a good place to start. Supplementation with natural binders can help remove mycotoxins from the body. Certain binders work better for some types of mycotoxins that others, so it is important to use a variety:

- **Glutathione** is particularly useful for pulling toxins out of fatty tissue, but does not necessarily bind toxins for removal from the body via stools. Dosage: 500-1000 mg two to three times daily. Use of glutathione is associated with few, if any, side effects.

- **Chlorella** is a type of freshwater algae that binds many organic toxins for removal from the body. It also provides wonderful healing properties for the gut. Reported side effects are rare. Dosage: 1000-3000 mg two to three times daily.

- **Bentonite clay** binds a variety of organic and biological toxins. Side effects include drying of the colon with regular use and constipation. Dosage: 1 tsp soaked in water for at least 30 minutes before use (or added to a smoothie), early in the morning or at bedtime.

- **Activated charcoal** is another strong toxin binder. It can be taken in capsule form. Dosage depends on the product.

  Do not take clay or charcoal with other supplements because they also bind beneficial substances. Bentonite clay and charcoal bind toxins much more strongly than chlorella, but also bind beneficial substances; therefore, they should be used only intermittently.

- Prescription medications for binding mycotoxins include **cholestyramine (Questran)** and **colesevelam (Welchol)**.

A f**ar infrared (FIR) sauna** is another way to rid the body of mycotoxins. Heat and sweating purge many types of toxins from the body, including mycotoxins. Start out slowly, and work up to 30 minutes a day over several weeks.

God Bless America

Greetings from Florida!

I'm sorry I didn't get this to you earlier, but I only recently discovered it and ordered it for you. Your name was on the add saying, "Order this for Bonnie." :)

Merry Christmas!

Love,
Dinah

28

Adrenals, Thyroid, and Menopause

Just living with an illness such as chronic Lyme is stressful enough — add in the responsibilities of day-to-day life, and stress can be overwhelming.

Your brain reacts to stress via your adrenal glands. You actually have two, one on top of each of your kidneys. The middle portion of the gland secretes the hormone epinephrine, better known as **adrenaline**. The outer portion of the adrenal gland secretes **cortisol**. These two stress hormones define how you will react to stress of any sort.

Adrenaline is the hormone that prepares you for confrontation. Just the thought of conflict accelerates pulse, quickens reflexes, and sharpens mental function. The chances of survival in a real emergency are dramatically increased with the changes initiated by adrenaline.

Adrenaline secretion is connected to the autonomic nervous system, which also includes the sympathetic (stimulating) and parasympathetic (calming) nervous systems. The autonomic nervous system regulates functions in the body, which happen automatically, such as heartbeat and breathing. It is heavily influenced by emotions and upper-level thought. If your brain is agitated, then your entire body becomes agitated.

If your body were a car, adrenaline would be your accelerator. If you ease up on the pedal most of the time and push it to the floor only when really necessary, stress is not going to be an issue. But if life causes you to push hard on the accelerator all the time, sooner or later it's going to catch up with you. Just having a chronic illness applies a certain amount of pressure to the accelerator that is beyond your control.

Cortisol is the hormone that directs the resources of the body to where they are needed for the given circumstances. When life is calm, cortisol secretion follows a gentle circadian (night and day) rhythm that balances all functions in the body. During acute stress, increased cortisol secretion follows surges of adrenaline. Increased cortisol prepares the body for stress by shifting resources away from everyday concerns (digesting food, repairing damage, immune function) toward handling imminent conflict.

The body is designed to handle normal day-to-day stresses that come and go, but when stress is unrelenting, the results can be quite destructive.

Constant adrenaline surges followed by sustained elevations in cortisol divert resources away from maintenance and healing functions. Immune functions become overwhelmed and dysfunctional. This inevitably causes the body to break down.

If stress doesn't let up, the adrenal glands become hyper-reactive (adrenal hyperactivity), and the stress response comes quicker and is more intense. **The end result is insomnia, fatigue, high blood pressure, anxiety, mental fatigue, and loss of ability to cope with stress**.

If you push down on the pedal hard enough and long enough, secretion of adrenal hormones becomes dysfunctional. The body continues to be driven by high adrenaline release, but cortisol secretion starts to wane, and the resources of the body can no longer keep up. Total collapse is inevitable. Some people call it "adrenal fatigue". **A person with dysfunctional cortisol secretion has absolutely no energy and sleeps too much. Fatigue no longer improves with rest or sleep. Low blood pressure, slow pulse, and depression of mood are typical.**

SOLUTIONS FOR ADRENAL DYSFUNCTION

If adrenal dysfunction describes your life, right now adrenaline is not your friend. It's like a car with a poorly tuned engine — the harder you push on the gas pedal, the more the engine is going to sputter and stall.

Let up on the pedal. Your approach to life needs to be calm and collected. Calm must be cultivated; it doesn't just happen. Note that the high points in life (being excited) can raise adrenaline just as much as the low points (feeling stressed out).

You have a stress threshold that precipitates symptoms. Try to maintain stress below that threshold. As your recovery progresses, you will be able to push down on the pedal a bit harder and enjoy a bit more freedom.

Shake off the little concerns, and let someone else worry about them. So many of the visible threats are not really threats at all. Let them go. Stop worrying about things you can do nothing about. Save your energy for the things that really matter.

Avoid arguments you can't win. Just walk away. Arguments raise your adrenaline levels and often waste your time. Pick your battles well — both at home and at work. This is a tough one, but you must learn to do it.

Make a pact with others close to you. Spouses, children, friends, and co-workers—**no arguments**. Work out disagreements civilly. Recognize that your illness can be as frustrating to them as it is to you.

Reduce unnecessary stimulation. Turn off the news, and filter media. What's happening on the other side of the world or possibly even down the street is not your concern if it does not directly affect your well-being or help you achieve your goal. Focus on things that enhance your motivation and raise your energy in a positive way.

Turn the volume down a notch. Literally. Listen only to quiet, relaxing music for a change. And sometimes just pure quiet is best.

Turn off your brain. Reducing the flow of thoughts and simultaneously relaxing the body takes practice. But practice pays off; your body and mind will learn to respond more rapidly and deeply. There are many resources available for learning these skills. Possibly one of the most comprehensive is *The Stress Reduction and Relaxation Workbook*, 6th edition, by Martha Davis, Elizabeth Robbins Eshelman, and Matthew McKay. The workbook catalogs and introduces most of the different techniques for learning relaxation. Also, there are almost unlimited smartphone and tablet apps that can help you master relaxation.

Take adaptogenic herbs. Adaptogens are a special class of herbal substances known for improving stress resistance. Adaptogenic herbs that are part of the core protocol include Cordyceps, Reishi, and eleuthero. The following adaptogenic herbs have special value for normalizing adrenal function (See **Appendix A** for dosing and more information on these and other beneficial herbs).

- **Ashwagandha** is one of the best adaptogens for balancing adrenal function. Native to India, ashwagandha is revered for its ability to balance and rejuvenate. Ashwagandha improves stress resistance, allows for better sleep, and reduces brain fog and fatigue. It reduces menopausal symptoms (especially hot flashes) and supports normal thyroid gland function. Ashwagandha also offers anti-inflammatory, antioxidant, anti-cancer, and immune-enhancing properties and is known to have antimicrobial properties against Chlamydia. Ashwagandha can be combined with l-theanine and other calming herbs for optimal benefit.

- **Asian Ginseng (*Panax ginseng*).** Ginseng is especially beneficial for adrenal fatigue associated with extreme lack of energy and excessive sleepiness. Ginseng supports normal adrenal function and improves energy. It may also improve mental alertness, concentration, and stamina. It is one of the most studied herbal substances in use. Ginseng is excellent for restoring normal adrenal function and balancing the HPA axis. **Because *Panax ginseng* is stimulating, it should be avoided by individuals with high blood pressure, insomnia, or anxiety.**

- **Licorice (*Glycyrrhiza glabra*).** Licorice would best be described as an adrenal tonic. Licorice specifically stimulates adrenal function. It will restore normal blood pressure if blood pressure is low and will restore normal cortisol rhythms. Licorice also offers potent antiviral properties and immune restoration. Licorice is a great synergist with other herbs. It should always be used in combination with other herbs and never alone. Use should be limited to short duration (less than 6 weeks); excessive or prolonged use can result in sodium retention and potassium loss with high blood pressure and swelling. **Licorice should be avoided by individuals experiencing high blood pressure, insomnia, or anxiety.**

One therapy you want to avoid for adrenal dysfunction is taking adrenal hormones. Some physicians routinely prescribe some form of cortisone and/or DHEA for adrenal dysfunction or insufficiency. Taking adrenal hormones eases symptoms initially, but in the long run, it suppresses natural secretion of adrenal hormones even further and worsens adrenal dysfunction. The only situation where chronic use of adrenal hormones is indicated is when adrenal tissue has been damaged to the point of being totally nonfunctional.

THE HPA AXIS

At a higher level, adrenal function is regulated by the hypothalamus, an almond-sized structure located at the base of the brain. The hypothalamus is responsible for regulating change; it's basically the thermostat of the body. The hypothalamus also exerts control over the thyroid gland and the ovaries/testes by way of the pituitary gland. **Together they make up the central hormonal pathway of the body called the hypothalamic-pituitary-adrenal axis, or HPA axis, for short.**

The autonomic nervous system and the HPA axis together control variations of normal functions in the body, including body temperature, thirst, hunger, weight, glucose and fat metabolism, physical manifestations of mood, sleep, fatigue, night and day rhythms, blood pressure, heart rate, and gastrointestinal function. Everything that happens in the body is connected to these two pathways.

The stress of chronic illness not only disrupts adrenal function, but also thyroid function and reproductive hormone functions. Though medical therapy is sometimes indicated, restoring balance in the entire HPA axis is important for normal health.

THYROID DYSFUNCTION

The thyroid gland controls metabolism in the body. The hypothalamus, via the pituitary gland, controls secretion of thyroid hormones. This connection makes thyroid function part of the HPA axis. Virtually everything that happens in the body is tied to the HPA axis, and balancing the HPA axis is extremely important for normal health and recovery from disease.

Hypothyroidism (low thyroid function) is the most common form of thyroid disease. It is a complex disorder, and dysfunction can occur in a variety of ways. The gland can basically burn out from exposure to stress factors. Also, antibodies can damage the gland and block thyroid hormone from working (an autoimmune condition called Hashimoto's thyroiditis). Iodine is necessary for the formation of thyroid hormones, and low iodine can lead to low thyroid hormone production and the formation of a goiter. Cysts and even cancer can form in the thyroid gland, compromising function.

Hypothyroidism is more common in women. There are hereditary tendencies that run in families. Associations have been made with wheat consumption and insulin resistance. Certain foods, known as goitrogens, can cause increased risk of hypothyroidism by blocking uptake of iodine. Common goitrogens include cruciferous vegetables, soy and soy products (including fermented soy), peanuts, and strawberries (mentioned in **Chapter 24**, Digestive Dysfunction). Generally, goitrogens are only a problem when frequently consumed raw.

Many toxins, including fluoride, chlorine, mercury, dioxins, and insecticides have been implicated as causative in thyroid disease. Toxins and the rise in nuclear radiation may be contributing to the steady rise in thyroid disease occurring over the past century. Stress is definitely a factor. Trauma to the neck and chest can initiate thyroid disease. A link with microbes, both viruses and bacteria, is certainly possible.

Possibly the most important factor in treating thyroid disease is finding a provider who understands the necessity of treating the patient, rather than just treating the numbers. If you are diagnosed with hypothyroidism, your healthcare provider may discuss the following options for therapy.

Prescription Medications for Hypothyroidism
Levothyroxine (Synthroid, Levoxyl, Tirosint). The most commonly used standard for treating hypothyroidism is levothyroxine. Though synthetically derived, levothyroxine is bio-identical human T_4, the most abundant thyroid hormone in the body. Most people do very well with this form of thyroid replacement, but some people do not convert T_4 into

the active thyroid hormone, T_3. These individuals tend to do better with natural porcine thyroid hormone.

Natural porcine thyroid (Armour Thyroid, Nature-Throid). This natural product is derived from the thyroid glands of pigs. The fact that it contains all forms of thyroid hormone in proper ratios provides an advantage for some patients. Porcine thyroid, however, is not bio-identical to human thyroid. With time, some people will develop antibodies to the porcine hormone, and the medication will lose effectiveness. Note that dosing of different thyroid medications is not equivalent — 100 mcg of levothyroxine is equal to 60-65 mg of porcine thyroid.

Human T_3 (Cytomel). Human T_3 is a good option for select patients. It is usually combined with levothyroxine to mimic normal balance of thyroid hormone secretion.

Natural Supplements Supporting Thyroid Function

Iodine supplements. Iodine supplementation is a controversial topic. Too little iodine (about 20% of Americans are considered deficient) can lead to goiter and hypothyroidism, but too much can actually aggravate thyroid disease. The current recommended daily allowance (RDA) is 150 mcg per day, but many experts recommend more, especially if you do not use iodized salt. Sea vegetables (seaweed) are commonly recommended as a natural iodine source, and it is true that sea vegetables offer the most bioavailable form of iodine, but the iodine content is highly variable between different sources. If you decide to supplement with more than the RDA, you may want to ask your healthcare provider about testing iodine levels, especially if you have active thyroid disease.

L-tyrosine. Thyroid hormone is made from iodine molecules attached to the amino acid, l-tyrosine. Supplements can help support normal thyroid function. L-tyrosine supplements are generally not necessary with a healthful diet.

Ashwagandha. This adaptogenic herb not only balances the HPA axis, but also stimulates thyroid gland activity (but does not act like thyroid hormone or interfere with thyroid medications). See **Appendix A** for complete information about Ashwagandha.

MENOPAUSE

Menopause is a natural process, not a disease. Even with the best of health habits, menopause still occurs. It is the natural consequence of midlife cessation of ovarian function.

The hormonal fluctuations associated with menopause disrupt the HPA axis and autonomic function. Resulting reactions include body thermostat variation, hot flashes, sleep disturbances, changes in fat distribution, heart rate changes, and often fatigue. Perimenopause, the stage leading up to menopause, can include all the above symptoms, but also irregular and sometimes heavy menstrual periods.

When menopause occurs on top of chronic illness, such as chronic Lyme, it can throw the body into a tailspin.

The best approach to menopause is a comprehensive approach. Good health practices in general ease the transition through menopause. Herbal therapies can make menopause more bearable. **Ashwagandha** reduces hot flashes and balances the HPA axis. The herb, **Vitex** (*Vitex agnus-castus*), restores progesterone secretion and normalizes the menstrual cycle. It also counteracts PMS. It is excellent for perimenopause (see **Appendix A** for more information about this herb).

Natural progesterone cream applied to the skin daily (available over-the-counter) opposes estrogen dominance and helps prevent heavy periods during perimenopause. Natural progesterone also reduces menopausal symptoms and slows bone loss.

pause, *bio-identical estrogen replacement* (with progester-one) properly administered in small doses can be life altering (it requires a prescription from a licensed healthcare provider).

ANDROPAUSE

The so-called cessation of testosterone production by males is less well defined. A healthy male is designed to maintain robust testosterone levels until the end of his life. Not being able to do so is a definite sign of poor health. It makes sense; if the body is not healthy, reproductive function is one of the first things to shut down.

Treating low testosterone production related to poor health with a driving anabolic steroid (testosterone) that pushes the body even harder can be downright dangerous. It is not surprising that testos-terone replacement therapy has been associated with many health con-cerns, including increased risk of stroke and heart attack.

Testosterone replacement should be approached carefully and with the lowest dose possible to achieve benefit. Testosterone replacement sup-presses natural testosterone secretion.

A better approach (albeit one that takes more time) is improving health habits and supporting normal glandular (testicular) function with herbal therapy. Most guys with low testosterone who change their way of life respond very favorably.

Herbs that support optimal testicular function and ideal male muscle mass (women can benefit from these same herbs also) include **epime-dium** and **rhaponticum** (see **Appendix A**). Wait until your recovery is well progressed before using these herbs, however, as they can be stimulating.

29

Active the Right Way

You must move to get well. It is essential for restoring immune function. How you move, however, matters in your recovery.

Exercise generates endorphins, the important feel-good chemicals that stimulate immune function and speed your recovery. Increased blood flow during exercise removes toxins from the body and normalizes hormones. Studies have shown that regular moderate exercise increases production of natural killer cells (Nieman 1993).

Exercise also stimulates formation of stem cells. Stem cells are cells that have the potential to become any kind of tissue. They are distributed throughout the body in small numbers to aid in tissue regeneration. Studies have shown that exercise increases the number of stem cells (Macaluso 2012).

To get well, you'll need all the endorphins and stem cells your body can generate, but excessive exercise can be counterproductive and even destructive. Using exercise to enhance recovery is about **achieving balance**. Regular gentle to moderate activity on a daily basis positively influences recovery. Intense exercise, especially before your body is ready, will set you back.

Moving causes friction. If joints, ligaments, and muscles are inflamed, this translates into tissue damage and pain. Early in recovery, this is rue because everything is very inflamed. **Any kind of movement will increase pain.** In addition, when your body is weak, maintaining posture and alignment is much more difficult during exercise, so injury is much more likely.

Start slowly. Even if the limit of your ability is walking around the living room three times, do it regularly until you can do more. Work up gradually. A regular walk around the block is a worthy goal. Set of goal of trying to some type of activity that involves movement every couple of hours of the time you are awake.

Give Qigong a try. Possibly the best movement exercise during recovery from chronic illness is the ancient Chinese art of Qigong (pronounced chi-gung). The slow, gentle movements of Qigong increase endorphins without adding to your pain. Qigong exercises also enhance posture, alignment, and balance. A class with an instructor is ideal for learning Qigong, but not totally necessary. The simple exercises can also be learned from a book, DVD, or YouTube videos.

Sign up for a yoga class. Yoga is perfect for restoring your body. Most anyone at any level of fitness and stamina can participate at some level. Classes are widely available in most every community. Private lessons are worth considering for muscle stiffness and back pain. Yoga postures stretch ligaments and improve posture. Yoga encourages blood flow to areas of the body where flow can be restricted, such as the spine. Yoga is also a great way to generate endorphins. People who practice yoga several times a week are typically more fit (and healthier) than people who pump weights at the gym several times a week.

Don't overdo it. Though exercise is beneficial, it is just as important not to overtax the body. Like hitting a wall, overdoing it can set you back a week or more. Learn your limits, and gradually increase as the healing process allows. Follow the 70% rule: Do not exceed 70% of your full capacity. Staying within your limit will prevent injury and compromising your recovery. Consistency is important. **Generating pain is not the goal.**

Warm up slowly. Increase activity very slowly so that your body has a chance to warm up. Exercise moderately as long as it feels good. Make sure you cool down adequately. If exercise results in a next-day exercise hangover, with pain and increased fatigue, allow time to recover and back down on the level of intensity.

Bounce back. A rebounder is a small personal trampoline. If doing any sort of exercise is a challenge, a rebounder provides a safe and easy way to ease back in. Simply bouncing 10-20 minutes a couple of times a day gets blood flowing, strengthens the autonomic nervous system, and increases lymphatic flow. Information about the benefits of rebounding can be found on the Internet.

Walking is a great place to start. In the beginning, that may just be around your house. As your strength improves, try to walk around your neighborhood. Stick to flat areas in the beginning. Follow the 70% rule for not overdoing it. Gradually build up to some inclines. Whenever you can, walk in natural areas, such as beaches and parks (being mindful of ticks, of course).

Add some resistance. Repetitions with light free weights systematically work muscle groups of the body. Start low with only 3-5 pounds, and gradually work up. Resistance training is designed to increase muscle tone and physical strength, not add bulk. Heavy weight lifting and bulking up is never necessary for robust health. Stay within your limits — injuring yourself is not the goal.

Body rolling. Body rolling is an interesting application of yoga poses using soft plastic balls to self-massage the spine and other parts of the body. This simple practice can dramatically reduce muscle aches and pains. It's like doing a self-massage to specific areas.

Make it fun. As health improves, embracing an athletic activity can be very rewarding. Pick a low-intensity activity, such as biking, hiking, golf, or kayaking.

Get outside. Whenever weather allows, do something active outside. Strive for an hour each day! It's great for your vitamin D level and your outlook on life! Barefoot contact with the ground also allows equalization of electrons between the body and the natural background (grounding). Moderate activities that work well for recovery include canoeing/kayaking, rowing, stand-up paddleboarding, biking, hiking, and gardening. Even cleaning out the garage or racking the yard counts as beneficial activity.

BOOSTING ENDORPHINS

Healthy levels of endorphins improve stress tolerance, boost immune function, enhance feelings of well-being, and reduce pain. Endorphins (opioid polypeptides) are chemical compounds produced by the hypothalamus and pituitary gland. Anything that balances or positively influences the hypothalamus generates endorphins — a positive attitude, vigorous massage, acupuncture, regular exercise, being calm, practicing yoga and Qigong/tai chi, and herbal adaptogens. Acute stress increases endorphin secretion, but chronic stress decreases secretion. Chronic Lyme, fibromyalgia, and other chronic illnesses are low-endorphin states. Restoring normal endorphin secretion is essential for restoring normal health.

Conclusion

Where do you see yourself a year from now?

Still searching for a new heroic cure, but living with cycles of chronic misery that never seem to end?

Or, are you on your way to being well?

Embracing a holistic approach to recovery takes commitment and effort, but the payoff is getting your life back. It's just a matter of being willing to take a different path.

Learn to follow your intuition; it will never steer you wrong. Everyone has intuition, but it often gets ignored or suppressed. What we want in life often contradicts what our intuition is telling us we need, so that little voice in the back of the head gets ignored.

To let your intuition be your guide, you have to give up on wants and expectations. You must live in the moment. Open up and let things happen. Give up the reins of control. Let go of fear. Intuition will bring you the information and things that you need to get well.

Negative emotions restrict intuition. Positive emotions promote it.

Opening up to intuition does not mean being complacent. On the contrary, you must keep searching and keep pushing forward, but with an open mind and an open heart.

Receive, don't take. The things you need will come to you if you let them.

I owe my recovery to intuition more than anything else.

EXPECTATIONS

About half of people who embrace natural herbal therapy alone will have a good response. Bump that up to two thirds for people who embrace a complete holistic approach to recovery.

In a short period of time, you could be enjoying some good days and looking forward to more. Most people start seeing benefit within as little as 3 months. How long it takes depends on the degree of your illness and how long you have been ill. Benefits accrue over time.

Some people will feel recovered within a year, and others will take longer. Age is a factor. Being recovered will be different for a 30-year-old than for a 70-year-old.

The remaining third of people will need to add on some type of heroic therapy. Pulsed antibiotics or some type of oxidative therapy are good first choices. **Remember: heroic therapies of any sort should always be balanced with restorative therapy options.** This allows for less toxic dosing of heroic therapies and shortened duration of use.

Note that "recovered" and "cured" have different implications. "Recovered" implies living a normal life. "Cured" implies that all offending microbes have been completely eradicated. While it may be possible to eradicate microbes, such as Borrelia, Mycoplasma, Bartonella, or

EBV, if you push hard enough for long enough, it is more likely that they will become dormant (no matter what route of therapy you choose). Maintaining a healthy immune system will be necessary to keep them that way.

PERSONAL JOURNEY

By the time I embraced herbal therapy, I had already cleaned up my diet and lifestyle significantly. I was still quite symptomatic, however. Within 3 months of starting a comprehensive regimen of herbs, I noticed significant reduction in all symptoms and improvement in energy. My recovery, however, was an up-and-down course of relapses and setbacks mixed with steady uphill progress.

Patience and persistence were necessary.
Every year, I got better and better, and every year I got more of my life back, but it took a full 5 years before I defined myself as recovered. It's now been more than 5 years since that point. I've continued with a healthy lifestyle, but I also continue taking a regular regimen of herbs.

I regularly try new herbs and lately have been exploring essential oils. I let both science and intuition guide my choices.

I still have the occasional setbacks, but I generally know why and how to correct them. I couldn't tell you if I've eradicated the offending microbes from my system — but I don't intend to let my guard down to find out.

By allowing intuition to be my guide and following a holistic approach to recovery, I am now living a normal life. I wish the same to anyone who struggles with chronic Lyme disease or any other chronic illness.

You can become well and you can get your life back!

Appendix A: More Herbs, Bioidenticals, and Essential Oils

ALTERNATIVE HERBS

One of the great things about herbal therapy is all the great herbs available. The herbal traditions of the world have supplied almost unlimited options. If, for some reason, you don't tolerate one herb, there are many others to put in its place.

Though having many choices seems complicated, it's really less so than you think. There are really no wrong choices — most well-known herbs provide benefit. Sometimes deciding whether a particular herb is right for you is a simple matter of just trying it!

While you would never do that with a drug, herbs have a much lower potential for toxicity. Trying a new one is generally quite safe. Start slow, and watch for side effects. While side effects are uncommon, some people experience stomach upset or excessive stimulation with some herbs.

Of course, knowing something about the herb is a good idea before you start taking it. The following section is a list of alternative options to consider to help you get started. For the herbs and natural substances listed in this chapter, dosages are provided when standard doses are known. When not listed, dosages are dependent on the product purchased.

If your interests carry you further, *Herbal Therapy & Supplements*, by Merrily A. Kuhn and David Winston, is a great little book to get started with herbal therapy. This basic handbook covers all of the most commonly used herbs. Both traditional use and scientific documentation are provided, along with dosages and potential side effects, for each herb discussed.

If you have a really healthy appetite for information, I encourage you to read all of Stephen Buhner's books on Lyme disease and coinfections. These books are well written and contain a wealth of valuable information. Note, however, that you do not have to take every herb mentioned for every coinfection to get well. There is a lot of cross-coverage between herbs.

Herbs have lower potential for toxicity than any other therapy, but allergic reactions and side effects are possible with any herb. Go slow when you first start taking herbs, and observe for effects, both positive or negative. Many herbs have antiplatelet properties (blood thinning). If you are taking blood thinners or have a history of coagulation problems, contact your healthcare provider before taking the herb. Herbs with immunomodulating properties should be avoided by individuals who are taking immunosuppressive drugs or who have had an organ transplant. Discontinue herbal therapy several days to a week before having major surgery. Use caution with herbal therapy if you are pregnant. Though most herbs pose less risk to pregnancy than most drugs, herbs should be used in pregnancy only if benefits outweigh potential risks.

ANTIMICROBIAL AND IMMUNOMODULATING HERBS

Anamu (*Petiveria alliacea*). An herb native to tropical regions of Central and South America that features potent medicinal properties. Also known as guinea hen weed, anamu has been traditionally used for colds, flu, pain, pneumonia, and arthritis. Potent sulfur compounds give anamu a garlic-like odor. These and other chemical compounds offer potent, broad-spectrum antimicrobial properties against bacteria, viruses, yeast, and fungi. Anamu is also immune enhancing and offers potent anti-inflammatory properties (inhibits COX-1) and anti-cancer properties. It increases cellular immunity and increases NK cells. Anamu is a great alternate antimicrobial herb. It is a good choice for providing extra coverage against Mycoplasma.

Suggested dosage: 1-2 grams (1000-2000 mg) of the whole herb, twice daily. Note that use of anamu will give urine and feces a distinct odor. **Regular use will deter mosquito and tick bites.**

Side effects: Safe and well tolerated. It should be avoided in pregnancy, however.

Artemisia (*Artemisia annua*). Artemisinin, the primary chemical compound found in artemisia, is a potent anti-parasitic (it kills parasites) that is commonly used for treatment of malaria. Activity is primarily limited to blood parasites; general antibacterial activity is limited. Artemisia is primarily indicated when Babesia is suspected as a coinfection in Lyme disease.

Suggested dosage: Depends on the preparation used. Artemisia should not be taken for longer than 7 days. Potency quickly declines with extended use. The dose can be repeated after 3 weeks.

Side effects: Significant risk of neurotoxicity (damage to nervous tissue) with extended use. Never use more than 1-2 months.

Chaga mushroom (*Inonotus obliquus*). Chaga is a powerful medicinal mushroom with immunomodulating properties. It contains potent anti-inflammatory substances and antioxidants. Chaga is strongly neuroprotective. It contains betulin, a potent anti-tumor (anti-cancer) substance. Consider adding a teaspoon of chaga mushroom powder to smoothies each day for added support. (All the medicinal mushrooms, including Reishi, shiitake, maitake, and lion's mane, have similar benefits.) Ground chaga mushroom can be used to make tea as an alternative to coffee and regular tea.

Side effects: Well tolerated. Avoid if mushroom allergies are present.

Cinchona bark is the original treatment for malaria. The primary active ingredient is quinine. It is an alternate for persistent Babesia outbreaks. The daily dose is 1000 mg twice daily.

Side effects: The recommended dose should not be exceeded because of potential cardiac toxicity, and the herb should not be used long term (more than a month).

Coptis (*Coptis chinensis*). Excellent source of berberine (other berberine plants include goldenseal, Oregon grape, and barberry). Berberine has strong antimicrobial properties, but is not well absorbed through the intestines when taking orally. Therefore, its primary value is restoring balance in gut microflora. According to Stephen Buhner, berberine also has value in destroying Chlamydia in the cecum of the intestine, a place used as a reservoir by the microbe. Coptis is also valuable as an eyewash for conjunctivitis (Bartonella, Chlamydia).

Side effects: Generally well tolerated. Side effects are mainly gastrointestinal. Can lower blood pressure.

Cryptolepis (*Cryptolepis sanguinolenta*). Traditionally used to treat malaria in Africa, Cryptolepis also demonstrates systemic antibacterial properties and antiprotozoal properties. Cryptolepis has also been found to have anti-inflammatory (blocks COX_2 and inflammatory cytokines) and anticancer properties. Provides antimicrobial activity against Babesia.

Side effects: Well tolerated.

Echinacea (*E. angustifolia, E. purpurea*). Immune stimulant with antiviral properties. Generally reserved for acute use with colds and flu. *E. angustifolia* is the most active. People with autoimmune illnesses should avoid echinacea.

Side effects: Caution is advised in autoimmune illness because of the immune-stimulating effects of this herb.

Houttuynia (*Houttuynia cordata*). Native to India and Nepal. Systemic antimicrobial with antibacterial and antiviral properties. Also, studies have shown anti-inflammatory, antihistamine/anti-allergy, and antioxidant properties. Houttuynia provides coverage for all the major bacterial and viral microbes associated with Lyme disease.

Side effects: Fishy smell. Otherwise well tolerated.

Isatis (*I. tinctoria, I. indigotica*). Native to Russia, but now a common invasive in the US, Europe, and Asia. It is a member of the broccoli family with antiviral/antibacterial properties. Can be used for suppressing herpes-type viruses. Can be used topically for conjunctivitis.

Side effects: Generally well tolerated orally. Long-term side effects include fatigue and feeling cold. Use should be limited to 3 weeks.

Licorice (*Glycyrrhiza glabra*). Licorice is an excellent herb for restoring and supporting adrenal function. It will restore normal blood pressure and normal cortisol rhythms. Licorice also offers potent antiviral properties and immune restoration. Licorice is a great synergist with other herbs and should always be used in combination with other herbs — never alone.

Suggested dosage: 500-mg capsules (standardized to 24% glycyrrhizic acids), one to two, up to three times daily.

Side effects: Elevated blood pressure. Stimulating. Excessive or prolonged use can result in sodium retention and potassium loss with high blood pressure and swelling. Use should be limited to short duration (less than 6 weeks), and recommended doses should not be exceeded. **Licorice should be avoided by individuals experiencing high blood pressure, insomnia, or anxiety.**

Lomatium (*Lomatium dissectum*). Native to China. Also known as Chinese honeysuckle. Strong antiviral/antibacterial properties. Excellent for suppressing relapses of herpes-type viruses (EBV, CMV, HHV).

Side effects: Low-grade fever and rash with long-term use.

Neem (*Azadirachta indica*). Native to India. Offers potent antibacterial, antiviral, antifungal, anti-inflammatory, and antioxidant properties. Also has been studied for potential anti-cancer properties and protective effects on the liver and kidneys. Very good for relapses of herpes-type viruses.

Side effects: Leaf and bark extracts are generally well tolerated. Supercritical CO_2 extracts and neem oil, if taken internally, can cause stomach and intestinal irritation. In a study of overdose in children, hepatic toxicity was noted.

Asian Ginseng (*Panax ginseng*). Stimulating adaptogen that has been used in China for at least 4000 years. Ginseng supports normal adrenal function and improves energy levels. It improves mental alertness, concentration, and stamina. It is one of the most studied herbal substances in use. Excellent for restoring normal adrenal function and balancing the HPA axis.

Suggested dosage: 300-500 mg of extract standardized to contain 4 to 7% ginsenosides one to two times daily.

Side effects: Stimulating—should be avoided in individuals with hypertension, heart disease, insomnia, or anxiety.

Pau D'Arco (*Tabebuia impetiginosa*). Antibacterial for bladder infections. Also useful for controlling Candida overgrowth. Contains quinones, which have natural antimicrobial properties.

Side effects: Nausea, pink urine, blood thinning at high doses. Long-term use should be avoided.

Prickly Ash (*Zanthoxylum clava-herculis*). Native to North America. Antibacterial. Commonly used in Lyme protocols. Enhances circulation. Relieves pain. Improves absorption of other herbs.

Side effects: Generally well tolerated.

Picrorhiza (*P. kurroa, P. scrophulariiflora*). Native to the Himalayas. Antibacterial and antiviral properties. Commonly used for hepatitis B. Immunomodulant for calming hyperimmune functions, including allergies and autoimmune phenomenon. Increases T-cell and B-cell functions. Powerfully protective of liver function (even better than milk thistle).

Side effects: Nausea and skin rash are possible, but uncommon. Avoid in pregnancy.

Red Root (*Ceanothus americanus*). Native to N. America. Clears lymphatics and improves lymphatic drainage. This may help reduce Herxheimer reactions by clearing debris from dead microbes.

Side effects: Enhances coagulation of blood — should not be used by individuals with risk of blood clots. Should only be used short term. Avoid in pregnancy. Avoid use with coagulant or anticoagulant drugs.

Red sage (*Salvia miltiorrhiza*). Native to Asia. Potent immunomodulator for normalizing immune functions. Important for protecting organ functions. May be useful for autoimmune illness. Used for cardiac pain. Reduces blood pressure.

Side effects: Generally well tolerated. Has blood-thinning and blood-pressure-lowering properties.

Rehmannia (*Rehmannia glutinosa*). A primary herb in traditional Chinese medicine, Rehmannia inhibits allergic responses and modulates immune functions. It is thought to be valuable for reducing autoimmune responses (lupus, rheumatoid arthritis, psoriatic arthritis, Sjogren's, and eczema). Considered an adrenal tonic, it supports adrenal function and relieves stress (adaptogenic). Rehmannia also demonstrates potent anti-inflammatory properties.

Side effects: Generally well tolerated. In higher doses, causes loose stools in some people. Avoid in pregnancy.

Rhodiola (*Rhodiola rosea*). A favorite adaptogen of Russian athletes and workers for decreasing fatigue, increasing alertness, and improving memory. It is primarily sourced to Siberia, but different species of rhodiola grow worldwide (including the Appalachian Mountains). Though it is mildly stimulating, natural sleep is restored in the face of stress. Rhodiola offers anti-depressant properties, providing a different option than St. John's wort (known for interactions with medications). Rhodiola enhances cardiovascular function and immune function and protects nerve and brain tissue. Traditionally, rhodiola was used to improve work tolerance at high altitudes, and research suggests that it may increase oxygen delivery to tissues, especially the heart. Rhodiola also offers significant immunomodulating properties.

Suggested dosage: 100-200 mg of standardized extract (2-3% rosavins, 0.8-1% salidroside) twice daily.

Side effects: For some people, the herb is mildly stimulating. In general, however, rhodiola is well tolerated.

Rosemary (*Rosmarinus officinalis*). Native to the Mediterranean. Both the herb and the essential oil have significant antimicrobial properties. Potent antioxidants. Traditionally, rosemary is often used for brain fog and depression.

Side effects: Leaf extract is generally well tolerated.

OTHER BENEFICIAL HERBS

Ashwagandha (*Withania somnifera*). Native to India and Africa, ashwagandha is revered for its ability to balance, energize, rejuvenate, and revitalize. Ashwagandha has been used for thousands of years as one of the most revered revitalizers in Ayurvedic medicine (traditional medicine of India). Ashwagandha is a calming adaptogen that is particularly useful in balancing the HPA axis in the brain (the control center for hormone regulation). By restoring balance in this important pathway, ashwagandha improves stress resistance, allows for improved sleep, reduces brain fog and fatigue, and eases the transition through menopause (especially hot flashes). These properties also lend to usefulness for controlling carbohydrate craving and weight loss. Ashwagandha also offers anti-inflammatory, antioxidant, antimutagenic, antiviral, antimicrobial, and immune-enhancing properties.

Dosage: Dependent on the preparation used.

Side effects: Ashwagandha has been used as both a food and a medicine for thousands of years. Side effects of any type are unusual and mild. Ashwagandha is appropriate for men, women, and adolescents. Occasionally, ashwagandha causes mild stimulation in some individuals. Ashwagandha does contain iron and should be avoided by individuals who retain iron (hemochromatosis).

Blue vervain (*Verbena hastata*). Calming herb. Beneficial for nervous spasm. Used for Bell palsy, PMS, and restless legs syndrome.

Side effects: Avoid in pregnancy.

Bacopa (*Bacopa monnieri*). Bacopa is considered a "tonic" for the nervous system. "Tonic" means that it has an overall balancing and restoring effect on that particular system. Native to India, bacopa has been used for thousands of years for treating sleep disturbances and anxiety. It specifically calms an overactive nervous system. It helps people sleep better and stay calmer, but does not have drug-like effects. Use of bacopa has demonstrated enhanced cognitive function in children with ADD, college students during exam time, and elderly dementia patients in controlled studies.

Dosage: 200-400 mg standardized to 50% bacosides at bedtime.

Side effects: Well tolerated with rare side effects. Some individuals notice more sedation than others. Sedation can be either decreased or enhanced by combining bacopa with other herbs.

Corydalis (*C. yanhusuo, C. ambigua*). Traditionally, corydalis has been used for relief of menstrual cramps, relief of abdominal pain and cramps, and invigoration of the blood. Corydalis exhibits a strong analgesic effect (but is a hundred times less potent than morphine). It has a slower onset of action than morphine. Evidence of dependence has not been noted with corydalis. The herb has pronounced sedative qualities and improves sleep. It also has marked anti-inflammatory properties and improves coronary blood flow.

Dosage: Highly dependent on the type of preparation used.

Side effects: Generally well tolerated. Avoid in pregnancy and while breastfeeding. Overdose can cause respiratory depression, sedation, and tremor. The potential for habituation dependence with Corydalis is much less than narcotics, but a small risk is still present. Should be avoided with active liver disease.

Epimedium (*E. grandiflorum*). Has a long history of use for restoring normal sexual function, but also provides strong adaptogenic qualities. Epimedium balances the HPA axis, improves coronary artery blood flow, and stimulates immune function. Known traditionally as a strong revitalizer. Combines well with rhaponticum and other herbs for rebuilding strength.

Side effects: mildly stimulating, but otherwise well tolerated.

Indian Pipe (*Monotropa uniflora*). Traditionally used for pain relief. Commonly combined with Corydalis.

Side effects: Vivid dreams.

Motherwort (*Leonurus cardiaca*). Motherwort has traditionally been used for relieving palpitations associated with menopause, menstrual mood changes, and nervous tension. It is calming and supports normal sleep at night, particularly when sleeplessness occurs at 3 am. Motherwort is strongly protective of nerve tissue and also protects mitochondria. It is a great supplement for maintaining normal blood pressure and providing general support for the cardiovascular system. Motherwort has been noted to have antiviral and anti-cancer properties. It is supportive of normal heart function and normalizes high blood pressure.

Dosage: 100-200 mg at bedtime (use higher doses of 400-500 mg if used alone).

Side effects: Well tolerated. Side effects are rare. Can lower blood pressure. Avoid in pregnancy.

Passionflower (*Passiflora incarnata*). For someone suffering from nervous tension and poor sleep, passion flower can be a real lifesaver. Passionflower has been long revered for its characteristic sedative properties. It has a reputation for restoring restful sleep without causing a next-day hangover. It also offers muscle relaxing and pain-relieving qualities.

Dosage: 150-300 mg of 10:1 extract at bedtime.

Side effects: Rare. Passionflower is listed under GRAS (Generally Recognized as Safe) status by the FDA. This means it is considered as safe as any food substance.

Rhaponticum (*R. carthamoides*). Adaptogenic herb known for improving stamina and strength. It is best known for promoting muscle mass. Rhaponticum also supports immune, neurological, and cardiovascular function.

Side effects: Mildly stimulating, but otherwise well tolerated. Avoid in late pregnancy.

Schisandra (*Schisandra chinensis*). Calming adaptogen with strong liver-protecting properties. Balances hormones. Immunomodulator.

Side effects: Safe and well tolerated.

Solomon's Seal (*Polygonatum biflorum*). Topical (cream and ointment) for enhancing healing for strains and sprains (joint, ligament, and cartilage injuries). Can be taken internally for the same purpose.

Side effects: Well tolerated.

Stephania (*S. tetrandra, S. cepharantha*). Immunomodulator reduces inflammatory cytokines. Especially good for reducing neural inflammation. Decreases vascular permeability (leaky vessels) from damage by inflammation and microbes (calcium-channel blocker). Good for eye conditions.

Side effect: Strong calcium-channel blocker — can lower blood pressure, and constipation can be a real problem with this herb.

St. John's wort (*Hypericum perforatum*). Naturally increases serotonin similarly to SSRI drugs. Serotonin is considered the "mood" hormone, but is also tied to pain pathways. Low serotonin is associated with chronic pain. Increasing serotonin with St. John's wort or drug therapy can benefit both mood and pain perception. Hypericum essential oil applied topically is very beneficial for painful joints. St. John's wort is also known to have antiviral and antibacterial properties.

Side effects: Can be stimulating in some individuals. Can affect metabolism of drugs and other herbs.

Vitex agnus-castus (chaste tree berry). Vitex acts as a tonic (hormonal modulator), specifically for the female reproductive system. It is thought to work by normalizing abnormal ovarian function by affecting the pituitary gland. Prolactin is decreased via dopamine antagonistic effect, FSH is inhibited, and LH is stimulated. This enhances corpus luteum function with an increase in progesterone and decrease in estrogen. By balancing hormonal function, almost any disorder associated with the female reproductive system is positively affected.

Dosage: depends on the preparation used.

Side effects: Generally very well tolerated. Side effects are rare and include mild stomach upset, itching, rash, fatigue, and hair loss. Caution is advised if used with drugs that affect dopamine, but no other drug interactions are known. Vitex can be used to enhance fertility, but should be discontinued after becoming pregnant. It can be used with breastfeeding.

OTHER BIOIDENTICALS

Bioidentical compounds generally do not provide the wide range of benefit found with herbs, but for specific indications, they can be valuable. Because most bioidentical compounds have been used therapeutically for a relatively short period of time, there is less information available about use of bioidentical substances. They have been used therapeutically for less than a hundred years.

L-carnitine (acetyl-l-carnitine). L-carnitine is important for metabolism of fatty acids in mitochondria. Antioxidant properties. Protective of mitochondrial function. Acetyl-l-carnitine crosses the blood-brain barrier more effectively than l-carnitine. Neuroprotective — may improve cognitive function.

Suggested dosage: 500-1000 mg acetyl-l-carnitine twice daily.

Side effects: none expected.

5-Hydroxytryptophan (5-HTP). 5-HTP is a precursor for both serotonin and melatonin in the brain. During the day, it has a mood-stabilizing effect, and during the night, it can promote improved sleep. Increased serotonin is associated with decreased perception of pain. 5-HTP is also metabolized as a normal substance in the body, and therefore there is no risk of dependence and tolerance.

Dosage: 100 mg two to three times daily. 100-300 mg at bedtime if used primarily for sleep.

Side effects: Not common, but some patients report nightmares or muscle aches when using it regularly. Use of 5-HTP should be avoided with SSRI drugs and St. John's wort because of the risk of serotonin syndrome, associated with excessive serotonin in the body.

Lipid-Replacement Therapy. Mitochondria and cells are surrounded by a membrane made of special fats called phospholipids. Eggs, liver, beef brain, and soy are the highest natural sources of phospholipids, but there is evidence that supplementing at higher levels (versus diet alone) can improve everything from fatigue to cognitive function. The three main phospholipids, phosphatidylcholine (PC), phosphatidylserine (PS), and glycerophosphocholine (GPC), are important for all cellular functions in the body, especially normal brain and muscle function.

Suggested dosage: PC - 1-3 grams (1000-3000 mg) twice daily, PS - 200-500 mg twice daily, GPC - 200-300 mg twice daily. Ingredients can be obtained separately. Loose powder is the most cost-effective and easily mixes with liquids. Dosage recommendations are purely an esti-mate based on studying products available and limited scientific studies available. Look for products free of GMO soy.

A healthful diet provides the raw materials for the body to make these fats, so lipid-replacement therapy should not be considered essential for your recovery. It may, however, provide some benefit and there is little potential for harm.

Side effects: None expected. Considered a functional food. Phospholipid supplements may actually enhance absorption of other supplements if taken together. Use with alpha-lipoic acid (and/or glutathione), NAC, and CoQ10 for complete mitochondrial support.

L-arginine. Clinical studies have shown that supplementation with the amino acid l-arginine spares loss of muscle mass. L-arginine enhances vascular function by increasing nitric oxide, which dilates blood ves-sels. Increased nitric oxide may also help suppress stealth microbes. It also helps clear ammonia from the body. L-arginine is a primary nutrient scavenged by Mycoplasma, and replacement may be beneficial.

Average dose is 3-6 grams (3000-6000 mg) daily.

Side effects: Generally well tolerated.

D-ribose. D-ribose is a five-sided sugar (pentose) that is the rate-limiting step in energy production. It is also important for synthesizing nucleic acids (DNA, RNA). Though d-ribose supplements do not appear to im-prove strength or athletic performance per se, they do appear to im-prove recovery. This is especially true in individuals with chronic Lyme disease or fibromyalgia. D-ribose can also reduce post-exertional pain.

Suggested dosage: 1 gram (1000 mg) two to three times daily. D-ribose will add sweetness to your smoothies.

Side effects: None expected. Considered a functional food.

L-theanine. L-theanine is a unique amino acid found only in green tea and certain mushrooms. It counteracts the effects of caffeine and not surprisingly, green tea is not as stimulating as coffee. L-theanine crosses into the brain and affects neurotransmitters in such a way as to induce calmness, support positive mood, and improve mental focus. It counters the negative effects of stress-induced adrenaline secretion and can lower blood pressure in hypertensive individuals. It does not cause sedation during the day, but does promote natural sleep at night.

Dosage: 200 mg one to two times daily.

Side effects: Almost unheard of. L-theanine is widely consumed in green tea by millions of people every day. Because l-theanine is metabolized by the same pathways as other amino acids in the body, there appears to be little risk of tolerance and dependence.

ESSENTIAL OILS

Essential oils are herbal plants from which the oil-based components have been extracted. Similar to herbs, essential oils provide many health benefits, including immunomodulation and antimicrobial, anti-inflammatory, antioxidant, and anticancer properties. Essential oils may be beneficial for helping to break down biofilms. Some plants can be used to make both water-alcohol based extracts or essential oils.

Essential oils, however, have higher potential for skin and mucous membrane irritation, along with higher potential for liver toxicity (some oils more than others). Therefore, essential oils should be used with more caution than herbal preparations. The most common way to use essential oils is by aromatherapy. Essential oils can be diffused into the air with a diffuser or a drop or so placed on clothing, skin, or a pillow at night. If used too aggressively, some essential oils, such as clove or cinnamon, diffused into the air can burn nasal passageways and the lungs.

Some essential oils can be massaged directly into skin for joint and muscle pain. Non-irritating essential oils for skin application include **frankincense, ginger, tea tree, grapefruit, helichrysum, sandalwood, rosemary, basil, chamomile, white birch, lavender, and peppermint**. These oils offer both anti-inflammatory and antimicrobial properties. Essential oils should be diluted in a carrier oil (jojoba, grapeseed, coconut) in a 4:1 ratio of the carrier to the essential oil. These oils also provide antimicrobial activity from chemical substances present in the oils absorbed through the skin.

The essential oils with the most significant antimicrobial properties include **clove, cinnamon, cassia, thyme, and oregano**. These oils have higher potential to irritate mucous membranes and skin. They therefore should be used in diluted concentrations or administered by aromatherapy. Drops of pure oil can also be applied to the soles of the feet several times a day. Skin irritation is less of a problem on the soles of the feet, and oils are quickly absorbed directly into the bloodstream. This method of administration is ideal for someone who has severe gastrointestinal problems and cannot take herbal therapy.

Essential oils can be used internally, but when absorbed through the intestines, some of the active oil-based chemical compounds are neutralized by the liver. Even so, people have reported positive benefits from using essential oils internally for Lyme disease. A few drops of different oils are placed in capsules and swallowed several times a day. Gastric and intestinal irritation from essential oils is the most common factor that limits use of therapy. Most protocols limit use of oils to 2 to 4 weeks at a time, with several weeks of rest in between.

Possibly the safest oil to use internally that has antimicrobial properties is tea tree oil (*Melaleuca alternifolia*). Other essential oils commonly used in Lyme protocols include frankincense, oregano, thyme, cassia, clove, lemon balm (Melissa), cinnamon, and 4 thieves (combination oil). Protocols can be found by searching for essential oils for Lyme disease on the Internet.

Appendix B: Protect the Integrity of Your Microbiome!

By this point, you may be a little bit paranoid about ticks and mosquitos — and you should be! Ticks and mosquitos transmit a wide range of different types of host-seeking microbes. Infection with a new microbe or reinfection with a microbe you've already been exposed to can throw your recovery into a tailspin.

Biting insects, of course, are not the only way to acquire new microbes. Microbes can gain access to your body by breathing them in, through food and liquid you consume, intimate contact with other people, and sometimes through the skin.

You want to add as few new microbes to your microbiome as possible. Stealth microbes are always waiting to slip in through a crack in the doorway — they are the ultimate opportunists — so don't leave your door cracked!

Everyday things you can do to protect your microbiome:

- **Wash your hands** or use hand sanitizers (these products contain only alcohol, which is toxic to microbes, but not toxic to you) after being in public and exposed to other people.

- **Avoid heavily crowded public places** as much as possible.

- **Stay home when you are sick.** Please.

- **Use precautions during intimate contact** with another person.

- **Avoid being a feast for biting insects.**

- **Cook or wash your food thoroughly.**

- **Drink filtered water.**

Having a history of Lyme disease doesn't mean that you have to stay inside…you just have to pick your outdoor adventures carefully. Open areas free of brush and low foliage reduce chances of tick exposure. If you enjoy hiking, pick trails that are well traveled and foliage that has been cut back. Mountain biking on trails reduces insect exposure. Beaches are tick free!

Mosquitos come out less in the daytime. If you enjoy camping, invest in a screened extension for your tent, and stay in after dark. Camp only in open areas. Campgrounds with bathrooms reduce exposure to ticks while using the bathroom (as opposed to going in the woods).

When you do venture into the outdoors, use protection.

- **DEET** is the most effective and longest acting insect repellant, but also the most toxic. Individuals with any chronic illness should avoid using DEET.

- **Permethrin** is an option for treating clothing (but not bare skin) before going outdoors. Permethrin is a synthetic form of natural pyrethrin that specifically targets the insect nervous system and has low toxicity to mammals.

- **Essential oils** are safe alternatives to synthetic chemicals. **Citronella** and **lemon eucalyptus** are the most well-known, but if you don't care for the smell, **lavender**, **juniper**, **oregano**, **clove**, and **geranium** work as well. These oils compare well with DEET in effectiveness, but do not last as long and must be reapplied frequently. They can be combined for increased effectiveness. Mix the oils in a 1:4 ratio with water and alcohol (50/50 mix), and shake before applying to skin and clothing. Oils can also be mixed with sunflower oil, but it may stain clothing. Commercial products containing these ingredients can be found with an Internet search.

- **Yarrow tincture** is a non-essential oil option that works as well as DEET. It can be applied to skin or clothing.

- **Skin-So-Soft and other perfume products** also compared well to DEET in one study. These are also good non-toxic choices, if you happen to enjoy that particular fragrance. This research suggested that the fragrances mask the scent of certain skin bacteria, which are attractors for mosquitos (ticks and mosquitos are more drawn to some people than others). However, there was no comment about the effectiveness of these products against ticks.

- **Be extremely vigilant about ticks.** When walking or hiking, whenever you brush by vegetation, stop and check for the possibility of a tick crawling up your legs or body.

- **Tick check.** When you come home from the woods, immediately place your clothes in the dryer for 30 minutes. Ticks perish quickly in dry heat. Then put them in the wash. Check yourself very thoroughly by feel and sight before hopping in the shower for a good scrub down.

- **Take herbs regularly.** My personal observation (also confirmed by others) is that many herbs make you less attractive to ticks and mosquitos. Since taking herbs, I have noticed that I am less likely to be bitten by mosquitos than people around me. Finding ticks on my body after spending time outdoors has been rare since starting herbs, and I can't remember the last time I had one embedded in my skin. All the antimicrobial herbs have value, but the best ones (in my opinion) are **garlic** and **anamu**.

- **Be aware that pets regularly bring ticks inside.** Have your pet regularly treated to reduce both ticks and fleas; all blood-sucking insects carry potential disease-causing microbes. The potential for harm to your pet is small compared to the misery they would have from being infested with fleas and other microbes from tick and mosquito bites. Protecting them also protects you.

If you do happen to be bitten by a tick:

- **Remove embedded ticks carefully.** The proper way to remove an embedded tick is by grasping it firmly with tweezers as close to the skin as possible and pulling it directly out. Do not use matches or other techniques.

- **After removing an embedded tick, give your doctor a call.** Antibiotics can help your immune system clear microbes, but may not eliminate them completely. The standard CDC recommendation for tick-bite prophylaxis is a single 200-mg dose of doxycycline, but only in high-risk areas. Considering that most anywhere there are ticks should be considered a high-risk area and ticks carry a wide variety of other microbes, this seems woefully inadequate. A more reasonable choice is **doxycycline 100 mg twice daily for 2-4 weeks**, especially if symptoms are present.

- **Doxycycline covers for all the primary tick-borne microbes except Babesia.** The medications used for treatment of Babesia infection are associated with significant side effects, so they are not ideal choices for prophylaxis. Metronidazole is an antiprotozoal drug that has been used successfully in veterinary medicine against certain species of Babesia. It is also well tolerated by humans and commonly used by humans for other purposes. If concern for Babesia is present, prophylaxis with **Metronidazole 500 mg twice daily for 1-2 weeks** may be a reasonable consideration (though this has not been tested in clinical studies). Metronidazole should not be used for more than 2 weeks.

- **Frequent tick bites.** If you happen to be in an environment where tick bites are a frequent occurrence, antibiotics with every tick bite is impractical. In this case, taking antimicrobial herbs continually may be your best protection.

- **Herbal insurance.** It's not usual for people to show up with chronic Lyme symptoms 6 months after taking a course of

antibiotics. Therefore, use of herbal therapy for a
period (3 months to a year) is not a bad idea. The best choices
are the primary antimicrobial herbs: **andrographis**, **cat's claw**,
Japanese knotweed, and **stabilized allicin (garlic)**.

What about vaccinations? Flu vaccines can protect you from coming
down with the flu, but they can also cause flare-ups of chronic Lyme
disease symptoms. Flu vaccines stimulate antibody production, but as a
tradeoff, may inhibit cellular immunity, allowing intracellular microbes to
flourish. It's really a personal choice. During mild years, the flu vaccine
may be best avoided; wait for the years when severe flu outbreaks with
new viruses are predicted. There is no effective vaccine against Lyme
disease (and there probably never will be).

Maintaining a healthy immune system is the most important thing that
you can do to protect yourself against all potential offenders and maintain a healthy microbiome!

Acknowledgements

I and the world owe a debt of gratitude to Stephen Buhner for his tireless research of both microbes that are associated with Lyme disease and the herbs that provide a solution for them. He also deserves credit for being a pioneer in the modernization of herbal medicine. He is joined by David Winston, Donald Yance, Leslie Taylor, and many others. Together, they are changing the way the world views herbal medicine.

This book and all the resources that surround it would not be possible without my daughter, Braden, and her efforts to establish Vital Plan. More than just a supplement company, it has become an essential resource for thousands of people.

I am very appreciative for all the support I received from the staff. A special thanks to Chris Turner for content editing and guiding the project. Also thanks to Esther Lee and Cari Farrell for design work and Ryan Burke for checking doses and standardization of supplement recommendations. And none of it would matter without Jon Hudson guiding marketing to make sure that the book reaches the people who need it most.

I would also like to thank the customer advisory board for pre-reading the book and giving constructive feedback. Thanks also to the customer support team, Tim Yarborough, Alec Widen, and Emily Grimes, for arranging that essential support, and Meghan Arnold for keeping up with social media.

Good editing is essential for any book to shine, and Ashley Cullen made the book much better with her outstanding job of doing the final edit on the book. Her diligent effort to pick up every one of the many typos I left behind and cross check all the references is very much appreciated.

Resources

When I transitioned my medical practice to include herbal medicine in 2005, one of the frustrations became finding reputable products to recommend to patients. Because availability of herbal products in my area was sparse, I began selling carefully selected products in the office. Profits from supplement sales helped compensate for low reimbursements from insurance companies. This allowed me to spend more time with patients and avoid ordering unnecessary procedures and labs.

Ultimately, I became fascinated with the modern supplement industry and started having supplements made to my exact specifications. That way I could control quality, potency, and to a certain extent, cost.

My daughter became involved, and in 2010, we formed an online supplement company. The goal from the beginning, however, was to do much more than provide herbal and natural supplements. Through the website, we could reach people and help guide them in the path back to wellness with support, resources, and programs. To date the company has enhanced the lives of thousands of people.

In 2015, the company proudly achieved **B-Corp** status. A **benefit corporation** is a for-profit company that provides positive impact on society, workers, the community and the environment.

Oddly, FDA and FTC regulations prohibit me from mentioning the name of that company in conjunction with any information that might help you overcome Lyme disease. You can, however, find book updates, extra information, webinars, and lots of other useful information at **RawlsMD. com.** You can also get download extras and updates for *Unlocking Lyme* at **UnlockingLyme.com/Extras.**

If you are interested in learning more about basic herbal medicine, I would highly recommend *Adaptogens, Herbs for Strength, Stamina, and Stress Relief* (2007), by David Winston RH(AHG) and Steven Maimes. Now a classic, it's an easy read that has introduced many people to herbal therapy. David Winston also co-wrote, with Merrily A. Kuhn, another little handbook on herbs, called *Herbal Therapy & Supplements, A Scientific and Traditional Approach* (2008).

For a deeper dive into adaptogens, consider a copy of *Adaptogens in Medical Herbalism* (2013), by Donald Yance CN MH RH(AHG). His primary professional focus is using herbal medicine to support cancer therapy, and he also wrote *Herbal Medicine, Healing, & Cancer* (1999).

If you have interest in studying the biochemical aspect of herbal medicine, I highly recommend *Medical Herbalism, The Science and Practice of Herbal Medicine* (2003), by David Hoffman. The first third of the book is devoted to describing the chemical components of the most common herbs and what they do. David Hoffman has also written a series of short herbal guides for specific problems, such as *Healthy Digestion*, in the Storey Medicinal Herb Guide Series.

For authoritative information about herbs from the Amazon basin, I recommend *The Healing Power of Rainforest Herbs* (2005), by Leslie Taylor, ND.

If you want to know absolutely everything about the microbes associated with Lyme disease and the herbs that can be used to treat Lyme disease, I highly recommend the 2015 edition of *Healing Lyme, Natural Healing of Lyme Borreliosis and the Coinfections Chlamydia and Spotted Fever Rickettsioses*, by Stephen Buhner. Buhner has also written a series of books about natural therapy for the known co-infections and other interesting books on a variety of topics.

Both David Winston and Donald Yance have their own quality lines of herbal products. Leslie Taylor did have an excellent line of herbal products that supported indigenous rainforest populations, but finally gave up sale of products because of frustrations with dealing the FDA. Stephen Buhner does not endorse specific products, but does list trusted resources at the end of his books.

Endorphins are essential for recovery from any chronic illness and the best way to generate endorphins is through moderate exercise. Early on in recovery, however, pain often prevents exercise. Many people have found that low dose naltrexone is useful for controlling pain and boosting endorphins. Information about low dose naltrexone and compounding pharmacies that source it can be found at lowdosenaltrexone.org.

The nonprofit, Environmental Working Group, at ewn.org, is an excellent resource for detoxifying the world you come in contact with and cleaning up your diet.

For finding healthful meat, eatwild.com is a great resource.

There are many companies that make excellent FIR saunas. If you decide to purchase one, get one made from wood (not plastic) and big enough for at least two people.

Medicinal cannabis will become much more prevalent on the landscape of treating chronic illness, but with the proliferation of new companies, it's hard to recommend specific companies or products. If you choose to use cannabis products, make sure supercritical CO_2 is used for the extraction process and not hexane. I am familiar with pure-CBD products from Blue Bird Botanicals and Stanley Brother's Charlotte's Web and I have confidence in the quality, but there are other reputable companies out there.

References

Chapter 1

Barbour AG, Hayes SF. Biology of Borrelia species. *Microbiol Rev.* 1986;50(4): 381-400.

Barbour AG, Burgdorfer W, Grunwaldt E, Steere AC. Antibodies of patients with Lyme disease to components of the Ixodes dammini spirochete. *J Clin Invest.* 1983 Aug;72(2):504-15.

Berghoff W. Chronic Lyme disease and co-infections: differential diagnosis. *Open Neurol J.* 2012;6: 158-178.

Brooks GF, Carroll KC, Butel JS, Morse SA. *Jawetz, Melnick, & Adelberg's Medical Microbiology.* 24th ed. McGraw-Hill/Lange; 2007.

Buhner SH. *Healing Lyme: Natural Healing of Lyme Borreliosis and the Coinfections Chlamydia and Spotted Fever Rickettsiosis.* 2nd ed. Raven Press; 2015.

Burgdorfer W. Discovery of the Lyme disease spirochete and its relation to tick vectors. *Yale J Biol Med.* 1984 Jul-Aug;57(4):515-20.

Burgdorfer W, Barbour AG, Hayes SF, Benach JL, Grunwaldt E, Davis JP. Lyme disease-a tick-borne spirochetosis? *Science.* 1982 Jun 18;216(4552):1317-9.

Burgdorfer W. How the discovery of Borrelia burgdorferi came about. *Clin Dermatol.* 1993 Jul-Sep;11(3):335-8.

Centers for Disease Control and Prevention. Lyme disease. http://www.cdc. gov/lyme/. Accessed July and September 2016.

Dietrich M, Gómez-Díaz E, McCoy KD. Worldwide distribution and diversity of seabird ticks: implications for the ecology and epidemiology of tick-borne pathogens. *Vector Borne Zoonotic Dis.* 2011 ;11(5):453-470.

Goering RV, Dockrell HM, Zuckerman M, Roitt IM, Chiodini PL. *Mims' Medical Microbiology.* 5th ed. Elsevier; 2013.

Hall SS. Iceman Unfrozen. *National Geographic.* November 2011.

Heylen D, Fonville M, van Leeuwen AD, Sprong H. Co-infections and transmission dynamics in a tick-borne bacterium community exposed to songbirds. *Environ Microbiol.* 2016;18(3):988-996.

Hvidsten D, Stordal F, Lager M, et al. Borrelia burgdorferi sensu-lato-infected Ixodes ricinus collected from vegetation near the Arctic Circle. *Ticks Tick Borne Dis.* 2015;6(6):768-773.

Levy S. The Lyme Disease Debate: Host Biodiversity and Human Disease Risk. *Environ Health Perspect.* 121:A120-A125 (2013).

Lloyd D. Circular letter #12-32. State of Connecticut, State Dept. of Health; 1976.

Masuzawa T. Terrestrial distribution of the Lyme borreliosis agent Borrelia burgdorferi sensu lato in East Asia. *Jpn J Infect Dis.* 2004;57(6):229-235.

McGarry JW. Travel and disease vector ticks. *Travel Med Infect Dis.* 2011;9(2):49-59.

Murray P, Rosenthal K, Pfaller M. *Medical Microbiology.* 8th ed. Elsevier; 2016.

Poinar Jr G. Spirochete-like cells in a Dominican amber Amblyomma tick (Arachnida: Ixodidae). *Historical Biology: An International Journal of Paleobiology.* 2015; 27(5):565-570.

Radolf JD, Caimano MJ, Stevenson B, Hu LT. Of ticks, mice and men: understanding the dual-host lifestyle of Lyme disease spirochaetes. *Nat Rev Microbiol.* 2012;10(2):87-99.

Steere AC, Coburn, Glickstein L. The emergence of Lyme disease. J Clin Invest. 2004;113(8)1093-1101.

Chapter 2

Antonara S, Ristow L, Coburn J. Adhesion mechanisms of Borrelia burgdorferi. *Adv Exp Med Biol.* 2011;715:35-49.

Barbour AG, Hayes SF. Biology of Borrelia species. *Microbiol Rev.* 1986;50(4): 381-400.

Brooks GF, Carroll KC, Butel JS, Morse SA. *Jawetz, Melnick, & Adelberg's Medical Microbiology*. 24th ed. McGraw-Hill/Lange; 2007.

Brorson Ø. Destruction of spirochete Borrelia burgdorferi round-body propagules (RBs) by the antibiotic Tigecycline. *Proc Natl Acad Sci U S A*. 2009 Nov 3; 106(44): 18656–18661.

Brown CR, Blaho VA, Loiacono CM. Treatment of mice with the neutrophil-depleting antibody RB6-8C5 results in early development of experimental Lyme arthritis via the recruitment of Gr-1- polymorphonuclear leukocyte-like cells. *Infect Immun*. 2004;72(9):4956-4965.

Buhner SH. *Healing Lyme: Natural Healing of Lyme Borreliosis and the Coinfections Chlamydia and Spotted Fever Rickettsiosis*. 2nd ed. Raven Press; 2015.

Cook MJ. Lyme borreliosis: a review of data on transmission time after tick attachment. *Int J Gen Med*. 2015; 8: 1–8.

Ebady R, Niddam AF, Boczula AE, et al. Biomechanics of Borrelia burgdorferi vascular interactions. *Cell Rep*. 2016;16(10):1-12.

Estrada-Peña A, Gray JS, Kahl O, Lane RS, Nijhof AM. Research on the ecology of ticks and tick-borne pathogens—methodological principles and caveats. *Front Cell Infect Microbiol*. 2013;3:29.

Goering RV, Dockrell HM, Zuckerman M, Roitt IM, Chiodini PL. *Mims' Medical Microbiology*. 5th ed. Elsevier; 2013.

Hajdušek O, Síma R, Ayllón N, et al. Interaction of the tick immune system with transmitted pathogens. *Front Cell Infect Microbiol*. 2013;3:26.

Hasler P, Giaglis S, Hahn S. Neutrophil extracellular traps in health and disease. *Swiss Med Wkly*. 2016 Oct 10;146:w14352.

Kazimírová M, Štibrániová I. *Tick salivary compounds: their role in modulation of host defences and pathogen transmission. Front Cell Infect Microbiol*. 2013;3:43.

Kugeler KJ, Griffith KS, Gould LH, et al. A review of death certificates listing Lyme disease as a cause of death in the United States. *Clin Infec Dis.* 2011;52(3):364-367.

Lantos PM, Auwaerter PG, Wormser GP. A systematic review of Borrelia burgdorferi morphologic variants does not support a role in chronic Lyme disease. *Clin Infect Dis.* 2014 Mar;58(5):663-71.

Lochhead RB, Sonderegger FL, Ma Y, et al. Endothelial cells and fibroblasts amplify the arthritogenic type I IFN response in murine Lyme disease and are major sources of chemokines in Borrelia burgdorferi-infected joint tissue. *J Immunol.* 2012;189(5):2488-2501.

Lusitani D, Malawista SE, Montgomery RR. Calprotectin, an abundant cytosolic protein from human polymorphonuclear leukocytes, inhibits the growth of Borrelia burgdorferi. *Infect Immun.* 2003;71(8):4711-4716.

McCoy KD, Léger E, Dietrich M. *Host specialization in ticks and transmission of tick-borne diseases: a review. Front Cell Infect Microbiol.* 2013;3:57.

Mead PS. Epidemiology of Lyme disease. *Infect Dis Clin North Am.* 2015;29(2):187–210.

Melaun C, Zottzman S, Santaella VG, et al. Occurrence of Borrelia burgdorferi s.l. in different genera of mosquitoes (Culicidae) in Central Europe. *Ticks Tick Borne Dis.*2016;7(2):256-263.

Menten-Dedoyart C, Faccinetto C, Golovchenko M, et al. Neutrophil extracellular traps entrap and kill Borrelia burgdorferi sensu stricto spirochetes and are not affected by Ixodes ricinus tick saliva. *J Immunol.* 2012;189(11):5393-5401.

Meriläinen L et al. Morphological and biochemical features of Borrelia burgdorferi pleomorphic forms. *Microbiology.* 2015 Mar;161(Pt 3):516-27.

Meriläinen L et al. Pleomorphic forms of Borrelia burgdorferi induce distinct immune responses. *Microbes Infect.* 2016 Jul-Aug;18(7-8):484-95.

Miklossy J et al. Persisting atypical and cystic forms of Borrelia burgdorferi and local inflammation in Lyme neuroborreliosis. *J of Neuroinflam.* 2008, 5:40

Montgomery RR, Lusitani D, de Boisfleury Chevance A, Malawista SE. Human phagocytic cells in the early innate immune response to Borrelia burgdorferi. *J Infect Dis.* 2002;185(12):1773-1779.

Petzke MM, Iyer R, Love AC, Spieler Z, Brooks A, Schwartz I. Borrelia burgdorferi induces a type I interferon response during early stages of disseminated infection in mice. *BMC Microbiol.* 2016;16:29.

Piesman J. Experimental acquisition of the Lyme disease spirochete, Borrelia burgdorferi, by larval Ixodes dammini (Acari: Ixodidae) during partial blood meals. *J Med Entomol.* 1991 Mar;28(2):259-62.

Radolf JD, Caimano MJ, Stevenson B, Hu LT. Of ticks, mice and men: understanding the dual-host lifestyle of Lyme disease spirochaetes. *Nat Rev Microbiol.* 2012;10(2):87-99.

Richter D, Matuschka FR, Spielman A, Mahadevan L. How ticks get under your skin: insertion mechanics of the feeding apparatus of Ixodes ricinus ticks. *Proc Biol Sci.* 2013;280(1773):20131758.

Schönrich G, Raftery MJ. Neutrophil Extracellular Traps Go Viral. *Front Immunol.* 2016 Sep 19;7:366.

Stibrániová I, Lahová M, Bartíková P. Immunomodulators in tick saliva and their benefits. *Acta Virol.* 2013;57(2):200-16.

Tilly K, Rosa P, Stewart P. Biology of Infection with Borrelia burgdorferi. *Infect Dis Clin North Am.* 2008 Jun; 22(2): 217–234.

Chapter 3

BORRELIA

de la Fuente J, Estrada-Pena A, Cabezas-Cruz A, Brey R. Flying ticks: anciently evolved associations that constitute a risk of infectious disease spread. *Parasit Vectors.* 2015;8:538.

Diakou A, Norte AC, Lopes de Carvalho I, et al. Ticks and tick-borne pathogens in wild birds in Greece. *Parasitol Res.* 2016;115(5):2011-2016.

Eisen RJ, Eisen L, Beard CB. *County-Scale Distribution of Ixodes scapularis and Ixodes pacificus (Acari: Ixodidae) in the Continental United States, J Med Entomol.* 2016;53(2):349-386.

Floris R, Menardi G, Bressan R, et al. Evaluation of a genotyping method based on the ospA gene to detect Borrelia burgdorferi sensu lato in multiple samples of Lyme borreliosis patients. *New Microbiol.* 2007;30(4):399-410.

Klaus C, Gethmann J, Hoffmann B, Ziegler U, Heller M, Beer M. Tick infestation in birds and prevalence of pathogens in ticks collected from different places in Germany. *Parasitol Res.* 2016;115(7):2729-2740.

Lyme History and Borrelia Species. http://www.lymeaustralia.com/history--borrelia-species.html. Accessed July 2016.

Margos G, Tsao JI, Castillo-Ramírez S, et al. Two boundaries separate Borrelia burgdorferi populations in North America. *Appl Environ Microbiol.* 2012;78(17):6059-6067.

Newman EA, Eisen L, Eisen RJ, et al. Borrelia burgdorferi sensu lato spirochetes in wild birds in northwestern California: associations with ecological factors, bird behavior and tick infestation. *PLoS One.* 2015;10(2): e0118146.

Rudenko N, Golovchenko M, Belfiore NM, Grubhoffer L, Oliver JH Jr. Divergence of Borrelia burgdorferi sensu lato spirochetes could be driven by the host: diversity of Borrelia strains isolated from ticks feeding on a single bird. *Parasit Vectors.* 2014;7:4.

Rudenko N, Golovchenko M, Clark K, Oliver JH, and Grubhoffer L. Detection of Borrelia burgdorferi sensu stricto in Amblyomma americanum ticks in the southeastern United States: the case of selective compatibility. *Emerg Microbes Infect.* 2016;5:e48. Published online 25 May 2016.

Rudenko N, Golovchenko M, Grubhoffer L, Oliver JH Jr. Updates on Borrelia burgdorferi sensu lato complex with respect to public health. *Ticks Tick Borne Dis.* 2011;2(3):123-128.

Schotthoefer AM, Frost HM. Ecology and epidemiology of Lyme borreliosis. *Clin Lab Med.* 2015;35(4):723-743.

Scott JD, Foley JE. Detection of Borrelia americana in the avian coastal tick, Ixodes auritulus (Acari: Ixodidae), collected from a bird captured in Canada. *Open J AnimSci.* 2016;6:207-216.

Scott JD, Lee MK, Fernando K, et al. Detection of Lyme disease spirochete, Borrelia burgdorferi sensu lato, including three novel genotypes in ticks (Acari: Ixodidae) collected from songbirds (Passeriformes) across Canada. *J Vector Ecol.* 2010;35(1):124-139.

Wodecka B, Skotarczak B. Identification of host blood-meal sources and Borrelia in field-collected Ixodes ricinus ticks in north-western Poland. *Ann Agric Environ Med.* 2016;23(1):59-63.

World Health Organization, International travel and health, distribution of Lyme Borreliosis, http://www.who.int/ith/diseases/lyme/en/. Accessed July 2016.

Yang J, Liu Z, Niu Q, et al. Tick-borne zoonotic pathogens in birds in Guangxi, Southwest China. *Parasit Vectors.* 2015; 8:637.

OTHER BORRELIA ILLNESSES

Barbour AG, Bunikis J, Travinsky B, et al. Niche partitioning of Borrelia burgdorferi and Borrelia miyamotoi in the same tick vector and mammalian reservoir species. *Am J Trop Med Hyg.* 2009;81(6):1120-1131.

Collares-Pereira M, Couceiro S, Franca I, et al. First isolation of Borrelia lusitaniae from a human patient. *J Clin Microbiol.* 2004;42(3):1316-1318.

Gil H, Barral M, Escudero R, Garcia-Perez A, Anda P. Identification of a new Borrelia species among small mammals in areas of northern Spain where Lyme disease is endemic. *Appl Environ Microbiol.* 2005;71(3):1336-1345.

Krause PJ, Fish D, Narasimhan S, Barbour AG. Borrelia miyamotoi infection in nature and in humans. *Clin Microbiol Infect.* 2015;21(7):631-639.

Masters EJ, Grigery CN, Masters RW. STARI, or Masters Disease: Lone Star tick–vectored Lyme-like Illness. *Infect Dis Clin North Am.* 2008;22(2):361-376.

Masuzawa T. Terrestrial distribution of the Lyme borreliosis agent Borrelia burgdorferi senso lato in East Asia. *Jpn J Infect Dis.* 2004;57(6):229-35.

Middelveen MJ, Bandoski C, Burke J, et al. Exploring the association between Morgellons disease and Lyme disease: identification of Borrelia burgdorferi in Morgellons disease patients. *BMC Dermatol.* 2015;15:1.

Middelveen MJ, Burugu D, Poruri A, et al. Association of spirochetal infection with Morgellons disease. *F1000Res.* 2013;2:25.

Middelveen MJ, Stricker RB. Filament formation associated with spirochetal infection: a comparative approach to Morgellons disease. *Clin Cosmet Investig Dermatol.* 2011;4:167-177.

Rudenko N, Golovchenko M, Grubhoffer L, Oliver JH Jr. Borrelia carolinensis sp. nov., a new (14th) member of the Borrelia burgdorferi Sensu Lato complex from the southeastern region of the United States. *J Clin Microbiol.* 2009;47(1):134-141. Epub 2008 Nov 19.

Rudenko N, Golovchenko M, Lin T, Gao L, Grubhoffer L, Oliver JH Jr. Delineation of a new species of the Borrelia burgdorferi Sensu Lato Complex, Borrelia americana sp nov. *J Clin Microbiol.* 2009:47(12):3875-3880. Epub 2009 Oct 21.

Sayler KA, Loftis AD, Beatty SK, et al. Prevalence of Tick-Borne Pathogens in Host-Seeking Amblyomma americanum (Acari: Ixodidae) and Odocoileus virginianus (Artiodactyla: Cervidae) in Florida. *J Med Entomol.* 2016. Epub ahead of print.

Telford SR 3rd, Goethert HK, Molloy PJ, et al. Borrelia miyamotoi Disease: Neither Lyme Disease Nor Relapsing Fever. *Clin Lab Med.* 2015;35(4):867-882.

Tick-borne relapsing fever (TBRF): transmission. http://www.cdc.gov/relapsing-fever/transmission/index.html. Accessed July 2016.

Wagemakers A, Staarink PJ, Sprong H, Hovius JW. Borrelia miyamotoi: a widespread tick-borne relapsing fevers spirochete. *Trends Parasitol.* 2015;31(6):260-269.

COINFECTIONS

Angelakis E, Billeter SA, Brietschwerdt EB, Chomel BB, Raoult D. Potential for tick-borne bartonelloses, *Emerg Infect Dis.* 2010;16(3):385-391.

Baneth G. Tick-borne infections of animals and humans: a common ground. *Int J Parasitol*. 2014;44(9):591-596.

Baseman JB, Tully JG. Mycoplasmas: sophisticated, reemerging, and burdened by their notoriety. *Emerg Infect Dis*. 1997;3(1):21-32.

Berghoff W. Chronic Lyme Disease and Co-infections: Differential Diagnosis. *Open Neurol J*. 2012; 6: 158-178.

Brites-Neto J, Duarte KM, Martins TF. Tick-borne infections in human and animal population worldwide. *Vet World*. 2015;8(3):301-315.

Buhner SH. *Healing Lyme: Natural Healing of Lyme Borreliosis and the Coinfections Chlamydia and Spotted Fever Rickettsiosis*. 2nd ed. Raven Press; 2015.

Cisak E, Wojcik-Fatla A, Zajac V, Sawczyn A, Sroka J, Dutkiewicz J. Spiroplasma— an emerging arthropod-borne pathogen? *Ann Agric Environ Med*. 2015;22(4):589-593.

Clinton RM, Carabin H, Little SE. Emerging zoonoses in the southern United States: toxocariasis, bovine tuberculosis and southern tick-associated rash illness. *Am J Med Sci*. 2010;340(3):187-193.

Edouard S, Nabet C, Lepidi H, Fournier PE, Raoult D. Bartonella, a common cause of endocarditis: a report on 106 cases and review. *J Clin Microbiol*. 2015;53(3):824-829.

Endresen GK. Mycoplasma blood infection in chronic fatigue and fibromyalgia syndromes. *Rheumatol Int*. 2003;23(5):211-215. Epub 2003 Jul 16.

Estrada-Peña A, de la Fuente J. The ecology of ticks and epidemiology of tick-borne viral diseases. *Antiviral Res*. 2014;108:104-128.

Gilroy CB, Keat A, Taylor-Robinson D. The prevalence of Mycoplasma fermentans in patients with arthritides. *Rheumatology*. 2001;40(12):1355-1358.

Hakkarainen K, Turrunen H, Miettinen A, Kaitik M, Jannson E. Mycoplasmas and arthritis. *Ann Rheum Dis*. 1992;51(10):1170-1172.

Ismail N, Bloch KC, McBride JW. Human ehrlichiosis and anaplasmosis. *Clin Lab Med*. 2010;30(1):261-292.

Moumène A, Meyer DF. Ehrlichia's molecular tricks to manipulate their host cells. *Microbes Infect.* 2016;18(3):172-179.

Moutailler S, Popovici I, Devillers E, Vayssier-Taussat M, Eloit M. Diversity of viruses in Ixodes ricinus, and characterization of a neurotropic strain of Eyach virus. *New Microbes New Infect.* 2016;11:71-81.

Moutailler S, Valiente Moro C, Vaumourin E, et al. Co-infection of Ticks: The Rule Rather Than the Exception. *PLoS Negl Trop Dis.* 2016;10(3):e0004539.

Mycoplasma pneumoniae infection. http://www.cdc.gov/pneumonia/atypical/mycoplasma/index.html. Accessed June 2016.

Narasimhan S, Fikrig E. Tick microbiome: the force within. *Trends Parasitol.* 2015;31(7):315-323.

Norman RA, Worton AJ, Gilbert L. Past and future perspectives on mathematical models of tick-borne pathogens. *Parasitology.* 2016143(7):850-859. Epub 2015 Dec 18.

Parola P, Paddock CD, Socolovschi C, et al. Update on tick-borne rickettsioses around the world: a geographic approach. *Clin Microbiol Rev.* 2013;26(4):657-702.

Pfäffle M, Littwin N, Muders SV, Petney TN. The ecology of tick-borne diseases. *Int J Parasitol.* 2013;43(12-13):1059-1077.

Pujalte GG, Chua JV. Tick-borne infections in the United States. *Prim Care.* 2013;40(3):619-635.

Razin S, Yogev D, Naot Y. Molecular biology and pathogenicity of mycoplasmas. *Microbiol Mol Biol Rev.* 1998;62(4):1094-1156.

Rivera-Tapia J, Rodriguez-Preval N. Possible role of mycoplasmas in pathogenesis of gastrointestinal diseases. *Rev Biomed.* 2006;17:132-139.

Roediger WE. Intestinal mycoplasma in Crohn's disease. *Novartis Found Symp.* 2004;263:85-93; discussion 93-98, 211-218.

Salinas LJ, Greenfield RA, Little SE, Voskuhl GW. Tickborne infections in the southern United States. *Am J Med Sci.* 2010;340(3):194-201.

Stromdahl EY, Hickling GJ. Beyond Lyme: aetiology of tick-borne human diseases with emphasis on the southeastern United States. *Zoonoses Public Health*. 2012;59(Suppl 2):48-64.

Taylor L (2001). Mycoplasmas—stealth pathogens. http://www.rain-tree.com/myco.htm#.V-v_wigrKUk. Accessed July 2016.

Tijsse-Klasen E, Koopmans MP, Sprong H. Tick-borne pathogen—reversed and conventional discovery of disease. *Front Public Health*. 2014;2:73.

Trout Fryxell RT, DeBruyn JM. The Microbiome of Ehrlichia-Infected and Uninfected Lone Star Ticks (Amblyomma americanum). *PLoS One*. 2016;11(1):e0146651.

Waites KB, Talkington DF. Mycoplasma pneumoniae and its role as a human pathogen. *Clin Microbiol Rev*. 2004;17(4):697-728.

Zhang S, Tsai S, Wu TT, Li B, Shih JW, Lo SC. Mycoplasma fermentans infection promotes immortalization of human peripheral blood mononuclear cells in culture. *Blood*. 2004;104(13):4252-4259.

Chapter 4

Angelakis E, Mediannikov O, Parola P, Raoult D. Rickettsia felis: The Complex Journey of an Emergent Human Pathogen. *Trends Parasitol*. 2016;32(7):554-64. Epub 2016 May 4.

Brites-Neto J, Duarte KM, Martins TF. Tick-borne infections in human and animal population worldwide. *Vet World*. 2015;8(3):301-315.

Buhner SH. *Healing Lyme: Natural Healing of Lyme Borreliosis and the Coinfections Chlamydia and Spotted Fever Rickettsiosis*. 2nd ed. Raven Press; 2015.

Casadevall A, Pirofski L. Host-pathogen interactions: the attributes of virulence. *J Infect Dis*. 2001;184(3)337-344. Epub 2001 Jun 27.

Casadevall A, Pirofski LA. Host-pathogen interactions: basic concepts of microbial commensalism, colonization, infection, and disease. *Infect Immun*. 2000;68(12):6511-6518.

Casadevall A, Pirofski LA. Host-pathogen interactions: redefining the basic concepts of virulence and pathogenicity. *Infect Immun.* 1999;67(8): 3703-3713.

Ebel GD. Update on Powassan virus: emergence of a North American tick-borne flavivirus. *Annu Rev Entomol.* 2010;55:95-110.

Faccini-Martínez ÁA, García-Álvarez L, Hidalgo M, Oteo JA. Syndromic classification of rickettsioses: an approach for clinical practice. *Int J Infect Dis.* 2014;28:126-139. Epub 2014 Sep 19.

Hermance ME, Thangamani S. Tick Saliva Enhances Powassan Virus Transmission to the Host, Influencing Its Dissemination and the Course of Disease. *J Virol.* 2015;89(15):7852-7860. Epub 2015 May 20.

Lloyd-Price J, Abu-Ali G, Huttenhower C. The healthy human microbiome. *Genome Med.* 2016;27:8(1):51.

National Geographic, Seeking the Source of Ebola, by David Quammen, July 2015.

Nelder MP, Russell CB, Sheehan NJ, et al. Human pathogens associated with the blacklegged tick Ixodes scapularis: a systematic review. *Parasit Vectors.* 2016;9:265.

Parola P, Paddock CD, Socolovschi C, et al. Update on tick-borne rickettsioses around the world: a geographic approach. *Clin Microbiol Rev.* 2013;26(4):657-702.

Petersen C, Round JL . Defining dysbiosis and its influence on host immunity and disease. *Cell Microbiol.* 2014;16(7):1024-1033

Petersen C, Round JL. Defining dysbiosis and its influence on host immunity and disease. *Cell Microbiol.* 2014;16(7):1024-1033. Epub 2014 Jun 2.

The Human Microbiome Project. http://hmpdacc.org/. Accessed August 2016.

Truchan HK, Seidman D, Carlyon J. Breaking in and grabbing a meal: Anaplasma phagocytophilum cellular invasion, nutrient acquisition, and promising tools for their study. *Microbes Infect.* 2013;15(14-15):1017-1025.

Chapter 5

Allen HB, Morales D, Jones K, Joshi S. Alzheimer's disease: a novel hypothesis integrating spirochetes, biofilm, and the immune system. *J Neuroinfect Dis.* 2016;7(1)

Beati L, Péter O, Burgdorfer W, Aeschlimann A, Raoult D. Confirmation that Rickettsia helvetica sp. nov. is a distinct species of the spotted fever group of rickettsiae. *Int J Syst Bacteriol.* 1993 Jul;43(3):521-6.

Benson-Bunch J (Aug 2016). Alzheimer's and Lyme Disease. Caldwell Lyme Web site. https://caudwelllyme.com/2016/08/25/alzheimers-and-lyme-disease/. Accessed August 2016.

Berer K, Krishnamoorthy G. Microbial view of central nervous system autoimmunity. *FEBS Lett.* 2014;588(22):4207-4213.

Bogdanos DP, Smyk DS, Invernizzi P, et al. Infectome: a platform to trace infectious triggers of autoimmunity. *Autoimmun Rev.* 2013;12(7):726-740. Epub 2012 Dec 22.

Campo L, Larocque P, La Malfa T, Blackburn WD, Watson HL. Genotypic and phenotypic analysis of Mycoplasma fermentans strains isolated from different host tissues. *J Clin Microbiol.* 1998;36(5):1371-1377.

Danzer C, Mattner J. Impact of microbes on autoimmune diseases. *Arch Immunol Ther Exp (Warsz).* 2013;61(3):175-186.

Ghosh S, Steere AC, Stollar BD, Huber BT. In situ diversification of the antibody repertoire in chronic Lyme *arthritis* synovium. *J Immunol.* 2005;174(5):2860-2869.

Goering RV, Dockrell HM, Zuckerman M, Roitt IM, Chiodini PL. *Mims' Medical Microbiology.* 5th ed. Elsevier; 2013.

Jansson E, Miettinen A, Hakkarainen K, et al. Cultivation of fastidious mycoplasmas from human arthritis. *Z Rheumatol.* 1983;42(2):66-69.

Kaiser C, Ernst M. *Organic Lettuce & Leafy Greens.* Cooperative Extension Service, University of Kentucky College of Agriculture, Food and Environment; July 2012.

Kim D, Yoo SA, Kim WU. Gut microbiota in autoimmunity: potential for clinical applications. *Arch Pharm Res*. 2016 Jul 22. Epub ahead of print.

Lehmer RR, Andrews BS, Robertson JA, Stanbridge EJ, de la Maza L, Friou GJ. Clinical and biological characteristics of Ureaplasma urealyticum induced polyarthritis in a patient with common variable hypogammaglobulinaemia. *Ann Rheum Dis*. 1991;50(8):574-576.

Logan AC, Venket Rao A, Irani D. Chronic fatigue syndrome: lactic acid bacteria may be of therapeutic value. *Med Hypotheses*. 2003;60(6):915-923.

Longman RS, Littman DR. The functional impact of the intestinal microbiome on mucosal immunity and systemic autoimmunity. *Curr Opin Rheumatol*. 2015;27(4):381-387.

Lowry S, Brent LH, Menaldino S, Kerr JR. A case of persistent parvovirus B19 infection with bilateral cartilaginous and ligamentous damage to the wrists. *Clin Infect Dis*. 2005;41(4): e42-e44. Epub 2005 Jul 14.

Luckey D, Gomez A, Murray J, White B, Taneja V. Bugs & us: the role of the gut in autoimmunity. *Indian J Med Res*. 2013;138(5):732-743.

MacDonald A. Alzheimer's neuroborreliosis with trans-synaptic spread of infection and neurofibrillary tangles derived from intraneuronal spirochetes. *Med Hypotheses*. 2007;68(4):822-825. Epub 2006 Oct 20.

MacDonald A. Cystic Borrelia in Alzheimer's disease and in non-dementia neuroborreliosis. *Alzheimer's & Dementia the Journal of the Alzheimer's Association*. 2006;2(3):S433.

MacDonald AB, Miranda JM. Concurrent neocortical borreliosis and Alzheimer's disease. *Hum Pathol*. 1987;18(7):759-761.

Maritsi DN, Zarganis D, Metaxa Z, Papaioannou G, Vartzelis G. Bartonella henselae Infection: An Uncommon Mimicker of Autoimmune Disease. *Case Rep Pediatr*. 2013;2013:726826. Epub 2013 Jan 17.

McMullen JE. *The Travel & Tropical Medicine Manual*. 2nd ed. Philadelphia, PA: WB Saunders; 1995.

Miklossy J. Alzheimer's disease—a spirochetosis? *Neuroreport*. 1993;4(7):841-848.

Murray P, Rosenthal K, Pfaller M. *Medical Microbiology*. 8th ed. Elsevier; 2016.

Namiki K, Goodison S, Porvasnik S, et al. Persistent exposure to Mycoplasma induces malignant transformation of human prostate cells. *PLoS One*. 20094(9):e6872.

Nicolson G. Chronic bacterial and viral infections in neurodegenerative and neurobehavioral diseases. *Lab Medicine*. 2008;39(5):291-299.

Petersen C, Round JL . Defining dysbiosis and its influence on host immunity and disease. *Cell Microbiol*. 2014;16(7):1024-1033

Pillar C. The Swiss Agent: Long-forgotten research unearths new mystery about Lyme Disease. *STAT, Reporting from the fronts of health and medicine*. October 12, 2016. www.statnews.com/2016/10/12/swiss-agent-lyme-disease-mystery/

Potgieter M, Bester J, Kell DB, Pretorius E. The dormant blood microbiome in chronic, inflammatory diseases. *FEMS Microbiol Rev*. 2015;39(4):567-591. Epub 2015 May 3.

Proal AD, Albert PJ, Marshall TG. Inflammatory disease and the human microbiome. *Discov Med*. 2014;17(95):257-265.

Rashid T, Ebringer A. Autoimmunity in Rheumatic Diseases Is Induced by Microbial Infections via Cross-reactivity or Molecular Mimicry. *Autoimmune Dis*. 2012;2012:539282. Epub 2012 Feb 20.

Razin S, Yogev D, Noat Y. Molecular biology and pathogenicity of Mycoplasmas. *Microbiol Mol Biol Rev*. 1998;62(4):1094-1156.

Root-Bernstein R, Fairweather D. Complexities in the relationship between infection and autoimmunity. *Curr Allergy Asthma Rep*. 2014;14(1):407.

Sandhya P, Danda D, Sharma D, Scaria V. Does the buck stop with the bugs?: an overview of microbial dysbiosis in rheumatoid arthritis. *Int J Rheum Dis*. 2016;19(1):8-20. Epub 2015 Sep 19.

Steed AL, Stappenbeck TS. Role of viruses and bacteria-virus interactions in autoimmunity. *Curr Opin Immunol*. 2014;31:102-107. Epub 2014 Oct 27.

Steiner G. Acute plaques in multiple sclerosis, their pathogenetic significance and the role of spirochetes as etiologic factor. *J Neuropathol Exp Neurol.* 1952;11(4):343-372.

Talkington J, Nickell SP. Borrelia burgdorferi spirochetes induce mast cell activation and cytokine release. *Infect Immun.* 1999;67(3):1107-1115.

Tully JG, Rose DL, Baseman JB, Dallo SF, Lazzell AL, Davis CP. Mycoplasma pneumoniae and Mycoplasma genitalium mixture in synovial fluid isolate. *J Clin Microbiol.* 1995;33(7):1851-1855.

Webster JP, Kaushik M, Bristow GC, McConkey GA. *Toxoplasma gondii* infection, from predation to schizophrenia: can animal behaviour help us understand human behaviour? *J Exp Biol.* 2013. 216 (Pt 1): 99–112.

Xu Y, Chen G. Mast cell and autoimmune diseases. *Mediators Inflamm.* 2015;2015:246126. Epub 2015 Apr 5.

Yandell K (Apr 1, 2016). Microbes meet cancer: Understanding cancer's relationship with the human microbiome could transform immune-modulating therapies. *The Scientist.*

Zárate-Bladés CR, Horai R, Caspi RR. Regulation of Autoimmunity by the Microbiome. *DNA Cell Biol.* 2016;35(9):455-458. Epub 2016 Jul 27.

Zhang L, Gough J, Christmas D, et al. Microbial infections in eight genomic subtypes of chronic fatigue syndrome/myalgic encephalomyelitis. *J Clin Pathol.* 2010;63(2):156-164. Epub 2009 Dec 2.

Chapter 9

Abbas AK, Lichtman AHH. *Basic Immunology, third edition.* St. Louis, MO: Elsevier; 2011.

Bralley A, Lord RS. *Laboratory Evaluations in Molecular Medicine.* Norcross, GA: The Institute for Advances in Molecular Medicine; 2001.

Castro C, Gourley M. Diagnostic testing and interpretation of tests for autoimmunity. *J Allergy Clin Immunol.* 2010;125(2 Suppl 2): S238-S247. Epub 2010 Jan 12.

Holtorf K. Innovative "alternative" therapies for chronic Lyme disease. 2016 ILADS Annual Conference.

Kumar P, Yadav U, Rai V. Methylenetetrahydrofolate reductase gene C677T polymorphism and breast cancer risk: Evidence for genetic susceptibility. *Meta Gene*. 2015 Oct 1;6:72-84.

Lab Tests Online. labstestsonline.org. Accessed July – September, 2016.

Lieberman J, Bell DS. Serum angiotensin-converting enzyme as a marker for the chronic fatigue-immune dysfunction syndrome: a comparison to serum angiotensin-converting enzyme in sarcoidosis. *Am J Med*. 1993 Oct;95(4):407-12.

Long S, Goldblatt J. MTHFR genetic testing: Controversy and clinical implications. *Aust Fam Physician*. 2016 Apr;45(4):237-40.

Moll S, Varga EA. Homocysteine and MTHFR Mutations. *Circulation*. 2015 Jul 7;132(1):e6-9

Murray P, Rosenthal K, Pfaller M. *Medical Microbiology*. 8th ed. Elsevier; 2016.

Myhill S, Booth NE, McLaren-Howard J. Chronic fatigue syndrome and mitochondrial dysfunction. *Int J Clin Exp Med*. 2009; 2(1): 1–16.

Ojo-Amaize EA, Conley EJ, Peter JB. Decreased natural killer cell activity is associated with severity of chronic fatigue immune dysfunction syndrome. *Clin Infect Dis*. 1994 Jan;18 Suppl 1:S157-9.

Oosting M et al. Recognition of Borrelia burgdorferi by NOD2 is central for the induction of an inflammatory reaction. *J Infect Dis*. 2010 Jun 15;201(12):1849-58.

Rai V. Methylenetetrahydrofolate Reductase A1298C Polymorphism and Breast Cancer Risk: A Meta-analysis of 33 Studies. *Ann Med Health Sci Res*. 2014 Nov-Dec; 4(6): 841–851.

Reynolds K. Small intestinal bacterial overgrowth (SIBO): an integrative approach. 2016 ILADS Annual Conference.

Wang XJ, Xu LH, Chen YM, Luo L, Tu QF, Mei J. Methylenetetrahydrofolate reductase gene polymorphism in endometrial cancer: A systematic review and meta-analysis. *Taiwan J Obstet Gynecol*. 2015 Oct;54(5):546-50.

Zandman-Goddard G, Shoenfeld Y. Hyperferritinemia in autoimmunity. *Isr Med Assoc J*. 2008;10(1):83-84.

Chapter 10

Barbour AG, Hayes SF. Biology of Borrelia species. *Microbiol Rev.* 1986;50(4): 381-400.

http://ispotlyme.com

Marques A, Brown MR, Fleisher TA. Natural killer cell counts are not different between patients with post-Lyme disease syndrome and controls *Clin Vaccine Immunol.* 2009;16(8):1249-1250.

Molins CR, Delorey MJ, Sexton C, Schriefer ME. Lyme Borreliosis Serology: Performance with Several Commonly Used Laboratory Diagnostic Tests and a Large Resource Panel of Well-Characterized Patient Samples. *J Clin Microbiol.* 2016; pii: JCM.00874-16. Epub ahead of print.

Murray P, Rosenthal K, Pfaller M. *Medical Microbiology.* 8th ed. Elsevier; 2016.

Nielsen CM, White MJ, Goodier MR, Riley EM. Functional Significance of CD57 Expression on Human NK Cells and Relevance to Disease. *Front Immunol.* 2013;4:422.

Stricker RB, Winger EE. Natural killer cells in chronic Lyme disease. *Clin Vaccine Immunol.* 2009;16(11):1704-1706.

www.advanced-lab.com/spirochete.php

www.cdc.gov/lyme/diagnosistesting/

www.ceresnano.com

www.galaxydx.com

www.igenex.com

www.labtestsonline.org

www.uab.edu/medicine/pathology/Mycoplasma-Home

Zhang L, Zong ZY, Liu YB, Ye H, LV XJ. PCR versus serology for diagnosing Mycoplasma pneumoniae infection: a systematic review & meta-analysis. *Indian J Med Res.* 2011;134(3): 270-280.

Chapter 12

Abrams Y. Complications of coinfection with Babesia and Lyme disease after splenectomy. *J Am Board Fam Med*. 2008;21(1):75-77.

Barnett ML, Linder JA. Antibiotic prescribing to adults with sore throat in the United States, 1997-2010. *JAMA Intern Med*. 2013;174(1):138-140.

Bartlett JG. Clinical practice. Antibiotic-associated diarrhea. *N Engl J Med*. 2002:346(5):334-339.

Berende A, ter Hofstede HJ, Vos FJ, et al. Randomized Trial of Longer-Term Therapy for Symptoms Attributed to Lyme Disease. *N Engl J Med*. 2016;374(13):1209-1220. [some benefit during use, but no overall benefit of prolonged antibiotic use 2 weeks IV ceftriaxone followed by 12 weeks doxycycline, clarithromycin, and hydroxychloroquine for 12 weeks versus placebo]

Berndtson K. Review of evidence for immune evasion and persistent infection in Lyme disease. *Int J Gen Med*. 2013;6:291-306.

Bork S et al. Growth-inhibitory effect of heparin on Babesia parasites. *Antimicrob Agents Chemother*. 2004 Jan;48(1):236-41.

Centers for Disease Control. Lyme disease: treatment. http://www.cdc.gov/lyme/treatment/index.html. Accessed July-October 2016.

Francino MP. Antibiotics and the Human Gut Microbiome: Dysbioses and Accumulation of Resistances. *Front Microbiol*. 2016;6:1543.

Fujimura KE, Slusher NA, Cabana MD, Lynch SV. Role of the gut microbiota in defining human health. *Expert Rev Anti Infect Ther*. 2010;8(4):435-454.

Infectious Diseases Society of America (Oct 4 2013). Antibiotics drastically overprescribed for sore throats, bronchitis. *Science Daily*. https://www.sciencedaily.com/releases/2013/10/131004105256.htm. Accessed September 2016.

Johnson L, Stricker RB. The Infectious Diseases Society of America Lyme guidelines: a cautionary tale about the development of clinical practice guidelines. *Philos Ethics Humanit Med*. 2010;5:9.

Jones SE, Versalovic J. Probiotic Lactobacillus reuteri biofilms produce antimicrobial and anti-inflammatory factors. *BMC Microbiol.* 2009;9:35.

Kalghatgi S, Spina CS, Costello JC, et al. Bactericidal antibiotics induce mitochondrial dysfunction and oxidative damage in Mammalian cells. *Sci Transl Med.* 2013;5(192):192ra85. [quinolones, aminoglycosides, beta-lactams]

Macfarlane S, Bahrami B, Macfarlane GT. Mucosal biofilm communities in the human intestinal tract. *Adv Appl Microbiol.* 2011;75:111-143.

Macfarlane S, Dillon JF. Microbial biofilms in the human gastrointestinal tract. *J Appl Microbiol.* 2007;102(5):1187-1196.

Macfarlane S, Woodmansey EJ, Macfarlane GT. Colonization of mucin by human intestinal bacteria and establishment of biofilm communities in a two-stage continuous culture system. *Appl Environ Microbiol.* 2005;71(11):7483-7492.

Morgun A, Dzutsev A, Dong X, et al. Uncovering effects of antibiotics on the host and microbiota using transkingdom gene networks. *Gut.* 2015;64(11):1732-1742. Epub 2015 Jan 22. [antibiotics destroy mitochondria; deplete microbiota causing immunodeficiency, and cause microbial resistance]

Moullan N, Mouchiroud L, Wang X, et al. Tetracyclines Disturb Mitochondrial Function across Eukaryotic Models: A Call for Caution in Biomedical Research. *Cell Rep.* 2015;10:1681-1691.

Perez-Cobas AE, Gosalbes MJ, Friedrichs A, et al. Gut microbiota disturbance during antibiotic therapy, a multi-omic approach. *Gut.* 2013;62(11):1591-1601. Epub 2012 Dec 12.

Rudenko N, Golovchenko M, Vancova M, et al. Isolation of live Borrelia burgdorferi senso lato spirochaetes from patients with undefined disorders and symptoms not typical for Lyme borreliosis. *Clin Microb Infect.* 2016;22(3):267. Epub 2015 Dec 8.

Shehab N, Patel P, Srinivasan A, Budnitz DS. Emergency department visits for antibiotic-associated adverse events. *Clin Infect Dis.* 2008;47(6):735-743.

Stricker RB, Johnson L. Lyme disease: the next decade. *Infect Drug Resist.* 2011;4:1-9.

Wormser GP, Dattwyler RJ, Shapiro ED, et al. The clinical assessment, treatment, and prevention of Lyme disease, human granulocytic anaplasmosis, and babesiosis: clinical practice guidelines by the Infectious Diseases Society of America. *Clin Infect Dis.* 2006;43(9):1089-1134. Epub 2006 Oct 2.

Chapter 13

Buhner SH. *Healing Lyme Disease Coinfections.* Rochester, VT: Healing Arts Press; 2013.

Buhner SH. *Healing Lyme: Natural Healing of Lyme Borreliosis and the Coinfections Chlamydia and Spotted Fever Rickettsiosis.* 2nd ed. Raven Press; 2015.

Buhner SH. *Herbal Antibiotics.* North Adams, MA: Storey Publishing; 2012.

Buhner SH. *Herbal Antivirals,.* North Adams, MA: Storey Publishing; 2013.

Halvorsen BL, Carlsen MH, Phillips KM, et al. Content of redox-active compounds in foods consumed in the United States. *Am J Clin Nutr.* 2006;84(1):95-135.

Hendler SS. *PDR for Nutritional Supplements.* 2nd ed. Montvale, NJ: Thomson Reuters; 2008.

Hoffmann D. *Medical Herbalism, the Science and Practice of Herbal Medicine.* Rochester, VT: Healing Arts Press; 2003.

Kuhn MA, Winston D. *Herbal Therapy & Supplements.* 2nd ed. Philadelphia, PA: Wolters Kluwer Health/Lippincott Williams & Wilkins; 2008.

Thomson Healthcare. *PDR for Herbal Medicines.* 4th ed. Montvale, NJ: Medical Economics Company; 2007.

Winston D, Maimes S. *Adaptogens: Herbs for Strength, Stamina, and Stress Relief.* Rochester, VT: Healing Arts Press; 2007.

Yance Jr D. *Adaptogens in Medical Herbalism.* Rochester, VT: Healing Arts Press; 2013.

Yance Jr. DR. *Herbal Medicine, Healing and Cancer: A Comprehensive Program for Prevention and Treatment.* Lincolnwood, IL: Keats Publishing; 1999.

Chapter 14

ANDROGRAPHIS

Arifullah M, Namsa ND, Mandal M, et al. Evaluation of anti-bacterial and anti-oxidant potential of andrographolide and echiodinin isolated from callus culture of Andrographis paniculata Nees. *Asian Pac J Trop Biomed.* 2013;3(8):604-610.

Chandrasekaran CV, Murali B, Deepak M, Agarwal A. In vitro comparative evaluation of non-leaves and leaves extracts of Andrographis paniculata on modulation of inflammatory mediators. *Antiinflamm Antiallergy Agents Med Chem.* 2012;11(2):191-197.

Chao WW, Kuo YH, Lin BF. Anti-inflammatory activity of new compounds from Andrographis paniculata by NF-kappaB transactivation inhibition. *J Agric Food Chem.* 2010;58(4):2505-2512.

Hua Z, Frohlich KM, Zhang Y, Feng X, Zhang J, Shen L. Andrographolide inhibits intracellular Chlamydia trachomatis multiplication and reduces secretion of proinflammatory mediators produced by human epithelial cells. *Pathog Dis.* 2015;73(1):1-11.

Lim JC, Chan TK, Ng DS, Sagineedu SR, Stanslas J, Wong WS. Andrographolide and its analogues: versatile bioactive molecules for combating inflammation and cancer. *Clin Exp Pharmacol Physiol.* 2012;39(3):300-310.

Mishra et al. Antibacterial activity of Andrographis paniculata (Burm. f.) Wall ex Nees leaves against clinical pathogens. *J Pharm Res.* 2013;7(5):459-462.

Mishra US, Mishra A, Kumari R, Murthy PN, Naik BS. Antibacterial Activity of Ethanol Extract of Andrographis paniculata. *Indian J Pharm Sci.* 2009;71(4):436-438.

Nanthini UR, Athinarayanan G, Ranjitsingh AJA, et al. Antimicrobial activity of leaf extracts of the medicinal plants Andrographis paniculata and Melia Azadirach L. *Int J Curr Res.* 2013;5(11):3563-3566.

Parichatikanond W, Suthisisang C, Dhepakson P, Herunsalee A. Study of anti-inflammatory activities of the pure compounds from Andrographis paniculata (burm.f.) Nees and their effects on gene expression. *Int Immunopharmacol.* 2010;10(11):1361-1373.

Salim E, Kumolosasi E, Jantan I. Inhibitory effect of selected medicinal plants on the release of pro-inflammatory cytokines in lipopolysaccharide-stimulated human peripheral blood mononuclear cells. *J Nat Med.* 2014;68(3):647-653.

Sheeja K, Kuttan G. Andrographis paniculata downregulates proinflammatory cytokine production and augments cell mediated immune response in metastatic tumor-bearing mice. *Asian Pac J Cancer Prev.* 2010;11(3):723-729.

Singha PK, Roy S, Dey S. Antimicrobial activity of Andrographis paniculata. *Fitoterapia.* 2003;74(7-8):692-694.

Sule et al. Screening for antibacterial activity of Andrographis paniculata used in Malaysian folkloric medicine: A possible alternative for the treatment of skin infections. *Ethnobotanical Leaflets.* 2010;14: 445-456.

Tang T, Targan SR, Li ZS, Xu C, Byers VS, Sandborn WJ. Randomised clinical trial: herbal extract HMPL-004 in active ulcerative colitis - a double-blind comparison with sustained release mesalazine. *Aliment Pharmacol Ther.* 2011;33(2):194-202. Epub 2010 Nov 30.

CAT'S CLAW

Allen-Hall L, Arnason JT, Cano P, Lafrenie RM. Uncaria tomentosa acts as a potent TNF-alpha inhibitor through NF-kappaB. *J Ethnopharmacol.* 2010;127(3):685-693.

de Paula LC, Fonseca F, Perazzo F, et al. Uncaria tomentosa (cat's claw) improves quality of life in patients with advanced solid tumors. *J Altern Complement Med.* 2015;21(1):22-30.

Domingues A, Sartori A, Valente LM, Golim MA, Siani AC, Viero RM. Uncaria tomentosa aqueous-ethanol extract triggers an immunomodulation toward a Th2 cytokine profile. *Phytother Res.* 2011;25(8):1229-1235.

Gonçalves C, Dinis T, Batista MT. Antioxidant properties of proanthocyanidins of Uncaria tomentosa bark decoction: a mechanism for anti-inflammatory activity. *Phytochemistry.* 2005;66(1):89-98.

Heitzman ME, Neto CC, Winiarz E, Vaisberg AJ, Hammond GB. Ethnobotany, phytochemistry and pharmacology of Uncaria (Rubiaceae). *Phytochemistry.* 2005;66(1):5-29.

Mammone T, Akesson C, Gan D, Giampapa V, Pero RW. A water soluble extract from Uncaria tomentosa (Cat's Claw) is a potent enhancer of DNA repair in primary organ cultures of human skin. *Phytother Res.* 2006;20(3):178-183.

Reis SR, Valente LM, Sampaio AL, et al. Immunomodulating and antiviral activities of Uncaria tomentosa on human monocytes infected with Dengue Virus-2. *Int Immunopharmacol.* 2008;8(3):468-476.

Rojas-Duran R, González-Aspajo G, Ruiz-Martel C, et al. Anti-inflammatory activity of Mitraphylline isolated from Uncaria tomentosa bark. *J Ethnopharmacol.* 2012;143(3):801-804.

Sandoval M, Okuhama NN, Zhang XJ, et al. Anti-inflammatory and antioxidant activities of cat's claw (Uncaria tomentosa and Uncaria guianensis) are independent of their alkaloid content. *Phytomedicine.* 2002;9(4):325-337.

Sandoval-Chacón M, Thompson JH, Zhang XJ, et al. Antiinflammatory actions of cat's claw: the role of NF-kappaB. *Aliment Pharmacol Ther.* 1998;12(12):1279-1289.

Williams JE. Review of antiviral and immunomodulating properties of plants of the Peruvian rainforest with a particular emphasis on Una de Gato and Sangre de Grado. *Altern Med Rev.* 2001;6(6):567-579.

CHINESE SKULLCAP

Butenko IG, Gladtchenko SV, Galushko SV. Anti-inflammatory properties and inhibition of leukotriene C4 biosynthesis in vitro by flavonoid baicalein from Scutellaria baicalensis georgy roots. *Agents Actions.* 1993;39 Spec No:C49-C51.

Chien CF, Wu YT, Tsai TH. Biological analysis of herbal medicines used for the treatment of liver diseases. *Biomed Chromatogr.* 2011;25(1-2):21-38.

Gasiorowski K, Lamer-Zarawska E, Leszek J, et al. Flavones from root of Scutellaria baicalensis Georgi: drugs of the future in neurodegeneration? *CNS Neurol Disord Drug Targets.* 2011;10(2):184-191.

Huang Y, Tsang SY, Yao X, Chen ZY. Biological properties of baicalein in cardiovascular system. *Curr Drug Targets Cardiovasc Haematol Disord.* 2005;5(2):177-184.

Jung HS, Kim MH, Gwak NG, et al. Antiallergic effects of Scutellaria baicalensis on inflammation in vivo and in vitro. *J Ethnopharmacol.* 2012;141(1):345-349.

Li-Weber M. New therapeutic aspects of flavones: the anticancer properties of Scutellaria and its main active constituents Wogonin, Baicalein and Baicalin. *Cancer Treat Rev.* 2009;35(1):57-68. Epub 2008 Nov 11.

Muluye RA, Bian Y, Alemu PN. Anti-inflammatory and Antimicrobial Effects of Heat-Clearing Chinese Herbs: A Current Review. *J Tradit Complement Med.* 2014;4(2):93-98.

Piao HZ, Jin SA, Chun HS, Lee JC, Kim WK. Neuroprotective effect of wogonin: potential roles of inflammatory cytokines. *Arch Pharm Res.* 2004;27(9):930-936.

Yune TY, Lee JY, Cui CM, Kim HC, Oh TH. Neuroprotective effect of Scutellaria baicalensis on spinal cord injury in rats. *J Neurochem.* 2009;110(4):1276-1287.

CORDYCEPS

Chang ST, Wasser SP. The role of culinary-medicinal mushrooms on human welfare with a pyramid model for human health. *Int J Med Mushrooms.* 2012;14(2):95-134.

Chen CY, Hou CW, Bernard JR, et al. Rhodiola crenulata and Cordyceps sinensis-based supplement boosts aerobic exercise performance after short-term high altitude training. *High Alt Med Biol.* 2014;15(3):371-379.

Chen S, Li Z, Krochmal R, Abrazado M, Kim W, Cooper CB. Effect of Cs-4 (Cordyceps sinensis) on exercise performance in healthy older subjects: a double-blind, placebo-controlled trial. *J Altern Complement Med.* 2010;16(5):585-590.

Guggenheim AG, Wright KM, Zwickey HL. Immune Modulation From Five Major Mushrooms: Application to Integrative Oncology. *Integr Med (Encinitas)*. 2014;13(1):32-44.

Jordan JL, Sullivan AM, Lee TD. Immune activation by a sterile aqueous extract of Cordyceps sinensis: mechanism of action. *Immunopharmacol Immunotoxicol*. 2008;30(1):53-70.

Nakamura K, Shinozuka K, Yoshikawa N. Anticancer and antimetastatic effects of cordycepin, an active component of Cordyceps sinensis. *J Pharmacol Sci*. 2015;127(1):53-56.

Ng TB, Wang HX. Pharmacological actions of Cordyceps, a prized folk medicine. *J Pharm Pharmacol*. 2005;57(12):1509-1519.

Shin S, Lee S, Kwon J, et al. Cordycepin Suppresses Expression of Diabetes Regulating Genes by Inhibition of Lipopolysaccharide-induced Inflammation in Macrophages. *Immune Netw*. 2009;9(3):98-105. Epub 2009 Jun 30.

Tuli HS, Sharma AK, Sandhu SS, Kashyap D. Cordycepin: a bioactive metabolite with therapeutic potential. *Life Sci*. 2013;93(23):863-869. Epub 2013 Oct 10.

Wang L, Hou Y. Determination of trace elements in anti-influenza virus mushrooms. *Biol Trace Elem Res*. 2011;143(3):1799-1807. Epub 2011 Feb 8.

Xiong Y, Zhang S, Xu L, et al. Suppression of T-cell activation in vitro and in vivo by cordycepin from Cordyceps militaris. *J Surg Res*. 2013;185(2):912-922. Epub 2013 Jul 22.

Yan F, Wang B, Zhang Y. Polysaccharides from Cordyceps sinensis mycelium ameliorate exhaustive swimming exercise-induced oxidative stress. *Pharm Biol*. 2014;52(2):157-161. Epub 2013 Sep 19.

Yue K, Ye M, Zhou Z, Sun W, Lin X. The genus Cordyceps: a chemical and pharmacological review. *J Pharm Pharmacol*. 2013;65(4):474-493. Epub 2012 Oct 23.

Zhang HW, Lin ZX, Tung YS, et al. Cordyceps sinensis (a traditional Chinese medicine) for treating chronic kidney disease. *Cochrane Database Syst Rev*. 2014;12:CD008353.

Zhou X, Luo L, Dressel W, et al. Cordycepin is an immunoregulatory active ingredient of Cordyceps sinensis. *Am J Chin Med.* 2008;36(5):967-980.

Zhu JS, Halpern GM, Jones K. The scientific rediscovery of a precious ancient Chinese herbal regimen: Cordyceps sinensis: part II. *J Altern Complement Med.* 1998;4(4):429-457. Review.

Zhu JS, Halpern GM, Jones K. The scientific rediscovery of an ancient Chinese herbal medicine: Cordyceps sinensis: part I. *J Altern Complement Med.* 1998;4(3):289-303.

GARLIC/ALLICIN

Borlinghaus J, Albrecht F, Gruhlke MC, Nwachukwu ID, Slusarenko AJ. Allicin: chemistry and biological properties. *Molecules.* 2014;19(8): 12591-12618.

Chan JY, Pang S, Lin J, Xia J, Wang Y. A review of the cardiovascular benefits and antioxidant properties of allicin. *Phytother Res.* 2013;27(5):637-646.

Coppi A, Cabinian M, Mirelman D, Sinnis P. Antimalarial activity of allicin, a biologically active compound from garlic cloves. *Antimicrob Agents Chemother.* 2006;50(5):1731-1737.

Corral MJ, Benito-Peña E, Jiménez-Antón MD, Cuevas L, Moreno-Bondi MC, Alunda JM. Allicin Induces Calcium and Mitochondrial Dysregulation Causing Necrotic Death in Leishmania. *PLoS Negl Trop Dis.* 2016;10(3):e0004525.

Feng Y, Zhu X, Wang Q, et al. Allicin enhances host pro-inflammatory immune responses and protects against acute murine malaria infection. *Malar J.* 2012;11:268.

Fratianni F, Ricardi R, Spigno P, et al. Biochemical Characterization and Antimicrobial and Antifungal Activity of Two Endemic Varieties of Garlic (Allium sativum L.) of the Campania Region, Southern Italy. *J Med Food.* 2016;19(7):686-691. Epub 2016 Jun 3.

Gonen A, Harats D, Rabinkov A, et al. The antiatherogenic effect of allicin: possible mode of action. *Pathobiology.* 2005;72(6):325-334.

Gu X, Wu H, Fu P. Allicin attenuates inflammation and suppresses HLA-B27 protein expression in ankylosing spondylitis mice. *Biomed Res Int.* 2013;2013:171573.

Guo N, Wu X, Yu L, et al. In vitro and in vivo interactions between fluconazole and allicin against clinical isolates of fluconazole-resistant Candida albicans determined by alternative methods. *FEMS Immunol Med Microbiol.* 2010;58(2):193-201. Epub 2009 Oct 5.

Harris JC, Cottrell SC, Plummer S, Lloyd D. Antimicrobial properties of Allium sativum (garlic). *Appl Microbiol Biotechnol.* 2001;57(3):282-286.

Jiang XW, Zhang Y, Song GD, et al. Clinical evaluation of allicin oral adhesive tablets in the treatment of recurrent aphthous ulceration. *Oral Surg Oral Med Oral Pathol Oral Radiol.* 2012;113(4):500-504.

Josling P. *Allicin: The Heart of Garlic.* HRC Publishing; 2005.

Kyung KH. Antimicrobial properties of allium species. *Curr Opin Biotechnol.* 2012;23(2):142-147.

Lawson LD, Gardner CD. Composition, stability, and bioavailability of garlic products used in a clinical trial. *J Agric Food Chem.* 2005;53(16):6254-6261.

Li XH, Li CY, Lu JM, Tian RB, Wei J. Allicin ameliorates cognitive deficits ageing-induced learning and memory deficits through enhancing of Nrf2 antioxidant signaling pathways. *Neurosci Lett.* 2012;514(1):46-50.

Liu C, Cao F, Tang QZ, et al. Allicin protects against cardiac hypertrophy and fibrosis via attenuating reactive oxygen species-dependent signaling pathways. *J Nutr Biochem.* 2010;21(12):1238-1250. Epub 2010 Feb 25.

Louis XL, Murphy R, Thandapilly SJ, Yu L, Netticadan T. Garlic extracts prevent oxidative stress, hypertrophy and apoptosis in cardiomyocytes: a role for nitric oxide and hydrogen sulfide. *BMC Complement Altern Med.* 2012;12:140.

Majewski M. Allium sativum: facts and myths regarding human health. *Rocz Panstw Zakl Hig.* 2014;65(1):1-8.

McMahon FG, Vargas R. Can garlic lower blood pressure? A pilot study. *Pharmacotherapy.* 1993;13(4):406-407.

O'Gara EA, Hill DJ, Maslin DJ. Activities of garlic oil, garlic powder, and their diallyl constituents against Helicobacter pylori. *Appl Environ Microbiol.* 2000;66(5):2269-2273.

Rana SV, Pal R, Vaiphei K, Sharma SK, Ola RP. Garlic in health and disease. *Nutr Res Rev.* 2011;24(1):60-71.

Ranjbar-Omid M, Arzanlou M, Amani M, Shokri Al-Hashem SK, Amir Mozafari N, Peeri Doghaheh H. Allicin from garlic inhibits the biofilm formation and ure-ase activity of Proteus mirabilis in vitro. *FEMS Microbiol Lett.* 2015;362(9). Epub 2015 Apr 2.

Salama AA, AbouLaila M, Terkawi MA, et al. Inhibitory effect of allicin on the growth of Babesia and

Theileria equi parasites. *Parasitol Res.* 2014;113(1):275-283. Epub 2013 Oct 31.

Shouk R, Abdou A, Shetty K, Sarkar D, Eid AH. Mechanisms underlying the antihypertensive effects of garlic bioactives. *Nutr Res.* 2014;34(2):106-115. Epub 2014 Jan 6.

Tsubura A, Lai YC, Kuwata M, Uehara N, Yoshizawa K. Anticancer effects of garlic and garlic-derived compounds for breast cancer control. *Anticancer Agents Med Chem.* 2011;11(3):249-253.

Viswanathan V, Phadatare AG, Mukne A. Antimycobacterial and Antibacterial Activity of Allium sativum Bulbs. *Indian J Pharm Sci.* 2014;76(3):256-261.

Wallock-Richards D, Doherty CJ, Doherty L, et al. Garlic revisited: antimicro-bial activity of allicin-containing garlic extracts against Burkholderia cepacia complex. *PLoS One.* 2014;9(12):e112726.

Wu X, Santos RR, Fink-Gremmels J. Analyzing the antibacterial effects of food ingredients: model experiments with allicin and garlic extracts on biofilm formation and viability of Staphylococcus epidermidis. *Food Sci Nutr.* 2015;3(2):158-168. Epub 2015 Feb 14.

Yang LJ, Fan L, Liu ZQ, et al. Effects of allicin on CYP2C19 and CYP3A4 activity in healthy volunteers with different CYP2C19 genotypes. *Eur J Clin Pharmacol.* 2009;65(6):601-608. Epub 2009 Jan 27.

Yoshida S, Kasuga S, Hayashi N, et al. Antifungal activity of ajoene derived from garlic. *Appl Environ Microbiol.* 1987;53(3):615-617.

GENERAL HERBS

Alzohairy MA. Therapeutics Role of Azadirachta indica (Neem) and Their Active Constituents in Diseases Prevention and Treatment. *Evid Based Complement Alternat Med.* 2016;2016: 7382506.

Ansah C, Mensah KB. A review of the anticancer potential of the antimalarial herbal cryptolepis sanguinolenta and its major alkaloid cryptolepine. *Ghana Med J.* 2013;47(3):137-147.

Blumenthal M (ed.). *The ABC Clinical Guide to Herbs.* Austin, TX: American Botanical Council; 2003.

Bonaccini L, Karioti A, Bergonzi MC, Bilia AR. Effects of Salvia miltiorrhiza on CNS Neuronal Injury and Degeneration: A Plausible Complementary Role of Tanshinones and Depsides. *Planta Med.* 2015;81(12-13):1003-1016.

Bone K, Mills S. *Principles and Practice of Phytotherapy.* 2nd ed. New York: Churchill/Livingston; 2013.

Borchardt J. Antimicrobial activity of native and naturalized plants of Minnesota and Wisconsin. *Planta Med.* 2008;2(5)98-110. [In vitro study tested 336 plants native and naturalized to the area of study with findings that 24% of them had significant antimicrobial activity against *Staph, E. coli, Pseudomonas,* and *Candida.*]

Buhner SH. *Healing Lyme Disease Coinfections.* Rochester, VT: Healing Arts Press; 2013.

Buhner SH. *Healing Lyme, Natural Healing and Prevention of Lyme Borreliosis and Its Coinfections.* Silver City, NM: Raven Press; 2005.

Buhner SH. *Healing Lyme.* 2nd ed. Silver City, NM: Raven Press; 2015.

Buhner SH. *Herbal Antibiotics.* North Adams, MA: Storey Publishing; 2012.

Buhner SH. *Herbal Antivirals.* North Adams, MA: Storey Publishing; 2013.

Chen JK, Chen TT. *Chinese Medical Herbology and Pharmacology.* City of Industry, CA: Art of Medicine Press; 2001.

Ganora L. *Herbal Constituents, Foundations of Phytochemistry.* Louisville, CO: Herbalchem Press; 2009.

Hendler SS. *PDR for Nutritional Supplements.* 2nd ed. Montvale, NJ: Thomson Reuters; 2008.

Hoffmann D. *Medical Herbalism, the Science and Practice of Herbal Medicine.* Rochester, VT: Healing Arts Press; 2003.

Hu S, Cai W, Ye J, Qian Z, Sun Z. Influence of medicinal herbs on phagocytosis by bovine neutrophils. *Zentralbl Veterinarmed A.* 1992;39(8):593-599.

Hudson T. *Women's Encyclopedia of Natural Medicine.* New Canaan, CT: Keats Publishing; 1999.

Isatis tinctoria monograph. *Altern Med Rev.* 2002;7(6):523-524.

Kuhn MA, Winston D. *Herbal Therapy & Supplements.* 2nd ed. Philadelphia, PA: Wolters Kluwer Health/Lippincott Williams & Wilkins; 2008.

Kumar M, Prasad SK, Hemalatha S. A current update on the phytopharmacological aspects of Houttuynia cordata Thunb. *Pharmacogn Rev.* 2014;8(15):22-35.

Medicines from the Earth. Lecture notes from multiple lectures. Annual Conference on Herbal Medicine; May 31-June 4, 2013. Black Mountain, NC.

Mills-Robertson FC, Tay SC, Duker-Eshun G, Walana W, Badu K. In vitro antimicrobial activity of ethanolic fractions of Cryptolepis sanguinolenta. *Ann Clin Microbiol Antimicrob.* 2012;11:16.

Pole S. *Ayurvedic Medicine: The Principles and Traditional Practice.* Philadelphia, PA: Churchill Livingstone/Elsevier; 2006.

Stamets P. *MycoMedicinals: An Informational Treatise on Mushrooms.* Olympia, WA: MycoMedia Productions; 2002.

Taylor L. *The Healing Power of Rainforest Herbs.* New Hyde Park, NY: Square One Publishers; 2005.

Tempesta MS. The clinical efficacy of cryptolepis sanguinolenta in the treatment of malaria. *Ghana Med J.* 2010;44(1):1-2.

Thomson Healthcare. *PDR for Herbal Medicines.* 4th ed. Montvale, NJ: Medical Economics Company; 2007.

Winston D, Maimes S. *Adaptogens: Herbs for Strength, Stamina, and Stress Relief.* Rochester, VT: Healing Arts Press; 2007.

Wood W. *The Practice of Traditional Western Herbalism.* Berkeley, CA: North Atlantic Books; 2004. Yance Jr D. *Adaptogens in Medical Herbalism.* Rochester, VT: Healing Arts Press; 2013.

Yance Jr. DR. *Herbal Medicine, Healing and Cancer: A Comprehensive Program for Prevention and Treatment.* Lincolnwood, IL: Keats Publishing; 1999.

GLUTATHIONE

Hagen TM, Bai C, Jones DP. Stimulation of glutathione absorption in rat small intestine by alpha-adrenergic agonists. *FASEB J.* 1991;5(12):2721-2727.

Hunjan MK, Evered DF. Absorption of glutathione from the gastro-intestinal tract. *Biochim Biophys Acta.* 1985;815(2):184-188.

L-glutathione white paper research review. www.kyowahakko-bio.co.jp/. Accesssed August 2016.

McKinley-Barnard S, Andre T, Morita M, Willoughby DS. Combined L-citrulline and glutathione supplementation increases the concentration of markers indicative of nitric oxide synthesis. *J Int Soc Sports Nutr.* 2015;12:27.

Richie JP Jr, Nichenametla S, Neidig W, et al. Randomized controlled trial of oral glutathione supplementation on body stores of glutathione. *Eur J Nutr.* 2015;54(2):251-263.

MARITIME PINE BARK

Bianchi S, Kroslakova I, Janzon R, Mayer I, Saake B, Pichelin F. Characterization of condensed tannins and carbohydrates in hot water bark extracts of European softwood species. *Phytochemistry*. 2015;120:53-61.

McGrath KC, Li XH, McRobb LS, Heather AK. Inhibitory Effect of a French Maritime Pine Bark Extract-Based Nutritional Supplement on TNF-α-Induced Inflammation and Oxidative Stress in Human Coronary Artery Endothelial Cells. *Evid Based Complement Alternat Med*. 2015;2015:260530.

Nakayama S, Kishimoto Y, Saita E, et al. Pine bark extract prevents low-density lipoprotein oxidation and regulates monocytic expression of antioxidant enzymes. *Nutr Res*. 2015;35(1):56-64.

OMEGA 3

Berge K, Musa-Veloso K, Harwood M, Hoem N, Burri L. Krill oil supplementation lowers serum triglycerides without increasing low-density lipoprotein cholesterol in adults with borderline high or high triglyceride levels. *Nutr Res*. 2014;34(2):126-133. Epub 2013 Dec 18.

Bunea R, Farrah K, Deutsch L. Evaluation of the effects of Neptune Krill Oil on the clinical course of hyperlipidemia. *Altern Med Rev*. 2004;9(4):420-428.

Deutsch L. Evaluation of the effect of Neptune Krill Oil on chronic inflammation of arthritic symptoms. *J Am Coll Nutr*. 2007;20(1):39-48.

Kidd PM. Omega-3 DHA and EPA for cognition, behavior, and mood: clinical findings and structural-functional synergies with cell membrane phospholipids. *Altern Med Rev*. 2007;12(3):207-227.

Maki KC, Reeves MS, Farmer M, et al. Krill oil supplementation increases plasma concentrations of eicosapentaenoic and docosahexaenoic acids in overweight and obese men and women. *Nutr Res*. 2009;29(9):609-615.

Nobili V, Alisi A, Musso G, Scorletti E, Calder PC, Byrne CD. Omega-3 fatty acids: Mechanisms of benefit and therapeutic effects in pediatric and adult NAFLD. *Crit Rev Clin Lab Sci*. 2016;53(2):106-120. Epub 2015 Oct 14.

Ramprasath V, Eyal I, Zchut S, Jones PJ. Enhanced increase of omega-3 index in healthy individuals with response to 4-week n-3 fatty acid supplementation from krill oil versus fish oil. *Lipids Health Dis.* 2013;12:178.

Rupp H, Wagner D, Rupp T, Schulte LM, Maisch B. Risk stratification by the "EPA+DHA level" and the "EPA/AA ratio" focus on anti-inflammatory and antiarrhythmogenic effects of long-chain omega-3 fatty acids. *Herz.* 2004;29(7):673-685.

Schuchardt JP, Schneider I, Meyer H, Neubronner J, von Schacky C, Hahn A. Incorporation of EPA and DHA into plasma phospholipids in response to different omega-3 fatty acid formulations—a comparative bioavailability study of fish oil vs. krill oil. *Lipids Health Dis.* 2011;10:145.

Tou JC, Jaczynski J, Chen YC. Krill for human consumption: nutritional value and potential health benefits. *Nutr Rev.* 2007;65(2):63-77.

Ulven SM, Kirkhus B, Lamglait A, et al. Metabolic effects of krill oil are essentially similar to those of fish oil but at lower dose of EPA and DHA, in healthy volunteers. *Lipids.* 2011;46(1):37-46. Epub 2010 Nov 2.

von Schacky C, Harris WS. Cardiovascular risk and the omega-3 index. *J Cardiovasc Med (Hagerstown).* 2007;8(Suppl 1):S46-S49.

RESVERATROL/JAPANESE KNOTWEED

Aluyen JK, Ton QN, Tran T, et al. Resveratrol: potential as anticancer agent. *J Diet Suppl.* 2012;9(1):45-56.

Cheng L, Jin Z, Zhao R, Ren K, Deng C, Yu S. Resveratrol attenuates inflammation and oxidative stress induced by myocardial ischemia-reperfusion injury: role of Nrf2/ARE pathway. *Int J Clin Exp Med.* 2015;8(7):10420-10428.

Chong E, Chang SL, Hsiao YW, et al. Resveratrol, a red wine antioxidant, reduces atrial fibrillation susceptibility in the failing heart by PI3K/AKT/eNOS signaling pathway activation. *Heart Rhythm.* 2015;12(5):1046-1056.

Cong X, Li Y, Lu N, et al. Resveratrol attenuates the inflammatory reaction induced by ischemia/reperfusion in the rat heart. *Mol Med Rep.* 2014;9(6):2528-2532.

Dolinsky VW, Dyck JR. Experimental studies of the molecular pathways regulated by exercise and resveratrol in heart, skeletal muscle and the vasculature. *Molecules.* 2014;19(9):14919-14947.

Ghanim H, Sia CL, Abuaysheh S, et al. An anti-inflammatory and reactive oxygen species suppressive effects of an extract of Polygonum cuspidatum containing resveratrol. *J Clin Endocrinol Metab.* 2010;95(9):E1-E8.

Han JH, Koh W, Lee HJ, et al. Analgesic and anti-inflammatory effects of ethyl acetate fraction of Polygonum cuspidatum in experimental animals. *Immunopharmacol Immunotoxicol.* 2012;34(2):191-195.

Joshi MS, Williams D, Horlock D, et al. Role of mitochondrial dysfunction in hyperglycaemia-induced coronary microvascular dysfunction: Protective role of resveratrol. *Diab Vasc Dis Res.* 2015;12(3):208-216.

Kakoti BB, Hernandez-Ontiveros DG, Kataki MS, Shah K, Pathak Y, Panguluri SK. Resveratrol and Omega-3 Fatty Acid: Its Implications in Cardiovascular Diseases. *Front Cardiovasc Med.* 2015;2:38.

Kirino A, Takasuka Y, Nishi A, et al. Analysis and functionality of major polyphenolic components of Polygonum cuspidatum (itadori). *J Nutr Sci Vitaminol (Tokyo).* 2012;58(4):278-286.

Kurita S, Kashiwaqi T, Ebisu T, Shimamura T, Ukeda H. Content of resveratrol and glycoside and its contribution to the antioxidative capacity of Polygonum cuspidatum (Itadori) harvested in Kochi. *Biosci Biotechnol Biochem.* 2014;78(3):499-502.

Lin CJ, Lin HJ, Chen TH, et al. Polygonum cuspidatum and its active components inhibit replication of the influenza virus through toll-like receptor 9-induced interferon beta expression. *PLoS One.* 2015;10(2):e0117602.

Lin SP, Chu PM, Tsai SY, Wu MH, Hou YC. Pharmacokinetics and tissue distribution of resveratrol, emodin and their metabolites after intake of Polygonum cuspidatum in rats. *J Ethnopharmacol.* 2012;144(3):671-676.

Liu Y, Ma W, Zhang P, He S, Huang D. Effect of resveratrol on blood pressure: a meta-analysis of randomized controlled trials. *Clin Nutr.* 2015;34(1):27-34.

Liu Z, Wei F, Chen LJ, et al. In vitro and in vivo studies of the inhibitory effects of emodin isolated from Polygonum cuspidatum on Coxsakievirus B_4. *Molecules*. 2013;18(10):11842-11858.

Meng C, Liu JL, Du AL. Cardioprotective effect of resveratrol on atherogenic diet-fed rats. *Int J Clin Exp Pathol*. 2014;7(11):7899-7906.

Mokni M, Hamlaoui S, Karkouch I, et al. Resveratrol Provides Cardioprotection after Ischemia/reperfusion Injury via Modulation of Antioxidant Enzyme Activities. *Iran J Pharm Res*. 2013;12(4):867-875.

Pasinetti GM, Wang J, Ho L, Zhao W, Dubner L. Roles of resveratrol and other grape-derived polyphenols in Alzheimer's disease prevention and treatment. *Biochim Biophys Acta*. 2015;1852(6):1202-1208.

Peng W, Qin R, Li X, Zhou H. Botany, phytochemistry, pharmacology, and potential application of Polygonum cuspidatum Sieb.et Zucc: a review. *J Ethnopharmacol*. 2013;148(3):729-745.

Piotrowska H, Kucinska M, Murias M. Biological activity of piceatannol: leaving the shadow of resveratrol. *Mutat Res*. 2012;750(1):60-82.

Rabassa M, Zamora-Ros R, Urpi-Sarda M, Andres-Lacueva C. Resveratrol metabolite profiling in clinical nutrition research—from diet to uncovering disease risk biomarkers: epidemiological evidence. *Ann N Y Acad Sci*. 2015;1348(1):107-115.

Raj P, Zieroth S, Netticadan T. An overview of the efficacy of resveratrol in the management of ischemic heart disease. *Ann N Y Acad Sci*. 2015;1348(1):55-67.

Singh CK, Liu X, Ahmad N. Resveratrol, in its natural combination in whole grape, for health promotion and disease management. *Ann N Y Acad Sci*. 2015;1348(1):150-160.

Song JH, Kim SK, Chang KW, et al. In vitro inhibitory effects of Polygonum cuspidatum on bacterial viability and virulence factors of Streptococcus mutans and Streptococcus sobrinus. *Arch Oral Biol*. 2006;51(12):1131-1140.

Su PW, Yang CH, Yang JF, Su PY, Chuang LY. Antibacterial Activities and Antibacterial Mechanism of Polygonum cuspidatum Extracts against Nosocomial Drug-Resistant Pathogens. *Molecules*. 2015;20(6):11119-11130.

Taraszkiewicz A, Fila G, Grinholc M, Nakonieczna J. Innovative strategies to overcome biofilm resistance. *BioMed Res Int*. 2013;2013: 150653.

Wang HL, Gao JP, Han YL, et al. Comparative studies of polydatin and resveratrol on mutual transformation and antioxidative effect in vivo. *Phytomedicine*. 2015;22(5):553-559.

Xie HC, Han HP, Chen Z, He JP. A study on the effect of resveratrol on lipid metabolism in hyperlipidemic mice. *Afr J Tradit Complement Altern Med*. 2013;11(1):209-212.

Yang X, Li X, Ren J. From French Paradox to cancer treatment: anti-cancer activities and mechanisms of resveratrol. *Anticancer Agents Med Chem*. 2014;14(6):806-825.

Yiu CY, Chen SY, Yang TH, et al. Inhibition of Epstein-Barr virus lytic cycle by an ethyl acetate subfraction separated from Polygonum cuspidatum root and its major component, emodin. *Molecules*. 2014;19(1):1258-1272.

Zheng H, Guo H, Hong Y, Zheng F, Wang J. The effects of age and resveratrol on the hypoxic preconditioning protection against hypoxia-reperfusion injury: studies in rat hearts and human cardiomyocytes. *Eur J Cardiothorac Surg*. 2015;48(3):375-381.

REISHI

Batra P, Sharma AK, Khajuria R. Probing Lingzhi or Reishi medicinal mushroom Ganoderma lucidum (higher Basidiomycetes): a bitter mushroom with amazing health benefits. *Int J Med Mushrooms*. 2013;15(2):127-43.

Collado Mateo D, Pazzi F, Domínguez Muñoz FJ, et al. GANODERMA LUCIDUM IMPROVES PHYSICAL FITNESS IN WOMEN WITH FIBROMYALGIA. *Nutr Hosp*. 2015;32(5):2126-2135.

Guggenheim AG, Wright KM, Zwickey HL. Immune Modulation From Five Major Mushrooms: Application to Integrative Oncology. *Integr Med (Encinitas).* 2014;13(1):32-44.

Kladar NV, Gavarić NS, Božin BN. Ganoderma: insights into anticancer effects. *Eur J Cancer Prev.* 2016:25(5):462-471.

Wang L, Hou Y. Determination of trace elements in anti-influenza virus mushrooms. *Biol Trace Elem Res.* 2011;143(3):1799-1807. Epub 2011 Feb 8.

SARSAPARILLA

Itharat A, Srikwan K, Ruangnoo S, Thongdeeying P. Anti-Allergic Activities of Smilax glabra Rhizome Extracts and Its Isolated Compounds. *J Med Assoc Thai.* 2015;98(Suppl 3):S66-S74.

Jiang J, Wu F, Lu J, Lu Z, Xu Q. Anti-inflammatory activity of the aqueous extract from Rhizoma smilacis glabrae. *Pharmacol Res.* 1997;36(4):309-314.

Jiang J, Xu Q. Immunomodulatory activity of the aqueous extract from rhizome of Smilax glabra in the later phase of adjuvant-induced arthritis in rats. *J Ethnopharmacol.* 2003;85(1):53-59.

Lu CL, Zhu W, Wang M, Xu XJ, Lu CJ. Antioxidant and Anti-Inflammatory Activities of Phenolic-Enriched Extracts of Smilax glabra. *Evid Based Complement Alternat Med.* 2014;2014:910438. Epub 2014 Nov 11.

Tse TW. Use of common Chinese herbs in the treatment of psoriasis. *Clin Exp Dermatol.* 2003;28(5):469-475.

Xu S, Shang MY, Liu GX, et al. Chemical constituents from the rhizomes of Smilax glabra and their antimicrobial activity. *Molecules.* 2013;18(5):5265-5287.

Chapter 16

BOSWELLIA

Gupta PK, Samarakoon SM, Chandola HM, Ravishankar B. Clinical evaluation of Boswellia serrata (Shallaki) resin in the management of Sandhivata (osteoarthritis). *Ayu.* 2011;32(4):478-482.

Kizhakkedath R. Clinical evaluation of a formulation containing Curcuma longa and Boswellia serrata extracts in the management of knee osteoarthritis. *Mol Med Rep.* 2013;8(5):1542-1548.

Prabhavathi K, Chandra US, Soanker R, Rani PU. A randomized, double blind, placebo controlled, crossover study to evaluate the analgesic activity of Boswellia serrata in healthy volunteers using mechanical pain model. *Indian J Pharmacol.* 2014;46(5):475-479.

ENZYMES

Conrozier T, Mathieu P, Bonjean M, et al. A complex of three natural anti-inflammatory agents provides relief of osteoarthritis pain. *Altern Ther Health Med.* 2014;20 Suppl 1:32-37.

Ja-Young Jang et al. Nattokinase improves blood flow by inhibiting platelet aggregation and thrombus formation. *Lab Anim Res.* 2013 Dec; 29(4): 221–225.

Sumi H, Hamada H, Nakanishi K, Hiratani H. Enhancement of the fibrinolytic activity in plasma by oral administration of nattokinase. *Acta Haematol.* 1990;84(3):139-43.

Walker AF, Bundy R, Hicks SM, Middleton RW. Bromelain reduces mild acute knee pain and improves well-being in a dose-dependent fashion in an open study of otherwise healthy adults. *Phytomedicine.* 2002;9(8):681-686.

GENERAL

Hoffmann D. *Medical Herbalism, the Science and Practice of Herbal Medicine.* Rochester, VT: Healing Arts Press; 2003.

Kuhn MA, Winston D. *Herbal Therapy & Supplements.* 2nd ed. Philadelphia, PA: Wolters Kluwer Health/Lippincott Williams & Wilkins; 2008.

Physician's Desk Reference. 69th ed. Montvale, NJ: PDR Network; 2014.

Yance Jr. DR. *Herbal Medicine, Healing and Cancer: A Comprehensive Program for Prevention and Treatment.* Lincolnwood, IL: Keats Publishing; 1999.

GLUCOSAMINE

Bruyère O, Altman RD, Reginster JY. Efficacy and safety of glucosamine sulfate in the management of osteoarthritis: Evidence from real-life setting trials and surveys. *Semin Arthritis Rheum.* 2016;45(4 Suppl):S12-S17.

Raynauld J-P, Pelletier J-P, Abram F, et al. Long-term effects of glucosamine/chondroitin sulfate on the progression of structural changes in knee osteoarthritis: 6-year follow-up data from the osteoarthritis initiative. *Arthritis Care Res (Hoboken).* 2016;68(10):1560-1566.

Roubille C, Martel-Pelletier J, Abram F, et al. Impact of disease treatments on the progression of knee osteoarthritis structural changes related to meniscal extrusion: Data from the OAI progression cohort. *Semin Arthritis Rheum.* 2015;45(3):257-267. Epub 2015 May 15.

Rovati LC, Girolami F, D'Amato M, Giacovelli G. Effects of glucosamine sulfate on the use of rescue non-steroidal anti-inflammatory drugs in knee osteoarthritis: Results from the Pharmaco-Epidemiology of GonArthroSis (PEGASus) study. *Semin Arthritis Rheum.* 2016;45(4 Suppl):S34-S41.

Runhaar J, Deroisy R, van Middelkoop M, et al. The role of diet and exercise and of glucosamine sulfate in the prevention of knee osteoarthritis: Further results from the PRevention of knee Osteoarthritis in Overweight Females (PROOF) study. *Semin Arthritis Rheum.* 2016;45(4 Suppl):S42-S48.

INFLAMMATION

Allen HB, Morales D, Jones K, Joshi S. A novel hypothesis integrating spirochetes, biofilm, and the immune system. *J Neuroinfect Dis.* 2016;7:1.

Cattano D, O'Connor B, Shakir R, Giunta F, Palazzo M. Acute inflammatory demyelinating polyneuropathy and a unilateral babinski/plantar reflex. *Anesthesiol Res Pract.* 2008;2008:134958. Epub 2007 Nov 12.

Chaudhry R, Ghosh A, Chandolia A. Pathogenesis of Mycoplasma pneumoniae: An update. *Indian J Med Microbiol.* 2016;34(1):7-16.

Garcia-Monco JC, Benach JL. Mechanisms of injury in Lyme neuroborreliosis. *Semin Neurol.* 1997;17(1):57-62.

Hughes RA, Hadden R, Gregson NA, Smith KJ. Pathogenesis of Guillain-Barré syndrome. *J Neuroimmunol.* 1999;100(1-2):74-97.

Iliopoulou BP, Alroy J, Huber BT. CD28 deficiency exacerbates joint inflammation upon Borrelia burgdorferi infection, resulting in the development of chronic Lyme arthritis. *J Immunol.* 2007;179(12):8076-8082.

Lesser RL. Ocular manifestations of Lyme disease. *Am J Med.* 1995;98(4A):60S-62S.

Ma Y, Sturrock A, Weis JJ. Intracellular localization of Borrelia burgdorferi within human endothelial cells. *Infect Immun.* 1991;59(2):671-678.

Narita M. Classification of Extrapulmonary Manifestations Due to Mycoplasma pneumoniae Infection on the Basis of Possible Pathogenesis. *Front Microbiol.* 2016;7:23.

Oosting M, Berende A, Sturm P, et al. Recognition of Borrelia burgdorferi by NOD2 is central for the induction of an inflammatory reaction. *J Infect Dis.* 2010;201(12):1849-1858.

Podbielska M, Dasgupta S, Levery SB, et al. Novel myelin penta- and hexa-acetyl-galactosyl-ceramides: structural characterization and immunoreactivity in cerebrospinal fluid. *J Lipid Res.* 2010;51(6):1394-1406.

Shimizu T. Inflammation-inducing Factors of Mycoplasma pneumoniae. *Front Microbiol.* 2016;7:414.

Sinkovics JG. Molecular biology of oncogenic inflammatory processes. I. Non-oncogenic and oncogenic pathogens, intrinsic inflammatory reactions without pathogens, and microRNA/DNA interactions (Review). *Int J Oncol.* 2012;40(2):305-349. Epub 2011 Nov 4.

Topcu Y, Bayram E, Karaoglu P, Yis U, Guleryuz H, Kurul SH. Coexistence of myositis, transverse myelitis, and Guillain Barré syndrome following Mycoplasma pneumoniae infection in an adolescent. *J Pediatr Neurosci.* 2013;8(1):59-63.

MONOLAURIN

Goc A, Niedzwiecki A, Rath M. Cooperation of Doxycycline with Phytochemicals and Micronutrients Against Active and Persistent Forms of Borrelia sp. *Int J Biol Sci.* 2016 Jul 22;12(9):1093-103.

Goc A, Niedzwiecki A, Rath M. In vitro evaluation of antibacterial activity of phytochemicals and micronutrients against Borrelia burgdorferi and Borrelia garinii. *J Appl Microbiol.* 2015 Dec;119(6):1561-72.

Schlievert PM, Peterson ML.Glycerol monolaurate antibacterial activity in broth and biofilm cultures. *PLoS One.* 2012;7(7):e40350.

Seleem D, Chen E, Benso B2, Pardi V, Murata RM. In vitro evaluation of antifungal activity of monolaurin against Candida albicans biofilms. *PeerJ.* 2016 Jun 22;4:e2148.

PEPTIDES

Cerovecki T et al. Pentadecapeptide BPC 157 (PL 14736) improves ligament healing in the rat. *J Orthop Res.* 2010 Sep;28(9):1155-61.

Holtorf K. Innovative "alternative" therapies for chronic Lyme disease. 2016 ILADS Annual Conference.

Klicek R et al. Stable gastric pentadecapeptide BPC 157 heals cysteamine-colitis and colon-colon-anastomosis and counteracts cuprizone brain injuries and motor disability. *J Physiol Pharmacol.* 2013 Oct;64(5):597-612.

Li J, Liu CH, Wang FS. Thymosin alpha 1: biological activities, applications and genetic engineering production. *Peptides.* 2010 Nov;31(11):2151-8.

Morozov VG, Khavinson VK. Natural and synthetic thymic peptides as therapeutics for immune dysfunction. *Int J Immunopharmacol.* 1997 Sep-Oct;19(9-10):501-5.

Sikiric P et al. Stable gastric pentadecapeptide BPC 157: novel therapy in gastrointestinal tract. *Curr Pharm Des.* 2011;17(16):1612-32. Review.

Yang X et al. Effect of thymosin alpha-1 on subpopulations of Th1, Th2, Th17, and regulatory T cells (Tregs) in vitro. *Braz J Med Biol Res.* 2012 Jan;45(1):25-32.

TURMERIC

Antony, et al. Relative bioavailability of BCM-95®CG (BCM-95). *Ind J Pharm Sci.* 2008;70(4):445-449.

Baum L, Lam CW, Cheung SK, et al. Six-month randomized, placebo-controlled, double-blind, pilot clinical trial of curcumin in patients with Alzheimer disease. *J Clin Psychopharmacol.* 2008;28(1):110-113.

Bengmark S, Mesa MD, Gil A. Plant-derived health: the effects of turmeric and curcuminoids. *Nutr Hosp.* 2009;24(3):273-281.

Chandran B, Goel A. A randomized, pilot study to assess the efficacy and safety of curcumin in patients with active rheumatoid arthritis. *Phytother Res.* 2012;26(11):1719-1725.

Ghosh S, Banerjee S, Sil PC. The beneficial role of curcumin on inflammation, diabetes and neurodegenerative disease: A recent update. *Food Chem Toxicol.* 2015;83:111-124. Epub 2015 Jun 9.

Goel A, Boland CR, Chauhan DP. Specific inhibition of cyclooxygenase-2 (COX-2) expression by dietary curcumin in HT-29 human colon cancer cells. *Cancer Letters.* 2001;172:111-118.

Ricciotti E, FitzGerald EA. Prostaglandins and inflammation. *Arterioscler Thromb Vasc Biol.* 2011;31(5):986-1000.

Sanmukhani J, Satodia V, Trivedi J, et al. Efficacy and safety of curcumin in major depressive disorder: a randomized controlled trial. *Phytother Res.* 2014;28(4):579-585. Epub 2013 Jul 6.

Sishu, et al. The bioavailability of curcumin from turmeric, BCM-95®. *Journal of Functional Foods.* 2010; 2(1):60-65.

Chapter 17

Akhondzadeh S, Naghavi HR, Vazirian M, Shayeganpour A, Rashidi H, Khani M. Passionflower in the treatment of generalized anxiety: a pilot double-blind randomized controlled trial with oxazepam. *J Clin Pharm Ther.* 2001;26(5):363-367.

Anderson JG, Kebaish SA, Lewis JE, Taylor AG. Effects of cranial electrical stimulation on activity in regions of the basal ganglia in individuals with fibromyalgia. *J Alt Complement Med.* 2014;20(3):206-207.

Auddy B, Hazara J, Mitra A, Abedon B, Ghosal S. A standardized withania somnifera extract significantly reduces stress-related parameters in chronically stressed humans. *JANA.* 2008;2(1):50-56.

Barclay TH, Barclay RD. A clinical trial of cranial electrotherapy stimulation for anxiety and comorbid depression. *J Affect Disord.* 2014;164:171-177.

Benson S, Downey LA, Stough C, Wetherell M, Zangara A, Scholey A. An acute, double-blind, placebo-controlled cross-over study of 320 mg and 640 mg doses of Bacopa monnieri (CDRI 08) on multitasking stress reactivity and mood. *Phytother Res.* 2014;28(4):551-559. Epub 2013 Jun 21.

Calabrese C, Gregory WL, Leo M, Kraemer D, Bone K, Oken B. Effects of a standardized Bacopa monnieri extract on cognitive performance, anxiety, and depression in the elderly: a randomized, double-blind, placebo-controlled trial. *J Altern Complement Med.* 2008;14(6):707-713.

Costello RB, Lentino CV, Boyd CC, et al. The effectiveness of melatonin for promoting healthy sleep: a rapid evidence assessment of the literature. *Nutr J.* 2014;13:106.

Elsas SM, Rossi DJ, Raber J, et al. Passiflora incarnata L. (Passionflower) extracts elicit GABA currents in hippocampal neurons in vitro, and show anxiogenic and anticonvulsant effects in vivo, varying with extraction method. *Phytomedicine.* 2010;17(12):940-949. Epub 2010 Apr 10.

Grundmann O, Wang J, McGregor GP, Butterweck V. Anxiolytic activity of a phytochemically characterized Passiflora incarnata extract is mediated via the GABAergic system. *Planta Med.* 2008;74(15):1769-1773. Epub 2008 Nov 12.

Kidd PM. Omega-3 DHA and EPA for cognition, behavior, and mood: clinical findings and structural-functional synergies with cell membrane phospholipids. *Altern Med Rev.* 2007;12(3):207-227.

Kirsch DL, Nichols F. Cranial electrotherapy stimulation for treatment of anxiety, depression, and insomnia. *Psychiatr Clin North Am.* 2013;36(1):169-176.

Lichtbroun AS, Raicer MM, Smith RB. The treatment of fibromyalgia with cranial electrotherapy stimulation. *J Clin Rheum.* 2001;7(2):72-78.

Ngan A, Conduit R. A double-blind, placebo-controlled investigation of the effects of Passiflora incarnata (passionflower) herbal tea on subjective sleep quality. *Phytother Res.* 2011;25(8):1153-1159. Epub 2011 Feb 3.

Otify A, George C, Elsayed A, Farag MA. Mechanistic evidence of Passiflora edulis (Passifloraceae) anxiolytic activity in relation to its metabolite fingerprint as revealed via LC-MS and chemometrics. *Food Funct.* 2015;6(12):3807-3817. Epub 2015 Oct 5.

Sarris J, McIntyre E, Camfield DA. Plant-based medicines for anxiety disorders, part 2: a review of clinical studies with supporting preclinical evidence. *CNS Drugs.* 2013;27(4):301-319.

Shikov AN, Pozharitskaya ON, Makarov VG, Demchenko DV, Shikh EV. Effect of Leonurus cardiaca oil extract in patients with arterial hypertension accompanied by anxiety and sleep disorders. *Phytother Res.* 2011;25(4):540-543. Epub 2010 Sep 13.

Shinomol GK, Muralidhara, Bharath MM. Exploring the role of "Brahmi" (Bocopa monnieri and Centella asiatica) in brain function and therapy. *Recent Pat Endocr Metab Immune Drug Discov.* 2011;5(1):33-49. Smith RB. *Cranial Electrotherapy Stimulation, Its First Fifty Years, Plus Three: A Monograph.* Mustang, OK: Tate Publishing & Enterprises; 2007.

Villet S, Vacher V, Colas A, et al. Open-label observational study of the homeopathic medicine Passiflora Compose for anxiety and sleep disorders. *Homeopathy.* 2016;105(1):84-91. Epub 2015 Aug 29.

Wohlmuth H, Penman KG, Pearson T, Lehmann RP. Pharmacognosy and chemotypes of passionflower (Passiflora incarnata L.). *Biol Pharm Bull.* 2010;33(6):1015-1018.

Chapter 18

Bergamaschi MM, Queiroz RH, Zuardi AW, Crippa JA. Safety and side effects of cannabidiol, a Cannabis sativa constituent. *Curr Drug Saf.* 2011;6(4):237-249.

Kuhn MA, Winston D. *Herbal Therapy & Supplements.* 2nd ed. Philadelphia, PA: Wolters Kluwer Health/Lippincott Williams & Wilkins; 2008.

lowdosenaltrexone.org Information about low dose naltrexone and resources for use.

Moore E, Wilkinson S. *The Promise of Low Dose Naltrexone Therapy.* Jefferson, NC: McFarland & Company, Inc; 2009.

Physician's Desk Reference. 69th ed. Montvale, NJ: PDR Network; 2014.

Porter RS. *The Merck Manual.* 19th ed. Whitehouse Station, NJ: Merck; 2011.

Russo E, Guy GW. A tale of two cannabinoids: the therapeutic rationale for combining tetrahydrocannabinol and cannabidiol. *Med Hypotheses.* 2006;66(2):234-246. Epub 2005 Oct 4.

Russo EB. Cannabinoids in the management of difficult to treat pain. *Ther Clin Risk Manag.* 2008; 4(1):245-259.

Russo EB. Taming THC: potential cannabis synergy and phytocannabinoid-terpenoid entourage effects. *Br J Pharmacol.* 2011;163(7):1344-1364.

Chapter 19

Alqutub AN, Masoodi I, Alsayari K, Alomair A. Bee sting therapy-induced hepatotoxicity: A case report. *World J Hepatol.* 2011;3(10):268-270. Epub 2011 Oct 27.

Barbault A, Costa FP, Bottger B, et al. Amplitude-modulated electromagnetic fields for the treatment of cancer: discovery of tumor-specific frequencies and assessment of a novel therapeutic approach. *J Exp Clin Cancer Res.* 2009;28:51.

Brandt LJ, Reddy SS. Fecal microbiota transplantation for recurrent Clostridium difficile infection. *J Clin Gastroenterol.* 2011;45(suppl):S159-S167.

Brandt LJ. Fecal transplantation for the treatment of Clostridium difficile infection. *Gastroenterol Hepatol (N Y)*. 2012;8(3):191-194.

Efrati S, Golan H, Bechor Y, et al. Hyperbaric oxygen therapy can diminish fibromyalgia syndrome – prospective clinical trial. *PLoS One*. 2015;10(5):e0127012.

Fife WP, Freeman DM. Treatment of Lyme disease with hyperbaric oxygen therapy [abstract]. Seattle, WA: The Undersea and Hyperbaric Medical Society Annual Meeting; 1998.

Holtorf K. Innovative "alternative" therapies for chronic Lyme disease. 2016 ILADS Annual Conference.

Janssen CW, Lowry CA, Mehl MR, et al. Whole-Body Hyperthermia for the Treatment of Major Depressive Disorder: A Randomized Clinical Trial. *JAMA Psychiatry*. 2016;73(8):789-795.

Lantos PM, Shapiro ED, Auwaerter PG, et al. Unorthodox alternative therapies marketed to treat Lyme disease. *Clin Infect Dis*. 2015;60(12):1783-1785. Epub 2015 Apr 6.

National Institutes of Health. National Center for Complementary and Integrative Health. Colloidal silver. https://nccih.nih.gov/health/silver. Accessed September 2016.

Ober C, Sinatra ST, Zucker M. *Earthing: The Most Important Health Discovery Ever?* Laguna Beach, CA: Basic Health Publications; 2010.

Shroff G. Human Embryonic Stem Cell Therapy in Crohn's Disease: A Case Report. *Am J Case Rep*. 2016;17:124-128.

Tonks A. Lyme wars. *BMJ*. 2007;335(7626):910-912.

Zhao C, Dai C, Chen X. Whole-body hyperthermia combined with hyperthermic intraperitoneal chemotherapy for the treatment of stage IV advanced gastric cancer. *Int J Hyperthermia*. 2012;28(8):735-741. Epub 2012 Nov 1.

Zimmerman JW, Jimenez H, Pennison MJ, et al. Targeted treatment of cancer with radiofrequency electromagnetic fields amplitude-modulated at tumor-specific frequencies. *Chin J Cancer*. 2013;32(11): 573-581.

Chapter 21

Crinnion WJ. Sauna as a valuable clinical tool for cardiovascular, autoimmune, toxicant-induced and other chronic health problems. *Altern Med Rev.* 2011;16(3):215-225.

Kihara T, Biro S, Ikeda Y, et al. Effects of repeated sauna treatment on ventricular arrhythmias in patients with chronic heart failure. *Circ J.* 2004;68(12):1146-1151.

Mero A, Tornberg J, Mäntykoski M, Puurtinen R. Effects of far-infrared sauna bathing on recovery from strength and endurance training sessions in men. *Springerplus.* 2015;4:321.

Sears ME, Kerr KJ, Bray RI. Arsenic, cadmium, lead, and mercury in sweat: a systematic review. *J Environ Public Health.* 2012;2012:184745.

Vatansever F, Hamblin MR. Far infrared radiation (FIR): its biological effects and medical applications. *Photonics Lasers Med.* 2012;4:255-266.

Chapter 22

Allen HB, Morales D, Jones K, Joshi S. Alzheimer's disease, a novel hypothesis integrating spirochetes, biofilm, and the immune system. *J Neuroinfect Dis.* 2016;7:1.

Costerton JW, Stewart PS, Greenburg EP. Bacterial biofilms: a common cause of persistent infections. *Science.* 1999;284(5418):1318-1322.

Fujimura KE, Slusher NA, Cabana MD, Lynch SV. Role of the gut microbiota in defining human health. *Expert Rev Anti Infect Ther.* 2010;8(4):435-454.

Hoyle BD, Costerton JW. Bacterial resistance to antibiotics: the role of biofilms. *Prog Drug Res.* 1991;37:91-105.

Jones SE, Versalovic J. Probiotic Lactobacillus reuteri biofilms produce antimicrobial and anti-inflammatory factors. *BMC Microbiol.* 2009;9:35.

Karatan E, Watnick P. Signals, regulatory networks, and materials that build and break bacterial biofilms. *Microbiol Mol Biol Rev.* 2009;73(2):310-347.

Kurtti TJ, Munderloh UG, Johnson RC, Ahlstrand GG. Colony formation and mor-phology in Borrelia burgdorferi. *J Clin Microbiol.* 1987;25(11):2054-2058.

Lennox J (2011). Biofilms: The Hypertextbook. http://biofilmbook.hypertext-bookshop.com/public_version/. Accessed August 2016.

Macfarlane S, Dillon JF. Microbial biofilms in the human gastrointestinal tract. *J Appl Microbiol.* 2007;102(5):1187-1196.

Macfarlane S, Woodmansey EJ, Macfarlane GT. Colonization of Mucin by Human Intestinal Bacteria and Establishment of Biofilm Communities in a Two-Stage Continuous Culture System. *Appl Environ Microbiol.* 2005;71(11):7483-7492.

Sapi A, Bastian SL, Mpoy CM, et al. Characterization of biofilm formation by Borrelia burgdorferi in vitro. *PLoS One.* 2012;7(10): e48277.

Sapi, MacDonald. Biofilms of Borrelia burgdorferi in chronic cutaneous borrelio-sis. *Am J Clin Pathol.* 2008;129:988-989.

Chapter 23

Borgermans L, Goderis G, Vandevoorde J, Devroey D. Relevance of chronic Lyme disease to family medicine as a complex multidimensional chronic dis-ease construct: A systematic review. *Int J Family Med.* 2014;2014:138016. Epub 2014 Nov 24.

Chapter 24

Concon J, Newburg D, Eades S. Lectins in wheat gluten proteins. *J Agric Food Chem.* 1983;31:939-941.

de Souza Ferreira C, Araújo TH, Ângelo ML, et al. Neutrophil dysfunction induced by hyperglycemia: modulation of myeloperoxidase activity. *Cell Biochem Funct.* 2012;30(7):604-610. Epub 2012 May 20.

Freed DL. Do dietary lectins cause disease? *BMJ.* 1999;318(7190):1023-1024.

Hamid R, Masood A. Dietary lectins as disease causing toxicants. *Pakistan J Nutr.* 2009;8(3):293-303.

Hollander D. Intestinal permeability, leaky gut, and intestinal disorders. *Curr Gastroenterol Rep.* 1999 Oct;1(5):410-6.

Javid A, Zlotnikov N, Pětrošová H, et al. Hyperglycemia impairs neutrophil-mediated bacterial clearance in mice infected with the Lyme disease pathogen. *PLoS One.* 2016;11(6):e0158019.

Liebman L, Al-Wahsh I. Probiotics and other key determinants of dietary oxalate absorption. *Adv Nutr.* 2011:(2):254-260

Majee SB, Biswas GR. Exploring plant lectins in diagnosis, prophylaxis, and therapy. *J Med Plant Res.* 2013;7(47):3444-3451.

Nachbar MS, Oppenheim JD. Lectins in the United States diet, a survey of lectins in commonly consumed foods and a review of the literature. *Am J Clin Nutr.* 1980;88(11):2338-2345.

Plant lectins. http://www.ansci.cornell.edu/plants/toxicagents/lectins.html. Accessed July 2016.

Rapin JR and Wiernsperger N. Possible links between intestinal permeability and food processing: A potential therapeutic niche for glutamine. *Clinics (Sao Paulo).* 2010;65(6):635-43.

Tagzirt M, Corseaux D, Pasquesoone L, et al. Alterations in neutrophil production and function at an early stage in the high-fructose rat model of metabolic syndrome. *Am J Hypertens.* 2014;27:1096-1104.

Chapter 25

ewn.org. The Environmental Working Group provides information about healthful food and lifestyle.

Hoffman D. *Healthy Digestion.* North Adams, MA: Storey Books; 2000.

VitalPlan.com/restore. Program designed to help implement healthful dietary and lifestyle modifications.

Chapter 26

ewn.org

Mutter J. Is dental amalgam safe for humans? The opinion of the scientific committee of the European Commission. *J OccupMed Toxicol.* 2011;6:2.

Rathore M, Singh A, Pant VA. The dental amalgam toxicity fear: a myth or actuality. *Toxicol Int.* 2012;19(2):81-88.

www.eatwild.com

Chapter 27

Aiko V, Mehta A. Occurrence, detection and detoxification of mycotoxins. *J Biosci.* 2015;40(5):943-954.

Nathan N. *Mold & Mycotoxins: Current Evaluation and Treatment 2016.*

Park SH, Kim D, Kim J, Moon Y. Effects of Mycotoxins on mucosal microbial infection and related pathogenesis. *Toxins (Basel).* 2015;7(11):4484-4502.

Shoemaker RC. *Mold Warriors.* Baltimore, MD: Gateway Press; 2005.

Chapter 29

Balchin R, Linde J, Blackhurst D, Rauch HL, Schönbächler G. Sweating away depression? The impact of intensive exercise on depression. *J Affect Disord.* 2016;200:218-221. Epub 2016 Apr 20.

Boehm K, Ostermann T, Milazzo S, Büssing A. Effects of yoga interventions on fatigue: a meta-analysis. *Evid Based Complement Alternat Med.* 2012;2012:124703. Epub 2012 Sep 6.

Busch AJ, Webber SC, Brachaniec M, et al. Exercise therapy for fibromyalgia. *Curr Pain Headache Rep.* 2011;15(5):358-367.

Carson JW, Carson KM, Jones KD, Lancaster L, Mist SD. Mindful Yoga Pilot Study Shows Modulation of Abnormal Pain Processing in Fibromyalgia Patients. *Int J Yoga Therap.* 2016 Sep 1. Epub ahead of print.

Lauche R, Cramer H, Häuser W, Dobos G, Langhorst J. A systematic overview of reviews for complementary and alternative therapies in the treatment of the fibromyalgia syndrome. *Evid Based Complement Alternat Med.* 2015;2015:610605.

Lynch M, Sawynok J, Hiew C, Marcon D. A randomized controlled trial of qigong for fibromyalgia. *Arthritis Res Ther.* 2012;14(4):R178.

Macaluso, F, Myburgh, K.H. Current evidence that exercise can increase the number of adult stem cells. *J Muscle Res Cell Motil.* 2012;33(3):187-198.

Mishra SK, Singh P, Bunch SJ, Zhang R. The therapeutic value of yoga in neurological disorders. *Ann Indian Acad Neurol.* 2012;15(4):247-254.

Mist SD, Firestone KA, Jones KD. Complementary and alternative exercise for fibromyalgia: a meta-analysis. *J Pain Res.* 2013;6:247-260. Epub 2013 Mar 27.

Muhammad CM, Moonaz SH. Yoga as Therapy for Neurodegenerative Disorders: A Case Report of Therapeutic Yoga for Adrenomyeloneuropathy. *Integr Med (Encinitas).* 2014;13(3):33-39.

Nieman DC, Miller AR, Henson DA, et al. Effects of high- vs moderate-intensity exercise on natural killer cell activity. *Med Sci Sports Exerc.* 1993;25(10):1126-1134.

Oka T, Tanahashi T, Chijiwa T, et al. Isometric yoga improves the fatigue and pain of patients with chronic fatigue syndrome who are resistant to conventional therapy: a randomized, controlled trial. *Biopsychosoc Med.* 2014;8(1):27.

Sawynok J, Lynch M. Qigong and fibromyalgia: randomized controlled trials and beyond. *Evid Based Complement Alternat Med.* 2014;2014:379715. Epub 2014 Nov 12.

Sinaei M, Kargarfard M.http://www.ncbi.nlm.nih.gov/pubmed/?term=Sinaei%20M%5BAuthor%5D&cauthor=true&cauthor_uid=24921622 The evaluation of BMI and serum beta-endorphin levels: the study of acute exercise intervention. *J Sports Med Phys Fitness.* 2015;55(5):488-494. Epub 2014 Jun 12.

Sutar R, Yadav S, Desai G. Yoga intervention and functional pain syndromes: a selective review. *Int Rev Psychiatry*. 2016;28(3):316-322. Epubd 2016 Jun 13.

Appendix A

Blumenthal M (ed.). *The ABC Clinical Guide to Herbs*. Austin, TX: American Botanical Council; 2003.

Bone K, Mills S. *Principles and Practice of Phytotherapy*. 2nd ed. New York: Churchill/Livingston; 2013.

Buhner SH. *Healing Lyme Disease Coinfections*. Rochester, VT: Healing Arts Press; 2013.

Buhner SH. *Healing Lyme: Natural Healing of Lyme Borreliosis and the Coinfections Chlamydia and Spotted Fever Rickettsiosis*. 2nd ed. Raven Press; 2015.

Buhner SH. *Herbal Antibiotics*. North Adams, MA: Storey Publishing; 2012.

Buhner SH. *Herbal Antivirals*. North Adams, MA: Storey Publishing; 2013.

Chen JK, Chen TT. *Chinese Medical Herbology and Pharmacology*. City of Industry, CA: Art of Medicine Press; 2001.

Ganora L. *Herbal Constituents, Foundations of Phytochemistry*. Louisville, CO: Herbalchem Press, 2009.

Hendler SS. *PDR for Nutritional Supplements*. 2nd ed. Montvale, NJ: Thomson Reuters; 2008.

Hoffmann D. *Medical Herbalism, the Science and Practice of Herbal Medicine*. Rochester, VT: Healing Arts Press; 2003.

Hudson T. *Women's Encyclopedia of Natural Medicine*. New Canaan, CT: Keats Publishing; 1999.

Kuhn MA, Winston D. *Herbal Therapy & Supplements*. 2nd ed. Philadelphia, PA: Wolters Kluwer Health/Lippincott Williams & Wilkins; 2008.

Lawless J. *The Illustrated Encyclopedia of Essential Oils*. Rockport, MA: Element Books Limited; 1995.

Medicines from the Earth. Lecture notes. Annual Conference on Herbal Medicine; May 31-June 4, 2014. Black Mountain, NC.

Pole S. *Ayurvedic Medicine: The Principles and Traditional Practice*. Philadelphia, PA: Churchill Livingstone/Elsevier; 2006.

Schnaubelt K. *The Healing Intelligence of Essential Oils*. Rochester, VT: Healing Arts Press; 2011.

Stamets P. *MycoMedicinals: An Informational Treatise on Mushrooms*. Olympia, WA: MycoMedia Productions; 2002.

Taylor L. *The Healing Power of Rainforest Herbs*. New Hyde Park, NY: Square One Publishers; 2005.

Thomson Healthcare. *PDR for Herbal Medicines*. 4th ed. Montvale, NJ: Medical Economics Company; 2007.

Winston D, Maimes S. *Adaptogens: Herbs for Strength, Stamina, and Stress Relief*. Rochester, VT: Healing Arts Press; 2007.

Wood W. *The Practice of Traditional Western Herbalism*. Berkeley, CA: North Atlantic Books; 2004.

Yance Jr D. *Adaptogens in Medical Herbalism*. Rochester, VT: Healing Arts Press; 2013.

Yance Jr. DR. *Herbal Medicine, Healing and Cancer: A Comprehensive Program for Prevention and Treatment*. Lincolnwood, IL: Keats Publishing; 1999.

Appendix B

Groves MN. Medicine chest, keeping bugs at bay. *Herb Quarterly*. 2016;Summer:20-22.

Rodriguez SD, Drake LL, Price DP, Hammond J, Hansen A. The Efficacy of Some Commercially Available Insect Repellents for Aedes aegypti (Diptera: Culicidae) and Aedes albopictus (Diptera: Culicidae). *J Insect Sci*. 2015;15:140.

Scent of a Woodsman. Ask Eddy column. *Canoe & Kayak*. 2016;Spring:22.

Suzuki K, Wakabayashi H, Takahashi M, et al. A possible treatment strategy and clinical factors to estimate the treatment response in Babesia gibsoni infection. *J Vet Med Sci.* 2007;69(5):563-568.